Supervision

Strategies for Successful Outcomes and Productivity

Susann Dowling

University of Houston

Allyn and Bacon

Boston ■ London ■ Toronto ■ Sydney ■ Tokyo ■ Singapore

To
Jerry Dowling—
life partner extraordinaire

Vice President: *Paul A. Smith*
Executive Editor and Publisher: *Stephen D. Dragin*
Editorial Assistant: *Barbara Strickland*
Marketing Manager: *Brad Parkins*
Editorial Production Service: *Chestnut Hill Enterprises, Inc.*
Manufacturing Buyer: *Chris Marson*
Cover Administrator: *Brian Gogolin*

Internet: www.abacon.com

Between the time Website information is gathered and published, some sites may have closed. Also, the transcription of URLs can result in typographical errors. The publisher would appreciate notification where these occur so that they may be corrected in subsequent editions.

Library of Congress Cataloging-in-Publication Data

Dowling, Susann
    Supervision : strategies for successful outcomes and productivity / Susann Dowling.
      p. cm.
    Includes bibliographical references and index.
    ISBN 0-205-31507-0
    1. Audiology—Study and teaching—Supervision.   2. Speech therapy—Study and teaching—Supervision.   I. Title.

RF291 .D69   2000
616.85'506'071—dc21

                                                            00-057616

Printed in the United States of America
10   9   8   7   6   5   4   3   2   1   05   04   03   02   01   00

CONTENTS

Introduction   xiii

Acknowledgments   xix

Appendix to the Introduction   xxi

PART ONE   Preparing the Stage   1

1   Creating Productivity and Professional Growth
within Organizations   3

Clinical Supervision Tasks Relevant to Creating Productivity
and Professional Growth within Organizations   3

Supervision and Organizational Culture   4
How to Motivate   5
What Motivates   7

Workplace Philosophy and Motivational Examples   9
Leadership   10
Leadership Styles   11
Value-Driven   14
Continuous Process Improvement   16
Critical Thinking   16

Application of Principles to Speech-Language
Pathology and Audiology   18
How to Motivate   18
What Motivates   20
Leadership Styles   20
Value-Driven   21
Continuous Process Improvement   22
Critical Thinking   23

Relationship of Creating Productivity and Professional
Growth and the Specified Supervision Tasks   23

Summary   24

References   25

PART TWO   Developing Tools and Strategies   27

2 Solving Puzzles: Setting the Stage for Growth   29

Clinical Supervision Tasks Relevant to Solving Puzzles, Setting Goals, Preparing for Growth   29

Data Collection and Performance Objectives as Supervisory Tools   29

Data Collection   31

Data Collection and Its Application to the Clinical Process   35
Individually Designed Systems   35
Supervisee Introduction to Data Collection   45

Professional Objectives in the Clinical Process   47
Literature   47
The Clinical Process   48

Data Collection: Its Application in the Supervisory Process   52
Data Collection Strategies   54
Implementation   54
Data Collection and Goal-Setting Options   61

Relationship of the Specified Supervision Tasks to Solving Puzzles, Setting Goals, Preparing for Growth   62

Summary   62

References   63

Appendix A: Clinical Data Collection Challenge   66

Appendix B: Supervisory Data Collection Challenge   70

3 Maximizing Feedback in the Supervisory Process   73

Clinical Supervision Tasks Relevant to Maximizing Feedback in the Supervisory Process   73
Literature   73
Nature and Effects   74
Effective Feedback Criteria   75
Supervisee Experiences   76

Feedback and Direct Observation   77
Narrative Feedback   78
Rating Scale Feedback   79
Objective Feedback   84
Competency-Based Assessment   85
Supervisee Feedback Involvement   86

Feedback Strategies   87
Feedback Techniques   87
Supervisee Observations   89
Verbal Feedback Strategies   90

Feedback Timing   91

Feedback on Written Material   92

Grades and Salary Increment Determination   94

Relationship of Maximizing Feedback in the Supervisory Process to the Specified Tasks of Supervision   95

Summary   96

References   96

Appendix A: Goal-Setting Criteria for the Student Clinician   100

Appendix B: A Guide for Clinical Practicum and Instructions for Implementation   103

Appendix C: Competency Based Objectives for Student Teaching in Speech-Language Pathology and Audiology   107

Appendix D: Clinical Competency Record and Student Evaluation Form   112

4 Structuring Effective Supervisory Conferences   118

Clinical Supervision Tasks Relevant to Structuring Effective Supervisory Conferences   118

Literature   119

Conference Reflections   120

Supervisee Expectations   120

Typical Conferences   122

Effective Conference Precursors   123
Preconference Planning: Supervisor   123
Preconference Planning: Supervisee   131

Conference Initiation   132

Facilitative Conference Behaviors   133
Verbal/Nonverbal Pacing   133
Positive Interpersonal Behaviors   135
Promotive Nonverbal Behaviors   138
Active Listening   138

Conference Content   139
Optimal Conference Summary   141
Conference Insights   141

**Relationship of Effective Conferencing
to the Specified Supervision Tasks   142**

Summary   143

References   143

Appendix: Guidelines for Supervisees on Preparing
for Supervision   147

PART THREE   Supervising People   149

5   Supervising Clinical Training   151

**Clinical Supervision Tasks Relevant to Supervision
in Clinical Training   151**

Supervisor Beginning Thoughts   152

Literature   152
Theory   152
Practice   153
Summary   154
Continuum of Supervision   154
Characteristics of Supervisees   156
Impressions of Supervisees   157
Potential for Bias   157

Supervision of the Beginning Clinician   158
Supervisee Acculturation   158
Goals   160
Strategies   160
Conference   161
Outcomes   161

Supervision of the Marginal Clinician   162
Identification   162
Goals   163
Strategies   163
Conference   165
Outcomes   166
Legal Implications   166

Supervision of the Average Clinician   167
Identification   167
Goals   168
Strategies   169

Conference 171
Outcomes 172
Legal Implications 172

Supervision of the Outstanding Clinician 172
Identification 172
Goals 173
Strategies 173
Conference 177
Outcomes 177
Legal Implications 177

Supervisor—Later Thoughts 178

Supervision of the Externship Experience 178
Supervisee Acculturation 179
Expectations 180
Feedback 180
Conference 180
Outcomes 181

Feedback about Supervision Experiences 181
Positive Perceptions 182
Negative Perceptions 182

Relationship of the Thirteen Tasks of Supervision to Supervising in Clinical Training 183

Summary 184

References 184

6 **Supervising Speech-Language Pathology Assistants 188**

Clinical Supervision Tasks Relevant to Supervising Speech-Language Pathology Assistants 188

The Speech-Language Pathology Assistant's Scope of Practice 189

Guidelines for Assistant Supervision 192
Nature of Assistants 194
Organizational Acculturation 195

Goals and Strategies for Attainment 196
Competent Performance 196
Responsibility and Client Service 196
Professional Behavior 197
Role Identification 197
Job Satisfaction 197

Supervisory Tools   198
Joint Planning and Role-Playing   199
Demonstration Therapy   199
Data Collection   199
Objective Setting   199
Structured Observations   200
Videotape and Audiotape   200
Selective Verbatim   201

Performance Documentation and Appraisal   201

Conference   202

Relationship of the Specified Supervision Tasks to Supervising Speech-Language Pathology Assistants   202

Summary   203

References   203

Appendix A: Sample Curriculum for the Speech-Language
Pathology Assistant   205
Speech-Language Pathology Assistant
Suggested Competencies   206
Approved Tasks for Communication Assistants   208

Appendix B: Decision Matrix for Amount and Type
of Monitoring   201
Assistant and Professional Planner   212
Client Review Table   213

7   Supervising in the Workplace   214

Clinical Supervision Tasks Relevant to Supervision in the Workplace   214

Supervision   215
Supervisor's Role Definition   215
Supervisee Interview   217
Job Initiation   218

Supervision Implementation   215
Supervisee Preparation   215
Supervisee Goals   220
Examples of Potential Objectives   221
Supervisory Techniques   222
Conference Strategies   224
Conference Issues   225
Effective Communication   225

Conference Evaluation   226
Supervision Benefits   226

Performance Evaluation   227
Bias   227
Three-Sixty Evaluation   228
Portfolio Assessment   229
Supervisor-Driven Evaluation   229
Format and Content   230

Organizational Effectiveness   231
Successful Workplaces   231
Job Satisfaction   236

**Relationship of Supervising in the Workplace
and the Specified Supervision Tasks   240**

Summary   241

References   241

P A R T   F O U R   Training Participants   245

**8   Preparing Supervisees for the
Supervisory Process   247**

**Clinical Supervision Tasks Relevant to Preparing
Supervisees for the Supervisory Process   247**

Context for Supervisee Preparation   248

Training Supervisees for the Supervisory Process   249

Supervisee Preparation   250
Supervision Continuum   251
Supervisory Process   254
Practicum Components   255

Supervisee Professional Growth   261
Self-Directed Growth   262
Outcomes   267

**Relationship of the Thirteen Tasks of Supervision
to Preparing the Supervisee for the
Supervisory Process   267**

Summary   268

References   268

9 **Creating Solutions: Supervisor Professional Growth**   **271**

   Clinical Supervision Tasks Relevant to the Professional Growth of the Supervisor   **271**

   Literature   **272**
      Speech-Language Pathology/Audiology   272
      Education   275
      Counseling   275
      Business   276
      Summary   278

   State of the Art   **278**
      Growth Opportunities   279
      Growth Decision   280
      Problem Identification   281
      Growth Commitment   281

   Self-Guided Growth   **282**
      Reading   282
      Reflecting   282
      Data-Collecting   282
      Modifying   283
      Goal-Setting   283
      Gathering Feedback   283
      Collaborating   284
      Taping   284
      Networking   284
      Meetings   284

   Formal Supervisor Training   **285**
      Coursework   285
      Problem-Solving   286
      Practicum   287
      Advanced   287

   Research-Directed Development   **288**

   Relevance of the Thirteen Tasks of Supervision to Supervisor Professional Growth   **289**

   Summary   **289**

   References   **290**

   Appendix A: Promotion Criteria for Supervisors and Clinical Staff   293

   Appendix B: Conference Analysis   296

Appendix C: Student Evaluation of Practicum Supervisor
Communication Disorders 298

PART FIVE Training Vehicles 301

10 Teaching Clinic: A Vehicle for Clinical and Supervisory Growth 303

Clinical Supervision Tasks Relevant to Developing Clinical and Supervisory Skills through the Teaching Clinic Methodology 303

Literature 303
Speech-Language Pathology 304
Social Work 304
Psychology 305
Education 306
New Directions 307

Teaching Clinic Method 308
Phases 309
Ground Rules 311
Training 311
Rationale for Training Components 312
Facilitation 313
Value 313
Applicability 314
New Directions Revisited 314

Teaching Clinic Adaptations 315
Professional Growth 317

Alternate Uses 318

Benefits 319

Liabilities 320

Research Summary 320

Teaching Clinic Summary 321

Relationship of the Teaching Clinic Approach to the Specified Supervision Tasks 322

Summary 323

References 323

Appendix A: Teaching Clinic Training Material 326

11   **Teaching Supervisory Skills through Role-Playing and Simulation   331**

Clinical Supervision Tasks Relevant to Teaching Supervisory Skills through Role-Playing and Simulation   331

Role-Playing and Simulation   333

Role-Playing: Literature   333
The Use of Role-Playing   333
The Impact of Role-Playing   335

Implementing Role-Playing   336
Advance Preparation   336
Application Strategies   336

Relationship of Role-Playing in Teaching Supervisory Skills to the Specified Supervision Tasks   333
Examples of Role-Playing   339

Role-Playing Summary   343

Simulation   343

Simulation: Literature   343
Teacher Education   343
Health-Care Education   344
Business Applications   345

Relationship of the Use of Simulation to the Specified Supervision Tasks   346

Simulation Game   347

Simulation Orientation   348
Example of Response   349
Cast of Characters   350

Simulation: Fall   352
School   352
University   354
Hospital   356

Simulation: Winter   359
School   359
University   362
Hospital   364

Simulation: Spring   367
School   367
University   369
Hospital   371

References   374

Index   377

INTRODUCTION

Healthcare professionals now face more opportunities and challenges than ever before. A variety of factors is the stimulus. First, graduate academic and clinical training continue to be the future of the profession. Second, shifts in health-care funding and managed care are changing the way clinical services are delivered. Third, speech-language pathology assistants are added to the array of professionals providing clinical services. Fourth, accountability and outcome measures are increasingly at the heart of clinical practice. Together, these create a complex context for the implementation of supervision.

This book is designed to make this task easier. It provides practical strategies for implementing the supervisory process. Information from the literature is provided for the reader as well. Thus, readers may pick and choose the information they find most helpful.

The 13 tasks of effective clinical supervision published as an American Speech-Language Hearing Association position statement (ASHA, 1985) and the Anderson (1988) Continuum of Supervision model serve as the synthesizing structures for this text. This former document appears in its entirety in Appendix A on page xxi. The supervision tasks and the related competencies identify the fundamentals of effective supervision. The Anderson model complements the 13 tasks. Anderson's continuum is a splendid tool for implementing and thinking about supervision and for adapting the process to the needs of the supervisee. Information regarding the development of the tasks and Anderson model follows to orient and prepare the reader for the body of this book.

Thirteen Task History

In the early 1960s, concerns about the quality of supervision in clinical training emerge in the literature in speech-language pathology (Perkins, 1962; Halfond, 1964; Kleffner, 1964; Villareal, 1964). Then, in 1974, Anderson calls for the American Speech-Language and Hearing Association to provide leadership in (1) defining the role of the supervisor, (2) identifying components of the supervisory process, and (3) encouraging the establishment of training programs for supervisors. In 1978, the ASHA Committee on Supervision publishes a position statement regarding the status of supervision in speech-language pathology and audiology (ASHA, 1978). This study documents the low status of supervisors in regard to visibility, salary, job security, and the lack of supervisory training for those performing this critical function. The report is intended as an impetus for change.

The work of the ASHA Committee on Supervision continues and, in 1980, minimum qualifications for supervisors are presented to the membership (Van-Demark, Borton, Dowling, Nelson, Rassi, Ulrich, & Vallon, 1980). They consist of the following:

1. Master's degree in speech pathology or audiology;
2. Three years of experience beyond the Clinical Fellowship Year (CFY);
3. Certificate of Clinical Competence (CCC) in the area to be supervised;
4. Six semester hours of academic coursework or its equivalent in continuing education credits.
5. 50 hours of practicum in supervision.

At least three of the semester hours are to be in supervision in speech-language pathology and/or audiology. Those remaining will pertain to the common body of supervision knowledge although they might be in speech-language pathology and audiology or a related discipline such as counseling, business management, social work, and education. The proposed requirements are presented at the annual convention of the American Speech-Language and Hearing Association and in *ASHA*. The response, in 1980 and 1981, from the membership is vigorous and overwhelmingly negative. Great concern is voiced regarding the potential emergence of specialty certification. As a result, the proposal is withdrawn.

Subsequently, with input from the Subcommittee on Supervision of the Council on Professional Standards in Speech-Language Pathology and Audiology, the ASHA Supervision Committee develops the tasks and competencies for supervision. The resulting report is approved by the Legislative Council and becomes an official position statement of the American Speech-Language and Hearing Association (ASHA, 1985).

The adoption of the supervision position statement by the American Speech-Language and Hearing Association is a monumental step toward quality supervision. However, the work is far from done. Position statements are official stances for recommended practice. But, they do not incorporate enforcement mechanisms to assure implementation.

The scholarly basis of and the interest in quality supervision continues to grow. There is now a solid body of supervision literature in speech-language pathology and audiology, education, social work, school counseling, psychology, and business. With the ongoing efforts of committed professionals, quality supervision will be the cornerstone in training and the workplace.

Supervisory Models

The second introductory topic that will assist the reader with the chapters of this book relates to supervisory models. The degree to which the specific tasks of supervision are realized is directly related to the supervisor and supervisee's training and their resulting philosophies regarding the process. Thus, a model to structure practice is critical.

Past research in speech-language pathology demonstrates that supervisors tend to be direct and use a telling style in the conference. This is thought to be particularly true of those without formal supervisory training. They are likely to dominate talk time, problem-solving, and strategy development, ask numerous questions, and use the same, unchanging style with all supervisees. These behaviors reflect a direct style of supervision and are thought to lead to passive supervisee involvement and dependence on the supervisor. Although some aspects of the thirteen tasks may be realized when this type of supervision is implemented, supervisee growth is significantly below the potential.

Optimal supervision, on the other hand, changes in response to the needs of the individuals involved. Supervisees are active participants in the process and grow toward the goal of self-supervision. They engage in data collection, problem-solving, and strategy development. Supervisees, as a result of their participation, do learn strategies for independent functioning.

This latter type of supervision is discussed in this text from the perspective of three theoretical models: Cogan (1973) *Clinical Supervision,* Anderson (1988) *Continuum of Supervision,* and Costa and Garmston (1994) *Cognitive Coaching.* Other theorists, such as Farmer and Farmer (1989), are also noted for their unique contributions.

Jean Anderson's *Continuum of Supervision* (1988) is the most widely recognized supervision model in speech-language pathology and audiology (Figure A). Anderson finds a theoretical soulmate in Morris Cogan. Cogan (1973), in education, introduces the concept of clinical supervision, which is designed to improve teaching behavior. His ongoing cycle of supervision consists of eight distinct phases. Colleagueship and supervision at the supervisee's level of need form the foundation of his method. Joint data collection, analysis, problem-solving, and strategy development are the basis of conferences.

Anderson extends and makes significant additions to Cogan's work. Anderson stresses the importance of modifying the supervisor's style in response to

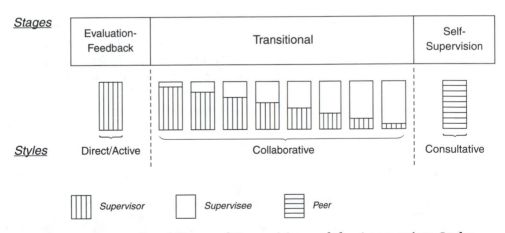

FIGURE A.   Composite of Stages of Supervision and the Appropriate Styles for Each Stage.

Anderson, J. *The Supervisory Process in Speech-Language Pathology and Audiology.* Austin, TX: Pro-Ed, 1988. Reprinted with permission of the author.

supervisee needs. She states that, depending on the level of the supervisee and the particular situation, a direct, collaborative, or consultative supervisory approach may be appropriate. Supervisees in the evaluation/feedback stage of development are most likely to need a direct, active method. As the supervisee begins to grow and moves into the transitional phase, collaboration becomes appropriate. When the supervisee is ready for self-supervision, the supervisor moves into a consultant role. Data collection, analysis, problem-solving and strategy development, with varying degrees of supervisor–supervisee involvement, occur as the clinician moves along the continuum of supervision toward increasing independence. In addition, this model actively fosters the supervisor's professional growth as well as that of the supervisee. The Anderson model will form the thread of supervisory theory that will weave throughout the chapters that follow.

Each chapter in the book begins by identifying the supervision tasks relevant to the topic. The content that follows is, then, designed to facilitate acquisition of the skills described. The continuum of supervision is addressed wherever appropriate throughout the text.

The first section of the book addresses organizational issues that provide the context for supervision. Ways are suggested to increase the effectiveness of supervision in training and work settings. The second section relates to tools and strategies for enhancing supervision. The hows and whys of data collection and goal setting and their use in the supervisory process are explored. In addition, fundamental aspects of supervision such as conferencing and providing feedback are addressed. The third section is devoted to the applications of the supervisory process to all levels of practitioners including clinical training, the working professional, and speech-language pathology assistants. The fourth section focuses on the training of participants, which includes preparing supervisees for active participation in the supervisory process and fostering lifelong supervisor professional growth. The final section presents training vehicles for use with present and future supervisors: the teaching clinic, role-play, and simulation.

The intended audience for this book is threefold. First, it is for those people enrolled in a clinical supervision or professional issues course or those participating in workshops on supervision. It also serves as a resource for working supervisors or those considering a supervisory position. Finally, it is for all supervisors and supervisees desiring ongoing professional growth. My hope is that readers will enjoy the book and find ways to use it to enhance their professional lives.

REFERENCES

American Speech-Language and Hearing Association. Committee on Supervision in Speech-language Pathology and Audiology. "Current status of supervision of speech-language pathology and audiology (special report)." *American Speech Hearing Association, 20* (1978): 478–486.

American Speech-Language and Hearing Association. Committee on Supervision in Speech-Language Pathology and Audiology. "Clinical supervision in speech-language pathology and audiology: A position statement." *American Speech Hearing Association, 27* (1985): 57–60.

Anderson, J. "Supervision of school speech, hearing and language programs—an emerging role." *American Speech Hearing Association, 16* (1974): 7–10.

Anderson, J. *The Supervisory Process in Speech-Language Pathology and Audiology.* Austin, TX: Pro-Ed., 1988.

Cogan, M. *Clinical Supervision.* Boston: Houghton Mifflin, 1973.

Costa, A., and Garmston, R. *Cognitive coaching: A foundation for renaissance schools.* Norwood, MA: Christopher Gordon Publishers, Inc. 1994.

Farmer, S. and Farmer, J., *Supervision in Communication Disorders,* Merrill, 1989.

Halfond, M.,"Clinical supervision—Stepchild in training." *American Speech Hearing Association, 6* (1964): 441–444.

Kleffner, F. (Ed.) *Seminar on Guidelines for the Internship Year.* Washington, DC: American Speech and Hearing Association, 1964.

Perkins, W. "Our profession—What is it?" *American Speech Hearing Association, 4* (1962): 339–344.

VanDemark, A., Borton, T., Dowling, S., Nelson, G., Rassi, J., Ulrich, S. and Vallon, J. "Qualifications for supervisors: A proposal for discussion." Miniseminar presented at the Annual Convention of the American Speech-Language and Hearing Association, Detroit, Michigan, 1980.

Villareal, J. (Ed.) *Seminar on Guidelines for Supervision of Clinical Practicum.* Washington, DC: American Speech and Hearing Association, 1964.

ACKNOWLEDGMENTS

This book could not have been completed without the contributions of numbers of wonderful individuals including the excellent editing and production staffs from Allyn and Bacon. The students in my supervision courses have continually challenged and shaped my views of the supervisory process as have those whom I have supervised. The same is true of Melissa Bruce, a valued colleague and partner in thought. Lynn Bliss, both friend and department chair, has found resources when needed and has provided ongoing support. Laura Porter and Julie Warner assisted with literature searches and Laura also helped in editing the references. Both Julie and Laura were competent, conscientious, and greatly appreciated. Debbie Romero provided thought-provoking ideas and was an excellent source of thoughtful feedback. The reviewers, Kristine Sbaschnig, Wayne State University, Deborah Romero, University of Houston, and Barbara Solomon, Purdue University, each provided comments that were helpful. I would also like to thank the individuals whose works have been reprinted in this text. Their contributions are unique and I appreciate their willingness to share their work. I take this opportunity to say thank you one and all.

In addition, I am deeply indebted to Jean Anderson, Professor Emeritus, from Indiana University. Her dedication and excitement sparked my initial interest in the supervisory process. The training program she directed cemented my commitment to furthering clinical supervision as a discipline. Further, many of the ideas in this work grew from those presented by her. During training and throughout my professional career, she has been a mentor and a valued friend.

And finally, Jerry, my husband, contributed in so many ways that I lose count. He trekked through library stacks searching, carrying and duplicating, created figures for the manuscript, assisted continuously as a computer resource, helped with editing, and aided in the organization and compilation of the manuscript. As always, he has been incredibly supportive throughout this work. He has my heartfelt thanks.

APPENDIX TO THE INTRODUCTION

The Thirteen Tasks of Supervision

Position Statement

Clinical Supervision in Speech-Language Pathology and Audiology*

The following position paper, developed by the Committee on Supervision, was adopted by the American Speech-Language-Hearing Association through its Legislative Council in November 1984 (LC 8-84). Members of the Committee included Elaine Brown-Grant, Patricia Casey, Bonnie Cleveland, Charles Diggs (*ex officio*), Richard Forcucci, Noel Matkin, George Purvis, Kathryn Smith, Peggy Williams (*ex officio*), Edward Wills, and Sandra Ulrich, Chair. Also contributing were the NSSLHA representatives Mary Kawell and Sheran Landis. The committee was under the guidance of Marianna Newton, Vice President for Professional and Governmental Affairs.

Contributions of members of the ASHA Committee on Supervision for the years 1976–1982 are acknowledged. The members of the 1978–1981 Subcommittee on Supervision (Noel Matkin, Chair) of the Council on Professional Standards in Speech-Language Pathology and Audiology are also acknowledged for their work from which the competencies presented herein were adapted.

> WHEREAS, the American Speech-Language-Hearing Association (ASHA) needs a clear position on clinical supervision, and
>
> WHEREAS, the necessity for having such a position for use in student training and in professional, legal, and governmental contexts has been recognized, and
>
> WHEREAS, the Committee on Supervision in Speech-Language Pathology and Audiology has been charged to recommend guidelines for the roles and responsibilities of supervisors in various settings (LC 14-74), and
>
> WHEREAS, a position statement on clinical supervision now has been developed, disseminated for both select and widespread peer review, and revised; therefore
>
> RESOLVED, that the American Speech-Language-Hearing Association adopts "Clinical Supervision in Speech-Language Pathology and Audiology" as the recognized position of the Association.

Introduction

Clinical supervision is a part of the earliest history of the American Speech-Language-Hearing Association (ASHA). It is an integral part of the initial training of speech-language

---

*Reprinted with permission from ASHA. "Clinical supervision in speech-language pathology and audiology." *American Speech Hearing Association* 27 (1985): 57–60.

American Speech-Language and Hearing Association. Committee on Supervision in Speech-Language Pathology and Audiology. "Clinical supervision in speech-language pathology and audiology: A position statement." *American Speech Hearing Association,* 27 (1985): 57–60.

pathologists and audiologists, as well as their continued professional development at all levels and in all work settings.

ASHA has recognized the importance of supervision by specifying certain aspects of supervision in its requirements for the Certificates of Clinical Competence (CCC) and the Clinical Fellowship Year (CFY) (ASHA, 1982). Further, supervisory requirements are specified by the Council on Professional Standards in its standards and guidelines for both educational and professional services programs (Educational Standards Board, ASHA, 1980; Professional Services Board, ASHA, 1983). State laws for licensing and school certification consistently include requirements for supervision of practicum experiences and initial work performance. In addition, other regulatory and accrediting bodies (e.g., Joint Commission on Accreditation of Hospitals, Commission on Accreditation of Rehabilitation Facilities) require a mechanism for ongoing supervision throughout professional careers.

It is important to note that the term **clinical supervision,** as used in this document, refers to the tasks and skills of clinical teaching related to the interaction between a clinician and client. In its 1978 report, the Committee on Supervision in Speech-Language Pathology and Audiology differentiated between the two major roles of persons identified as supervisors: clinical teaching aspects and program management tasks. The Committee emphasized that although program management tasks relating to administration or coordination of programs may be a part of the person's job duties, the term **supervisor** referred to "individuals who engaged in clinical teaching through observation, conferences, review of records, and other procedures, and which is related to the interaction between a clinician and a client and the evaluation or management of communication skills" (*ASHA,* 1978, p. 479). The Committee continues to recognize this distinction between tasks of administration or program management and those of clinical teaching, which is its central concern.

The importance of supervision to preparation of students and to assurance of quality clinical service has been assumed for some time. It is only recently, however, that the tasks of supervision have been well-defined, and that the special skills and competencies judged to be necessary for their effective application have been identified. This Position Paper addresses the following areas:

■ tasks of supervision
■ competencies for effective clinical supervision
■ preparation of clinical supervisors

Tasks of Supervision

A central premise of supervision is that effective clinical teaching involves, in a fundamental way, the development of self-analysis, self-evaluation, and problem-solving skills on the part of the individual being supervised. The success of clinical teaching rests largely on the achievement of this goal. Further, the demonstration of quality clinical skills in supervisors is generally accepted as a prerequisite to supervision of students, as well as of those in the Clinical Fellowship Year or employed as certified speech-language pathologists or audiologists.

Outlined in this paper are 13 tasks basic to effective clinical teaching and constituting the distinct area of practice which comprises clinical supervision in communication disorders. The committee stresses that the level of preparation and experience of the supervisee, the particular work setting of the supervisor and supervisee, and client variables will influence the relative emphasis of each task in actual practice.

The tasks and their supporting competencies which follow are judged to have face validity as established by experts in the area of supervision, and by both select and widespread peer review. The committee recognizes the need for further validation and strongly encourages ongoing investigation. Until such time as more rigorous measures of validity are established, it will be particularly important for the tasks and competencies to be reviewed periodically through quality assurance procedures. Mechanisms such as Patient Care Audit and Child Services Review System appear to offer useful means for quality assurance in the supervisory tasks and competencies. Other procedures appropriate to specific work settings may also be selected.

The tasks of supervision discussed above follow:

1. establishing and maintaining an effective working relationship with the supervisee;
2. assisting the supervisee in developing clinical goals and objectives;
3. assisting the supervisee in developing and refining assessment skills;
4. assisting the supervisee in developing and refining clinical management skills;
5. demonstrating for and participating with the supervisee in the clinical process;
6. assisting the supervisee in observing and analyzing assessment and treatment sessions;
7. assisting the supervisee in the development and maintenance of clinical and supervisory records;
8. interacting with the supervisee in planning, executing, and analyzing supervisory conferences;
9. assisting the supervisee in evaluation of clinical performance;
10. assisting the supervisee in developing skills of verbal reporting, writing, and editing;
11. sharing information regarding ethical, legal, regulatory, and reimbursement aspects of professional practice;
12. modeling and facilitating professional conduct; and
13. demonstrating research skills in the clinical or supervisory processes.

Competencies for Effective Clinical Supervision

Although the competencies are listed separately according to task, each competency may be needed to perform a number of supervisor tasks.

1.0 Task: Establishing and maintaining an effective working relationship with the supervisee.

Competencies required:

1.1 Ability to facilitate an understanding of the clinical and supervisory processes.
1.2 Ability to organize and provide information regarding the logical sequences of supervisory interaction, that is, joint setting of goals and objectives, data collection and analysis, evaluation.
1.3 Ability to interact from a contemporary perspective with the supervisee in both the clinical and supervisory process.
1.4 Ability to apply learning principles in the supervisory process.
1.5 Ability to apply skills of interpersonal communication in the supervisory process.
1.6 Ability to facilitate independent thinking and problem solving by the supervisee.
1.7 Ability to maintain a professional and supportive relationship that allows supervisor and supervisee growth.
1.8 Ability to interact with the supervisee objectively.
1.9 Ability to establish joint communications regarding expectations and responsibilities in the clinical and supervisory processes.
1.10 Ability to evaluate, with the supervisee, the effectiveness of the ongoing supervisory relationship.

2.0   Task: Assisting the supervisee in developing clinical goals and objectives.

Competencies required:

2.1   Ability to assist the supervisee in planning effective client goals and objectives.

2.2   Ability to plan, with the supervisee, effective goals and objectives for clinical and professional growth.

2.3   Ability to assist the supervisee in using observation and assessment in preparation of client goals and objectives.

2.4   Ability to assist the supervisee in using self-analysis and previous evaluation in preparation of goals and objectives for professional growth.

2.5   Ability to assist the supervisee in assigning priorities to clinical goals and objectives.

2.6   Ability to assist the supervisee in assigning priorities to goals and objectives for professional growth.

3.0   Task: Assisting the supervisee in developing and refining assessment skills.

Competencies required:

3.1   Ability to share current research findings and evaluation procedures in communication disorders.

3.2   Ability to facilitate an integration of research findings in client assessment.

3.3   Ability to assist the supervisee in providing rationale for assessment procedures.

3.4   Ability to assist supervisee in communicating assessment procedures and rationales.

3.5   Ability to assist the supervisee in integrating findings and observations to make appropriate recommendations.

3.6   Ability to facilitate the supervisee's independent planning of assessment.

4.0   Task: Assisting the supervisee in developing and refining management skills.

Competencies required:

4.1   Ability to share current research findings and management procedures in communication disorders.

4.2   Ability to facilitate an integration of research findings in client management.

4.3   Ability to assist the supervisee in providing rationale for treatment procedures.

4.4   Ability to assist the supervisee in identifying appropriate sequences for client change.

4.5   Ability to assist the supervisee in adjusting steps in the progression toward a goal.

4.6   Ability to assist the supervisee in the description and measurement of client and clinician change.

4.7   Ability to assist the supervisee in documenting client and clinician change.

4.8   Ability to assist the supervisee in integrating documented client and clinician change to evaluate progress and specify future recommendations.

5.0   Task: Demonstrating for and participating with the supervisee in the clinical process.

Competencies required:

5.1   Ability to determine jointly when demonstration is appropriate.

5.2   Ability to demonstrate or participate in an effective client-clinician relationship.

5.3   Ability to demonstrate a variety of clinical techniques and participate with the supervisee in clinical management.

5.4 Ability to demonstrate or use jointly the specific materials and equipment of the profession.

5.5 Ability to demonstrate or participate jointly in counseling of clients or family/guardians of clients.

6.0 Task: Assisting the supervisee in observing and analyzing assessment and treatment sessions.

Competencies required:

6.1 Ability to assist the supervisee in learning a variety of data collection procedures.

6.2 Ability to assist the supervisee in selecting and executing data collection procedures.

6.3 Ability to assist the supervisee in accurately recording data.

6.4 Ability to assist the supervisee in analyzing and interpreting data objectively.

6.5 Ability to assist the supervisee in revising plans for client management based on data obtained.

7.0 Task: Assisting the supervisee in development and maintenance of clinical and supervisory records.

Competencies required:

7.1 Ability to assist the supervisee in applying record-keeping systems to supervisory and clinical processes.

7.2 Ability to assist the supervisee in effectively documenting supervisory and clinically related interactions.

7.3 Ability to assist the supervisee in organizing records to facilitate easy retrieval of information concerning clinical and supervisory interactions.

7.4 Ability to assist the supervisee in establishing and following policies and procedures to protect the confidentiality of clinical and supervisory records.

7.5 Ability to share information regarding documentation requirements of various accrediting and regulatory agencies and third-party funding sources.

8.0 Task: Interacting with the supervisee in planning, executing, and analyzing supervisory conferences.

Competencies required:

8.1 Ability to determine with the supervisee when a conference should be scheduled.

8.2 Ability to assist the supervisee in planning a supervisory conference agenda.

8.3 Ability to involve the supervisee in jointly establishing a conference agenda.

8.4 Ability to involve the supervisee in joint discussion of previously identified clinical or supervisory data or issues.

8.5 Ability to interact with the supervisee in a manner that facilitates the supervisee's self-exploration and problem solving.

8.6 Ability to adjust conference content based on the supervisee's level of training and experience.

8.7 Ability to encourage and maintain supervisee motivation for continuing self-growth.

8.8 Ability to assist the supervisee in making commitments for changes in clinical behavior.

8.9 Ability to involve the supervisee in ongoing analysis of supervisory interactions.

9.0   Task: Assisting the supervisee in evaluation of clinical performance.

Competencies required:

9.1   Ability to assist the supervisee in the use of clinical evaluation tools.
9.2   Ability to assist the supervisee in the description and measurement of his/her progress and achievement.
9.3   Ability to assist the supervisee in developing skills of self-evaluation.
9.4   Ability to evaluate clinical skills with the supervisee for purposes of grade assignment, completion of Clinical Fellowship Year, professional advancement, and so on.

10.0 Task: Assisting the supervisee in developing skills of verbal reporting, writing, and editing.

Competencies required:

10.1 Ability to assist the supervisee in identifying appropriate information to be included in a verbal or written report.
10.2 Ability to assist the supervisee in presenting information in a logical, concise, and sequential manner.
10.3 Ability to assist the supervisee in using appropriate professional terminology and style in verbal and written reporting.
10.4 Ability to assist the supervisee in adapting verbal and written reports to the work environment and communication situation.
10.5 Ability to alter and edit a report as appropriate while preserving the supervisee's writing style.

11.0 Task: Sharing in formation regarding ethical, legal, regulatory, and reimbursement aspects of the profession.

Competencies required:

11.1 Ability to communicate to the supervisee a knowledge of professional codes of ethics (e.g., ASHA, state licensing boards, and so on).
11.2 Ability to communicate to the supervisee an understanding of legal and regulatory documents and their impact on the practice of the profession (licensure, PL 94-142, Medicare, Medicaid, and so on).
11.3 Ability to communicate to the supervisee an understanding of reimbursement policies and procedures of the work setting.
11.4 Ability to communicate a knowledge of supervisee rights and appeal procedures specific to the work setting.

12.0 Task: Modeling and facilitating professional conduct.

Competencies required:

12.1 Ability to assume responsibility,
12.2 Ability to analyze, evaluate, and modify own behavior.
12.3 Ability to demonstrate ethical and legal conduct.
12.4 Ability to meet and respect deadlines.
12.5 Ability to maintain professional protocols (respect for confidentiality, etc).
12.6 Ability to provide current information regarding professional standards (PSB, ESB, licensure, teacher certification, etc.).

12.7 Ability to communicate information regarding fees, billing procedures, and third-party reimbursement.

12.8 Ability to demonstrate familiarity with professional issues.

12.9 Ability to demonstrate continued professional growth.

13.0 Task: Demonstrating research skills in the clinical or supervisory processes.

Competencies required:

13.1 Ability to read, interpret, and apply clinical and supervisory research.

13.2 Ability to formulate clinical or supervisory research questions.

13.3 Ability to investigate clinical or supervisory research questions.

13.4 Ability to support and refute clinical or supervisory research findings.

13.5 Ability to report results of clinical or supervisory research and disseminate as appropriate (e.g., in-service, conferences, publications).

Preparation of Supervisors

The special skills and competencies for effective clinical supervision may be acquired through special training which may include, but is not limited to, the following:

1. Specific curricular offerings from graduate programs; examples include doctoral programs emphasizing supervision, other postgraduate preparation, and specified graduate courses.

2. Continuing educational experiences specific to the supervisory process (e.g., conferences, workshops, self-study).

3. Research-directed activities that provide insight in the supervisory process.

The major goal of training in supervision is mastery of the "Competencies for Effective Clinical Supervision." Since competence in clinical services and work experience sufficient to provide a broad clinical perspective are considered essential to achieving competence in supervision, it is apparent that most preparation in supervision will occur following the preservice level. Even so, positive effects of preservice introduction to supervision preparation have been described by both Anderson (1981) and Rassi (1983). Hence, the presentation of basic material about the supervisory process may enhance students' performance as supervisees, as well as provide them with a framework for later study.

The steadily increasing numbers of publications concerning supervision and the supervisory process indicate that basic information concerning supervision now is becoming more accessible in print to all speech-language pathologists and audiologists, regardless of geographical location and personal circumstances. In addition, conferences, workshops, and convention presentations concerning supervision in communication disorders are more widely available than ever before, and both coursework and supervisory practicum experiences are emerging in college and university educational programs. Further, although preparation in the supervisory process specific to communication disorders should be the major content, the commonality in principles of supervision across the teaching, counseling, social work, business, and health care professions suggests additional resources for those who desire to increase their supervisory knowledge and skills.

To meet the needs of persons who wish to prepare themselves as clinical supervisors, additional coursework, continuing education opportunities, and other programs in the supervisory process should be developed both within and outside graduate education programs. As noted in an earlier report on the status of supervision (ASHA, 1978), supervisors themselves expressed a strong desire for training in supervision. Further, systematic study and investigation of the supervisory process is seen as necessary to expansion of the data base from which increased knowledge about supervision and the supervisory process will emerge.

The "Tasks of Supervision" and "Competencies for Effective Clinical Supervision" are intended to serve as the basis for content and outcome in preparation of supervisors. The tasks and competencies will be particularly useful to supervisors for self-study and self-evaluation, as well as to the consumers of supervisory activity, that is, supervisees and employers.

A repeated concern by the ASHA membership is that implementation of any suggestions for qualifications of supervisors will lead to additional standards or credentialing. At this time, preparation in supervision is a viable area of specialized study. The competencies for effective supervision can be achieved and implemented by supervisors and employers.

Summary

Clinical supervision in speech-language pathology and audiology is a distinct area of expertise and practice. This paper defines the area of supervision, outlines the special tasks of which it is comprised, and describes the competencies for each task. The competencies are developed by special preparation, which may take at least three avenues of implementation. Additional coursework, continuing education opportunities and other programs in the supervisory process should be developed both within and outside of graduate education programs. At this time, preparation in supervision is a viable area for specialized study, with competence achieved and implemented by supervisors and employers.

Bibliography

American Speech and Hearing Association. (1978). Current status of supervision of speech-language pathology and audiology [Special Report] *Asha, 20,* 478–486.

American Speech-Language-Hearing Association. (1980). *Standards for accreditation by the Education and Training Board.* Rockville, MD: ASHA.

American Speech-Language-Hearing Association. (1982). *Requirements for the certificates of clinical competence* (Rev.). Rockville, MD: ASHA.

American Speech-Language-Hearing Association. (1983). New standards for accreditation by the Professional Services Board. *Asha, 25,* 6, 51–58.

Anderson, J. (Ed.) (1980, July). *Proceedings: Conference on Training in the Supervisory Process in Speech-Language Pathology and Audiology.* Indiana University, Bloomington.

Anderson, J. (1981). A training program in clinical supervision. *Asha, 23,* 77–82.

Culatta, R., & J. Helmick. (1980). Clinical supervision: The state of the art—Part I. *Asha, 22,* 985–993.

Culatta, R., & J. Helmick. (1981). Clinical supervision: The state of the art—Part II. *Asha, 23,* 21–31.

Laney, M. (1982). Research and evaluation in the public schools. *Language, Speech, and Hearing Services in the Schools, 13,* 53–60.

Rassi, J. (1983, September). *Supervision in audiology.* Seminar presented at Hahnemann University, Philadelphia.

PART ONE

Preparing the Stage

Creating Productivity and Professional Growth within Organizations

Clinical Supervision Tasks Relevant to Creating Productivity and Professional Growth within Organizations

Task 1: Establishing and maintaining an effective working relationship;

Task 3: Assisting the supervisee in developing and refining assessment skills;

Task 4: Assisting the supervisee in developing and refining clinical management skills;

Task 6: Assisting the supervisee in observing and analyzing assessment and treatment sessions;

Task 9: Assisting the supervisee in evaluation of clinical performance;

Task 12: Modeling and facilitating professional conduct;

Task 13: Demonstrating research skills in the clinical or supervisory process.

Changes in the health care industry, managed care, and demands for accountability are altering how clinical services are delivered. The workplace and society are also facing the challenge and effects of a world economy. Corporations and health care organizations are downsizing and streamlining to remain competitive in the marketplace. Many organizations, including those in medicine, are multinational: They now have subsidiaries and/or working partners in other countries (Drucker, 1998). Today's dynamic environment presents supervisors in all work settings with a unique set of challenges and opportunities.

The practice of supervision permeates society. It exists in varying forms whenever one person monitors and facilitates the performance of another. The core aspects of supervision are similar independent of discipline and/or service delivery setting. Each setting is likely to have unique aspects as well. Supervision also takes place in a variety of organizational contexts, for example, universities, schools, hospitals, long-term care facilities, private practices, businesses, and government agencies. Within the field of speech-language pathology, individuals tend to become supervisors soon after acquiring appropriate certification or licensure.

In the context of business communities, there has been active concern about the impact of organizational climate/culture on worker productivity and satisfaction. These cultures vary markedly from one organization to another. The most successful companies are value-driven, with an overriding organizational philosophy, a mission, forming the basis for decision making. Consideration of organizational issues, including values, would enhance most service delivery settings.

Drucker (1998) states that for organizations to thrive in today's and future climates, they must be well-managed entrepreneurs. This means innovating, practicing continuous process improvement, and eliminating nonproductive products and practice. Successful innovation is based on tapping into unmet consumer needs: predicting the product or service they will want and then striving to meet that need. According to Lipton (1997), organizations with a value-driven vision are better prepared to innovate and respond quickly to changes in the environment.

This chapter will explore organizational issues that affect productivity and job satisfaction and are the context for effective supervision. These ideas will then be applied to the fields of speech-language pathology and audiology as the basis for implementing the thirteen Tasks of Supervision (ASHA, 1985). The six factors to be considered are integrally related to the success of a supervisor, to supervisee satisfaction, and to quality service delivery: (1) how to motivate, (2) what motivates, (3) leadership styles, (4) value-driven, (5) continuous process improvement, and (6) effective decision making. Each of these has the potential to improve outcomes in organizations that vary in purpose from training programs to service delivery settings.

Supervision and Organizational Culture

Dilemma

Kendra Anderson, supervisor, is thinking about one of her supervisees, Dennis Jones. She feels that his clinical work is sound but that he has the potential to be outstanding. He did complain last month about Maplewood School. He says that when he arrives they begin looking for a place for him to work that day. Often, he has to sit and wait while the secretary finishes a task before she even begins to look for a space for him. Kendra also overheard him tell one of the other clinicians that he resents having to wait to meet with her because she has been late a couple of times. She thinks she needs to talk to him about these issues. It annoys her that he is complaining. Sometimes, it seems he is only here for a paycheck. She tries to give him as much positive feedback as she can, but feels like their relationship is going downhill.

Kendra is voicing real concern about Dennis and her interactions with him. Is it a problem with Dennis? Is it a problem with the relationship? Is it the dynamics of the job? The sections that follow on *how* and *what* motivates will be helpful in providing strategies to understand this situation.

How to Motivate

Maslow's Hierarchy

The work of Maslow (1954) lays the foundation for much of what has subsequently emerged in the area of motivation. He states that workers have five hierarchial sets of needs, each of which must be achieved to free the individual to consider the next. The lowest level relates to *basic physical survival* such as hunger, thirst, sleep, and so on. These are followed by *safety and security* concerns. The latter includes comfort and an absence of danger, both physical and psychological, on the job. The third subset, according to Maslow, includes the drive for *social inclusion,* which means that workers want to be accepted as part of a group. Feelings such as belonging, love, affection, and participation are, therefore, important. Someone who works in an environment that meets these first three requirements is then likely to have concerns relating to Maslow's level four: *esteem and knowledge.* Here the employee works to earn recognition and prestige through achievement-oriented activities. A sense of confidence, competence, success, and intelligence becomes significant to the individual. The highest tier in the Maslow hierarchy is *self-actualization.* In implementation, a person functioning at this level represents the essence of the motto, "Be the best you can be." According to Maslow, the self-actualizing person, (1) strives to achieve his/her potential, (2) is challenged by work, (3) seeks intellectual stimulation, and (4) exhibits creativity.

Today, the majority of organizations consistently provide for basic human requirements described in the two lowest levels of Maslow's hierarchy. Adequate lighting, ventilation, air conditioning, water fountains, and restrooms are furnished. In regard to safety and security, the physical environments are typically free of health-threatening contaminants and adequate personal safety is provided along with, in many settings, reasonable job security. Recent changes in the health care industry are a threat to the latter in speech-language pathology. Even with that caveat, the majority of workers' proclaimed needs fall in the three higher Maslow categories: social, esteem, and self-actualization. To address the social aspects, an optimal organization will supply opportunities for social contact and interaction among employees. A centrally located area for coffee breaks, team projects, or periodic company social outings are beneficial. Further, the recognition of competence and achievement enhances esteem as does being treated as a professional. To foster self-actualization, the highest level of development, workers benefit from increased autonomy and control as well as the opportunity to engage in challenging but achievable work.

Recent societal changes, in part due to the impact of the world economy, changes in the health care industry, and, in part, to the influx of a new generation of workers, pose a serious threat to organizational loyalty and increase the complexities of supervision. First, economic pressure to compete with companies with low labor costs in other parts of the world and the stiff competition arising from overseas markets makes some companies lose sight of their most valuable asset, people. The drive to reduce the cost of health care and public school service is having the same impact in speech-language pathology and audiology. Downsizing and layoffs have become commonplace. Second, individuals entering the work-place within the last ten years represent a generation that is more self-focused than those preceding them. They have also observed organizational disloyalty among those around them. Third, the number of skilled laborers and knowledge workers is insufficient to meet the needs of organizations. The result of all these combined factors is a workforce clamoring for the highest bidder and one that frequently changes jobs. In fact, many people with specialized skills have left permanent positions to become consultants with a higher salary, no job security, and, often, no health or retirement benefits. From the viewpoint of organizational culture, two negative events have occurred: (1) the absence of loyalty or commitment to an organization, and (2) a threat to Maslow's need for safety and security (level 2). The result is that it is more difficult for a supervisor to motivate workers, to increase productivity, and to create an environment that fosters job satisfaction.

McGregor's Theory X and Y

McGregor's (1960) Theory X and Y is often referred to in the literature. It identifies two different orientations to management based on two contrasting perceptions of workers. Theory X parallels the classical view of man (Smith, 1939): Employees are innately lazy, hate work, must be coerced to perform, and respond only to external control. The opposing view, Theory Y, perceives people as goal-oriented, seeking achievement, taking initiative and responsibility, and deriving satisfaction from performing well, if given the opportunity. Theory Y workers demonstrate self-control and self-direction (McGregor, 1961). McGregor indicates that a company's fundamental assumptions about people, either X or Y, dictate management strategies.

Herzberg's Two-Factor Theory

Herzberg (1966) proposes that two sets of factors affect job satisfaction: *satisfiers* and *dissatisfiers*. He refers to the former as "motivators" and the latter as "hygienic factors." According to Kreitner and Kinicki (1989), dissatisfiers parallel the first three levels of Maslow's hierarchy and include factors such as basic safety, job security, salary, working conditions, and company policy. Bittel (1985) adds insurance/pension plans, good working conditions, congenial colleagues, and vacation time to this list. These hygienic issues, then, must be addressed in the work setting and provided at a level perceived as acceptable. Enhancing these variables significantly beyond this point, however, provides little benefit, as it has no further impact on output. Therefore, to truly stimulate the productivity of an individual, the dissatisfiers must be neutralized and additional circumstances provided that really do motivate, such as recognition, interesting work, and chances for personal growth. Bittel suggests the following are motivators: "challenging work, utilization of one's capabilities, opportunity to do something meaningful, recognition for achievement, sense of importance to organization, access to information, involvement in decision making" (1985).

Both employers and employees often mistakenly view salary as a key motivator. Instead, it is a hygienic factor. There is no question that if salaries are so low as to be an extreme dissatisfier, employees will leave an organization. But above that level, the impact of salary increases are short-lived. An employee may be elated/disturbed by a specific raise for a short time but will soon adopt the attitude of "The salary increment was last month, what will you do for me today?" The exception to the characterization of money as a dissatifier may occur if salary affects the higher level need of esteem. Prestige is a Maslow level four concern and salary, as compared to others similarly placed in an organization, has the potential to impact the perception of relative self-worth and could, therefore, influence one's self-esteem. For example, if employees of similar rank and experience receive markedly different salaries, the people earning less might feel that the level of compensation reflects their worth to the organization. Consequently, in addition to being a dissatisfier, under certain circumstances relative salary level might motivate.

McClelland's Need for Achievement

Early work by Murray (1938) identifies three specific drives thought to be prime motivators: the desire for achievement, affiliation, and power. The strength of the drive for a given individual varies on each of these parameters. Much of McClelland's (1973) work has focused on the achievement aspect. According to Blakeney (1983), people with a high need in this area thrive on task completion and prefer tasks of moderate difficulty (Kreitner and Kinicki, 1989). These individuals tend to want immediate, concrete performance feedback and will use the information to improve. In addition, they like tasks in which quality of performance is directly related to effort. The interest here in the achievement component is the role it plays later in the life-cycle theory of leadership.

How to motivate encompasses several components. Human needs and their developmental hierarchical ordering are an important key. Optimal performance is thought to be exhibited by individuals functioning at the highest Maslow (1954) level, self-actualization. According to Alderfer (1972), an unmet yearning may serve as a primary driver for a given individual. Thus, it is in the best interest of organizations to remove barriers to development and then actively foster growth by tapping into workers' desires for achievement, affiliation, and power. Efforts should be made to minimize job-related dissatisfiers and to emphasize those factors likely to enhance job satisfaction. In addition, management is likely to be more effective if managers assume that people want to achieve (McGregor's theory Y).

What Motivates

The theories of reinforcement, expectancy, and equity have emerged relative to "what motivates." An employee engaging in appropriate work behavior receives monetary and social rewards. The tenets of learning theory apply: (1) actions reinforced are likely to increase in frequency, (2) the shorter the delay between the event and the reinforcer, the greater the potency (Skinner, 1969). Expectancy, a second component, is also a factor. People expect to be rewarded for work efforts. The worker also assumes greater striving and output on the job will be compensated accordingly. Therefore, the more one labors, the greater the prize. Thus, individuals assess the situation, decide what they want, and then work at a consciously selected productivity level. Finally, employees anticipate equity or fairness: Two individuals with comparable training and/or experience who perform similarly will receive equivalent compensation.

Goal-setting is also thought to be a motivational strategy (Phillips & Gully, 1997). The setting of goals appears to affect an individual's motivation on two levels: pride or disappointment in specific achievement and in one's self-determination of overall ability to perform. Evans (1986) states that goals stimulate and guide behavior. Locke, Shaw, Saari, & Latham (1981) indicate that the acceptance of an objective prompts four sets of behaviors: (1) directing attention to relevant aspects of the task, (2) mobilizing effort, (3) generating persistence in behavior, and (4) developing strategies for effective performance. Phillips and Gully (1997) note that specific, difficult goals lead to better performance. Also, if goals are explicit, steady improvements in complex task performance occur (DeShon & Alexander, 1996). Success also makes the worker feel competent and able to do the job. An added benefit of this procedure is that feedback followed by the development of objectives increases work satisfaction and organizational commitment (Nelson, 1997). Finally, Dowling (1993) finds that achievement of supervisor conference talk behavior objectives increases confidence in one's ability to continue to develop as a supervisor.

Although people will accept goals imposed from above, Earley and Kanfer (1985) indicate that goal acceptance, goal satisfaction, and performance are highest for those given a choice in goal selection and in the decision of how to attain the end. They also report that employee performance is enhanced by the provision of a high-performing role model. The strong role model results in increased work performance, a greater acceptance of goals, and greater job satisfaction.

In regard to the issue of "what motivates," several theories are advanced. Reinforcement, expectancy, and equity are motivational factors. Goal-setting is also seen as a key factor.

Solution

After reading and thinking about how and what motivates, Kendra Anderson identifies several factors that may be contributing to Dennis's behavior. Not having a specific space available for him to work at Maplewood suggests that his services are not valued. In addition, having to wait for a secretary to finish her work before she tries to find a space and Kendra's being late to conferences says everyone's time is more valuable than his. He might also view it as a lack of respect for him as a person. Kendra also realizes that she has been seeing him through a theory X view of man, believing that money is the primary motivator. She continues to feel good about the amount of positive reinforcement she has been giving him but realizes she hasn't been setting objectives for growth with any of her staff and maybe hasn't been doing enough to encourage people to self-actualize. She is planning to meet with Dennis and develop a plan to begin to resolve these issues.

Workplace Philosophy and Motivational Examples

Supplemental to the theoretical issues of "how" and "what" motivates, reports from the workplace highlight the concepts. Stoffman (1987), reporting on the motivational insights noted by the president of Island Pacific Brewing Co., states that money is not a primary driver. Workers feel that recognition, responsibility, and pride in the company are more important. To stimulate productivity, the president uses memos to cite excellence, gives cash prizes, and includes employees in profit sharing. Stoffman also states that regularly scheduled performance evaluations are important in enhancing employee job satisfaction. This appraisal optimally includes a consideration of achievements, strengths, weaknesses, career goals, and strategies the company may use to assist the employee in reaching personal objectives. Finally, he reports that manager behavioral consistency is a basic element in worker motivation.

Drucker (1998) observes that a key to motivating knowledge workers is that they need to like their jobs. People want to be challenged. Knowing and believing in the organization's mission is important to them. Finally, they need to see that their efforts make a difference.

Birnbach notes that many people do indeed "work for money but not because of it" (1988, p. 14). She reports that people derive satisfaction from their jobs for a variety of reasons. Some employees express pride in the products or work produced by their companies (Lieber, 1998). Others revel in their job because it allows them to express their personal creativity or they have been successful in finding a position that parallels their own interests. In addition, many employees identify team membership as a job satisfier.

Popp, Davis, and Herbert (1986) examine the types of work-related reinforcement found to be most meaningful to employees. Opportunity for growth is identified as the most preferred work reward, followed by achievement, and then responsibility. Previous research, cited by these authors, demonstrates that preferences for motivators differ from occupation to occupation. Thus, the optimal circumstance may be to allow individuals or groups of employees to select the form of compensation most significant to them. These incentives would, then, be more effective as motivators.

Evans reflects on enhancing motivation from the viewpoint of management. He says that the manager "has to be a diagnostician when trying to improve performance" (1986, p. 218). As part of this process "the manager has to find out what aspects of motivation are missing and work on replacing them. These could include: setting difficult goals; setting comprehensive goals; helping people reach their goals; ensuring that people can reach their goals; boosting, not destroying confidence; developing an ideology of goal attainment; rewarding high performance due to effort; punishing sustained poor performance due to lack of effort; coaching, if poor performance is due to lack of ability; reinforcing attributions held by subordinates that failure is due to lack of effort; reinforcing attributions held by subordinates that success is due to ability; removing barriers to achievement; and seeking small wins" (1986, p. 218).

Nelson (1996) says that management's use of personal congratulations for good work is highly motivating to employees. An example is starting meetings with praise for those who deserve it (Nelson, 1997). Verbal praise is ranked first among sixty-seven possible incentives. Next in importance was a written note of congratulations. Barrow (1999) also underscores the effectiveness of personal notes of appreciation. Nelson (1997) says that an accolade is most effective when it immediately follows the good work. He defines strategies for giving praise effectively: (1) identify what the employee did, (2) let the person know the work was appreciated, (3) tell them why what they did was important, and (4) communicate how the effort has made the manager feel.

Nelson (1997) talks about the fact that "what motivates" is highly individual. He suggests asking employees to write down types of rewards they would find motivating. Finding out more about employees in terms of job, family, and personal desires allows the supervisor to adjust rewards to an employee's personal needs. Greenfield (1997) states, in general, that what people value most is control over their own time. Spitzer (1995) says that there are eight human needs underlying the successful motivation of others: activity, ownership, power, affiliation, competence, achievement, recognition, and meaning. Supervisors will want to address as many of these as possible when designing reward systems.

Some organizations use a broader range of motivational strategies, including telecommuting, flexibility in an employee's use of sick time, and offering personal services at work such as subsidized lunches, health clubs, and day care (Greenfield, 1997). Other options include annual incentive programs such as bonuses and employee stock options (Lewis, 1997). Some companies have employee dinners and outside activities that foster team building (Zuber, 1997). An example of the latter would be the organization's planning and implementation of a charity event or a weekend company conference at a resort. Firms that use outside events feel that they are very effective in increasing workers' motivation and productivity.

Leadership

In considering leadership, it is important to look at the context of supervision in speech-language pathology and audiology. For example, in a university training program, guidance is needed for students in classes, faculty, staff, and student providers of service delivery. In a hospital, rehabilitation facility, nursing home, public school, or private practice, the supervisor is likely to be managing varying numbers of professionals and support staff. The professional staff may include a speech-language pathology assistant, people in their clinical fellowship year, and others with several years and types of experience. The numbers of individuals being supervised may range from one to many. In addition, theoretical models of supervision, in particular that of Anderson, suggest that a supervisor's style should change in response to the needs of the supervisee. Combined, these variables make effective leadership a complex issue. Issues relating to leadership and the topics that follow are highlighted in the scenario that follows.

Dilemma

Roland has been the supervisor at Marcor Hospital for five years. During the first two years, a lot of staff turnover occurred. For the last three years his staff of five has been stable. He has always believed that an autocratic style of leadership with reasonable input from employees is the best way to get the job done. To maintain his interest in the job, he has implemented some major changes each year so that the programmatic and resource emphasis varies depending on the focus. His primary yardstick of success was the revenue generated. Things had gone smoothly until about two months ago. He announced to his staff that the emphasis for this year was going to be pediatrics. They would continue the other services but the goal was to build services for children. Roland thought that they would be excited about this new direction, but one of his staff members exploded in the meeting, saying "after all the effort we have put into building exemplary swallowing services, you expect us to push it into the corner?" He also noticed several other head nods and heard sounds of exasperation. He then told them he would come in and tell them how to adjust their treatment to the pediatric group. The meeting ended on a sour note. About a month later, Roland's boss told him that his departmental revenues had been down for the last six months and that he was having a hard time seeing where Roland's program was going, because his department is always doing something different. Because of the frequent changes, Roland's boss couldn't identify the program's purpose. After talking to his boss and thinking about his employees' reactions, Roland sensed that the program might be on rocky ground.

Roland is concerned about the drop in his departmental revenues and the feedback he perceived as negative from his boss. The meeting with his staff and their apparent frustration also surprised him. He is doing what he has always done and doesn't understand why it's not working. The material that follows may give Roland some insight into ways to turn the situation around.

Leadership Styles

Leadership theory, prior to the 1950s, was simplistic in focus. In the early 1900s, it was thought that exceptional leaders had certain characteristics such as charisma, forcefulness, decisiveness, and honor. Later, the idea developed that leaders varied along a continuum ranging from autocratic to democratic to laissez-faire. During the 1950s, concern surfaced about the simplicity of unidimensional leadership styles and their inability to explain the complexities of organizational command. With this realization came the notion that leadership has, at minimum, a dual focus. One component related to the individuals involved and the other to the nature of the task itself.

Leadership Grid   The Leadership Grid (Blake and McCanse, 1991) is a prime example of a leadership theory that encompasses both a task and person orientation. Their model, in grid format, reflects a concern for people on one axis and a concern for results on the other. Various leadership styles thus emerge, depending on the intersection of the points selected on the two dimensions. For example, a high production orientation, coupled with low concern for people, would result in task-oriented supervision with minimal interest in the individuals involved. In contrast, a high focus on both parameters results in an intense interest in productivity achieved through individuals committed to the organization. Blake and Mouton (1981) suggest that the high results/high people orientation is likely to be the most effective.

Roland, whose dilemma was described in Box 1.3, is an example of a high production, low people-oriented leader, which may not be appropriate given the length of time his staff has been at Marcor. In addition, he does not have a mission and makes almost no effort to foster supervisee professional growth. These key issues may underlie the frustration the supervisees are feeling, be the cause of his boss's concern, and be a factor in the reduced revenues. Clearly, he does not adapt his supervision to either supervisees or the situation.

Situational Leadership   The second cluster of theories suggests that there is a situational aspect to leadership. In some circumstances, one style is appropriate while in another an alternative may be more effective. One example is the Hersey and Blanchard (1982) Life-Cycle Model, a situational model of leadership, presented as a grid, much like Blake & McCanse's Leadership Grid. Hersey and Blanchard say that leadership style must take into account both the task to be completed and the individuals involved. The life-cycle model, in a grid format, has the relationship on one axis and task orientation on the other. Depending on the interplay of these factors, alternative supervisory styles may be adopted to produce maximal output. Four quadrants or primary supervisory styles are suggested: (1) *telling*—high task and low relationship, (2) *consulting*—high task and high relationship, (3) *participating*—high relationship and low task, and (4) *delegating*—low relationship and low task. The style changes as the situation evolves. The primary consideration in selecting an approach is the maturity of the worker, which is defined relative to three parameters: personal level of development, need for achievement, and past experience relevant to the current task. A given individual is assessed with regard to the above factors and is then assigned a level along the continuum of maturity ranging from 1 (low) to 4 (high). A worker identified as 1, low in maturity, is theorized to benefit from quadrant 1 supervision, high task and low relationship. This means that the efforts of the leader would be directed to teaching the employee how to perform the task with essentially no concern about that person as an individual. In contrast, for a supervisee diagnosed as a 4 (high) in maturity, the best strategy would be to increase the workers' independence with little emphasis on either the task or the interpersonal relationship. This would be true because s/he knows how to do the job and the employee/leader relationship has already been well developed. The key point that Hersey and Blanchard (1982) makes is that, as individuals grow, the effective leadership style changes. Thus, the skilled supervisor must continuously assess the employee to determine the optimal management style.

Mawdsley and Scudder (1989) extend the Life-Cycle Model to the field of speech-language pathology. The adaptation is called the Integrative Task-Maturity Model of Supervision (ITMMS). The intent is to modify supervisory style as a function of supervisee maturity. Similar to the life-cycle model, four levels of maturity are defined relating to the amount of perceived technical and emotional support required by the supervisee. Mawdsley and Scudder suggest assigning an initial level by considering the trainee's past clinical and academic experiences and then using the Wisconsin Procedure of Appraisal of Clinical Competence (W-PACC) (Shriberg, Filley, Hayes, Kwiatkowski, Schatz, Simmons, & Smith, 1975) as an ongoing measure of clinical independence. Thus, as the maturity levels of the supervisees change, supervisors alter their supervisory style. The four identified styles are telling, selling, participating, and delegating. For example, beginning clinicians are likely to need a telling style as they often are lacking in competence, confidence, and willingness, which means that a direct, telling style with a task focus is most beneficial. Supervisees in externships who are later in their training and are more mature benefit from a participating supervisory style. These supervisees are viewed as competent and willing but lacking in confidence. Therefore, in the conference, supervisors may give clinical suggestions and guidance but will focus more on providing support that will enhance the supervisees' level of self-assurance. Thus, the style changes in response to the needs of the supervisee. In addition, Mawdsley and Scudder discuss the implementation of their Integrative Task-Maturity Model in conjunction with the Cogan (1973) cycle of supervision. They suggest concrete ways to implement aspects of the Cogan model, such as conferencing and observing to reflect the style of supervision—telling, selling, participating, and delegating—for a given supervisee.

Other situational models exist. In speech-language pathology and audiology, the Anderson Continuum of Supervision is a prime example. Supervision is adapted to the situation and the needs of the supervisee (Anderson, 1988). In other disciplines, the situational approaches vary in regard to specifics but have many similarities. Each suggests that the most effective supervisory style is determined by the task, the characteristics of the worker or group of employees, and their perception and their support of the leader.

Leadership styles, whether unidimensional or situational, are intimately tied to worker motivation and productivity. Management teams are yet another factor in this equation. According to Cohen, Chang, and Ledford (1997), the use of self-managing teams increases employee job satisfaction. An example of a team is a natural work group. It consists of people with a common job focus. For example, a rehabilitation team makes a logical cluster as does a supervisor and those who directly report to this individual. The groups meet regularly to identify opportunities for improvement and to solve problems (Bowman, 1988). Some other types of teams are: parallel, project, and management (Cohen & Bailey, 1997). Even when teams are widely used, there remains a need for a supervisor/ manager to coordinate team work and to make final decisions when it is appropriate. In particular, the leader will sift through and integrate the work from various teams and be available for decision making in the event of a crisis (Drucker, 1998).

Leadership Skill   According to Scherer and Rogers (1999), if organizations are to be successful, leaders need to acknowledge and deal with not only events but how people feel about an action and its consequences. Many organizations ignore the "felt" component and, as a result, are not as successful as they could be. Scherer & Rogers suggest that individuals confront a problem, be it a circumstance or a person, when they first perceive it rather than letting negative emotions build. They advise being open about a predicament, letting others know how it makes one feel, and then working toward a constructive resolution. Focusing on the felt as well as the doing is likely to increase organizational productivity by minimizing barriers between people.

Value-Driven

In the historical development of organizational theory, in addition to "how" and "what" motivates and leadership styles, the idea of "value-driven" has emerged as an important aspect underlying effective management. This factor relates to the mission of an organization. Once the mission is defined it becomes the overriding value that permeates and guides all effort. It determines resource allocation and hiring patterns and shapes decision making. It also provides a consistent direction for organizational efforts.

The mission of an organization needs to be more than just lip service. It must be an enduring commitment to stated ideals (Lipton, 1997). It requires members to sit down and discuss their purpose, what they want the organization to be, and where they want it to go. Once this is decided and the mission is stated, everyone in the organization needs to know what the goals are and how they, individually, will contribute to attainment. Whenever decision making occurs, intended actions need to be viewed in the context of the organizational goals to be sure that they are consistent with the stated mission. Kotter (1997) says that values motivate people to work in the desired direction.

The number of organizations that have mission statements is increasing. The most successful use these goals as corporate values. Drucker (1998) says that Health Maintenance Organizations are leaders in managing the entire stream of health-care delivery. He also points out that their goal of cutting costs rather than focusing on quality health care is why they are struggling. Other organizations are more successful in identifying values that enhance both their internally and externally perceived success.

In sifting through companies that excel, Peters and Waterman (1982) look for the commonalities in values underpinning excellence. They report eight such characteristics. The first is a bias for action, a tendency to move forward with the company's best effort and then to make modifications if it doesn't work. The second is a customer orientation, with strong efforts to work with and for the consumer. Third, successful companies reward innovation and encourage entrepreneurship. Fourth, they feel that productivity emerges from individual employees and treat each contributor as a valuable member of the team. Fifth, the organizations are guided by corporate values. Management has "hands on" involvement at all levels of the organization. Sixth, excellent companies do what they do best. They don't branch out into areas in which they do not have sufficient expertise. Seventh, the strong companies tend to have flatter companies with fewer levels between top management and a given worker. Finally, there is a mix of a centralized and decentralized structure within the company and sufficient flexibility to shift the composition as needed. Fisher (1989), in describing high-commitment workplaces, adds to this list of components for excellence. He suggests the following: institutionalize continuous improvement, develop people, eliminate barriers to success, and demonstrate that work is an important part of life.

Celebrating winning is also stressed by Peters and Waterman. Excellent companies acknowledge achievement and give credit when it is due. They often give prizes or special recognition for successful performance. They actively strive to assist workers in feeling good about themselves, give them a sense of belonging, and let them know they are valued members of the corporate team.

Southwest Airlines is a consistently profitable service provider, even when their competitors are struggling. Barlow (1998) attributes this success the fact that Southwest puts its employees first and views them as valuable assets. Levering and Moskowitz (1998) quote a Southwest Airlines employee: "Working here is truly an unbelievable experience. They treat you with respect, pay you well, and empower you. They use your ideas to solve problems. They encourage you to be yourself. I love going to work."

Hewlett-Packard is a company cited as excellent by Peters and Waterman (1982). More than fifteen years later, it remains as one of the top one hundred companies to work for in the United States (Levering & Moskowitz, 1998). This organization is described as a people-oriented company. The guiding motto is the "the Hewlett-Packard way." Bill Hewlett has been quoted as saying: "I feel that in general terms it is the policies and actions that flow from the belief that men and women want to do a good job, a creative job, and that if they are provided with the proper environment they will do so. It is the tradition of treating every individual with consideration and respect and recognizing personal achievement. . . . The dignity and worth of the individual is a very important part, then, of the Hewlett-Packard way" (Peters and Waterman, 1982).

Continuous Process Improvement

Drucker (1998) has said that, if organizations are to flourish, they must be innovative entrepreneurs. The implementation of continuous process improvement is the basis of innovation. In quality improvement, desired outcomes are first identified, planning occurs, strategies are then implemented, and the results are assessed to determine if goals are met. If the objectives are not met, adjustments are made so that better results are achieved the next time. Leebov & Ersoz (1991) call this the plan, do, study, act cycle.

Continuous process improvement may involve the whole of an organization or a specific component. For example, if an organizational goal is accurate patient diagnosis, a first step is assessing the approach being used to determine if the outcome is being achieved or if there is a way to improve on what is being done. A plan is then developed, along with a method to determine if the goal is achieved. The strategy is then implemented and the success in increasing the accuracy of patient diagnosis is determined. Planning is then renewed. In general, quality improvement is a systematic way to move in the direction of organizational goals. It is also a healthy mindset for employees because individuals who are striving constantly to grow will feel a sense of accomplishment and take pride in their jobs.

Shingo (1988) suggests several steps in planning and implementing improvement. The first is to identify the problem. He wisely points out that individuals often accept a standard procedure as a given without questioning how it could be improved and/or streamlined. The next step is to gather accurate information through experimentation. He points out that there are multiple ways to achieve a goal; workers are seriously mislead if they assume that there is only one correct strategy. Often it is necessary to try several methods before rejecting any. Once the problem has been identified and related information has been collected, the next step is to formulate a solution through brainstorming. The final phase in innovation is actual implementation.

Deming's (1986) approach to continuous process improvement has been applied by a variety of organizations, including the American Speech-Language and Hearing Association. Bruce (Dowling & Bruce, 1996) discusses quality improvement as a mechanism to improve diagnosis and treatment in clinical service delivery. The goal is to continually refine the process. She implements the plan, do, study, act cycle and then assists supervisees in developing an action plan to improve performance. This includes the identification of additional knowledge or skills needed by the supervisee as well as a plan and time frame for acquisition.

Critical Thinking

A final factor that contributes organizational effectiveness is the ability of participants to engage in critical thinking. The complexity or styles of thought used in decision making are believed to be developmental in nature (Perry, 1970; Moses & Shapiro, 1996). According to Perry (1970) the most simplistic type of thought is binary in nature: Something is either right or wrong and there is no middle ground. At the next level of thought if there isn't a clear-cut answer, then the individual assumes that it is just a matter of opinion. This kind of thinking is followed by logical decision making based on the formation of supporting arguments. The highest level is an awareness that truth is conditional, that a solution correct in one circumstance may not be appropriate in another. The goal in implementing a critical thinking model is to have supervisees functioning at their highest levels of thought.

Critical thinking enhances organizational effectiveness. People at the two lowest levels, binary and relativistic thinking, may have only minimal clinical competency levels. They will be able to do what they have been specifically taught to do but will have difficulty functioning in novel situations. In contrast, logical thinkers are able to construct arguments and will be able to see the causal link between objective setting and performance and reward systems. They will have the tools to engage in clinical problem-solving. They will also be able to accurately assess whether a decision is consistent with organizational values. Clinicians with even more complex thinking, who understand that strategies and interpretations may vary depending on the context, will be able to implement diagnosis and treatment that is sensitive to individual needs and the circumstance.

The reader has now had the opportunity to read about leadership style, value-driven, continuous process improvement, and critical thinking as they relate to the supervisory process. Roland, the supervisor described at the start of this section has also read this section and has been thinking about these ideas in relation to the problems that have emerged in his department.

Solution

Roland is reflecting on the way he has been managing his department. He thinks about the fact that he has always used the same leadership approach, autocratic. He does a lot of telling with his staff when he observes and conferences with them. He further notes that there seems to be a change at the hospital in terms of what is expected of departments. He thinks the changing times may demand a different style of leadership. He concludes that varying his leadership style will be a challenge he will enjoy. He wants to talk to his staff about involving them in more of the decision making. Maybe his constant need for change doesn't work as well for the rest of the staff. By shifting direction so often, maybe there hasn't been an opportunity to assess the ongoing effects of treatment or to really refine it. He thinks that as a group, maybe we need to come up with a mission statement with specific values to steer any changes we make. Roland also thinks he would like to begin implementing continuous process improvement on a small scale and give staff members more control over planning and evaluating what they do. He also realizes that he has probably limited the professional growth of the staff because he tended to step in rather than encourage them to solve problems and make decisions. More collaboration would be helpful, too. He wonders if all of these factors have reduced staff productivity and job satisfaction. He is eager for the next staff meeting to get feedback about his ideas and to get the department back on track.

Application of Principles to Speech-Language Pathology and Audiology

How to Motivate

Considerations of Maslow's (1954) hierarchy and Herzberg's (1966) dissatisfiers are a good place to begin in thinking about supervisee motivation. The goal is to enhance supervisee self-esteem and to foster efforts toward self-actualization. To do so, the lower level Maslow concerns and Herzberg's dissatisfiers must be minimized or eliminated. These relate to basic working conditions. In most situations, although not always, water fountains, restrooms, and adequate heating, air conditioning, and lighting are provided as a matter of course, providing for physiological needs. Additional working conditions elements include adequate clinical facilities, materials, equipment, and reasonable workloads in terms of both volume and scheduling. Knowledge of departmental policies, due process procedures, and regularly scheduled and objectified evaluation procedures, are also a factor as they address fundamental security needs. Thus, supervisees benefit from knowing they will not arbitrarily or abruptly lose their jobs or space. In addition, a personal locker, desk, or locked drawer in which to store materials and personal items deals with safety issues and creates a sense of belonging, thereby meeting Maslow level 3 social needs. In training programs, the provision of study carrels or a room in which the supervisee has an individual space is helpful. In work settings, an office or designated personal workspace is desirable. For itinerant professionals, creating a sense of belonging is more difficult. A workspace for them to use, even if it is shared with other traveling professionals, increases their sense of being valued members of the team. In general, a place assigned to a supervisee increases self-esteem because it conveys the message that the organization respects the individual and recognizes the importance of personal space.

Social needs, Maslow's level 3, benefit from consideration in both training program and work environments. Humans are social animals and are more content in a place that encourages interaction and a sense of fun. A minimal step is to provide a lunch or coffee-break area. It is particularly helpful if it is centrally located and is used by all personnel. The elbow-rubbing stimulates a feeling of warmth and belonging. The workplace needs to be perceived as a pleasant place to be. Other methods to address social needs are to have informal functions such as potlucks, dinners, periodic social gatherings, meetings to welcome and/or acknowledge new employees and/or students, and other more formal occasions, as appropriate. Fostering organizations such as the National Student Speech, Language, Hearing Association (NSSLHA) and group assignments tends to enhance relationships among students and address the need for social interaction. These exchanges stimulate a sense of inclusion. In other settings such as private practices, schools, and hospitals, encouragement of staff to participate in team projects, committee work, and professional organizations may serve the same purpose.

Maslow's Level 4, esteem needs, can be meet in several ways. Recognition, perceived prestige, feelings of competence, confidence, and success all fall within the parameters of self-esteem. The Peters and Waterman (1982) strategy of celebrating winning serves as a good starting point. An annual award acknowledging the outstanding student, the exceptional speech pathologist, audiologist, or professional staff member is a step in the right direction. These individuals might be honored at a formal dinner or at an in-house reception. Publication of their excellence and a permanent memento to their efforts would further commemorate their competence. In reality, large awards go to a select few, but the concept of winning can be incorporated on a smaller scale on a regular basis. The "winner" of the week or month might earn a close parking spot, a special badge, lunch with a colleague or administrator. In most cases, opportunities for recognition are limited only by the imagination. The size or actual form of the award is unimportant. That which is of value is the recognition itself and its contribution to the individual's feeling of self-worth. Barrow (1999) notes that a reward most valued by supervisees is a personal note of thanks from a superior.

Supervisors, on a daily basis, have the opportunity to build supervisee self-esteem through the documentation and recognition of achievement and overall competence. Small celebrations of winning, such as a note to the supervisee or verbal reinforcement, go a long way in augmenting a feeling of personal well-being. Conveying respect for individuals has a similar effect. Assistance in the writing of realistic professional objectives and then collecting data to identify the presence or absence of growth is also excellent. Evolving clinicians then will have evidence to support their feelings of competence and a tool for further development. Similarly, the supervisor needs to convey confidence in the supervisee by acknowledging successes, giving feedback, and being supportive. It is important to share confidence in the clinician's ability to resolve problems. Even in the worst of circumstances, one in which the supervisee/employee is failing, the damage to the supervisee's self-esteem can be minimized by the supervisor who lets this person know that in spite of the ongoing events, s/he is a valuable human being.

As esteem and recognition needs are met, the desire for self-actualization is likely to emerge. It can be fostered in training programs and work settings in a variety of ways. For example, a supervisor, teacher, or program head who models a desire for continuous professional growth sets the standard for the supervisee. This is particularly true if supervisees are continually encouraged to perform better than they did the day before. Assigning cases that challenge professionals also stimulates growth, as does variety in case assignment. Further, advocating risk-taking and creativity stimulates the drive toward self-actualization. Giving supervisees responsibility, independence, and as much control as possible advances self-growth. The process is perpetuated by the supervisor who provides specific opportunities for supervisee growth such as workshop attendance, observing surgery, or visiting another professional or facility.

Shingo (1988) states that self-actualization is more likely to occur if the supervisor assumes that trainees and employees embody the theory Y view of man. That is, if given the opportunity, people want to achieve, will take initiative and responsibility, and will derive satisfaction from having done so. Within this context, it is important to always treat the supervisee as a responsible, worthwhile adult. In addition, continuous monitoring may be needed to determine the level at which the person is expending efforts. Alderfer (1972) points out that a blocked need causes regression to the next lower level. If an individual is not functioning at the self-esteem or self-actualization level, it may be important for the supervisor to identify and remove the barriers impeding that person's growth.

What Motivates

In this area, the issues of concern are reinforcement, contingency, expectancy, and objective setting. The use of both positive and negative feedback, with a conscious effort to realistically highlight success, is the goal. This is of particular value when combined with the setting of professional objectives, which causes the supervisee to continually stretch toward growth. Data collection, which will be discussed in another chapter, may be used to document achievement efforts and may also be used to encourage the supervisee to self-identify "wins" and, thus, build self-esteem.

An important part of reviewing objectives with supervisees is to identify ways the organization can assist the individual's development. This may include specific strategies that the supervisor might use during observation, data collection, and the conference. In the work environment, this may even extend to facility concerns. For example, if the treatment environment is not conducive to effective therapy, a room change, partitions, or scheduling changes may be necessary to eliminate barriers to success.

It is also vital to incorporate expectancy and contingency into the supervisory process. Discussions with supervisees about what is important to them and what they would find motivating sets the stage for a productive reward system. In this regard, rewarding successes, punishing continuing failure, and exhibiting consistency in supervisor behavior are critical. Supervisees should be rewarded if they work hard and put forth their best effort. As discussed earlier, verbal praise and written notes acknowledging successes are potent rewards. Announcements in meetings and notices recognizing good work are also valuable as tools to increase supervisee self-esteem and job satisfaction. Bonuses or opportunities to attend professional training are useful if they are available.

Leadership Styles

If the theoretical models postulated by Cogan and Anderson are considered from a leadership viewpoint, they would be best characterized as collaborative in focus. Cogan's prompts to supervise at the supervisee's level of readiness and Anderson's conception of the continuum of supervision both reflect a situational/contingency style of management.

In addition, the Mawdsley and Scudder Integrative Task Maturity Model and the Anderson continuum have a person and a task orientation that can be used to select the appropriate supervisory style. Anderson talks about levels of supervisor and supervisee readiness, as well as specific treatment knowledge as factors in determining whether the optimal style should be *direct, collaborative,* or *consultative.* Similarly, Mawdsley and Scudder suggest four styles, *telling, selling, participating,* and *delegating,* depending on the supervisee's level of task maturity, which is based on skills and personal willingness. A consistent high task/high person orientation with the total volume varying with the supervisee's needs is another alternative (Nicholls, 1986; Blake and McCanse, 1991). The important point here is that optimal supervision necessitates both a task and person focus (Scherer & Rogers, 1999). The amount of effort expended toward each, whether totally or proportionally, will depend on the individual supervisee and the given circumstance.

Value-Driven

The value-driven area has not been widely incorporated in speech-language pathology and audiology either in training programs or work environments. Isolated aspects may and do occur, but the concept, except in rare instances, is not incorporated in a holistic, integrated manner.

Value-drive has the potential to enhance training programs and work environments. A first step in beginning the process is to identify a value(s) compatible within a given organization. It must first be discussed, then selected, and finally installed as the formative guide. To work, everyone involved needs to "own" the mission. In addition, new workers or trainees should be selected on the basis of their potential for contibuting to the defined goals. Any of the following, as well as many other mottos identifying organizational missions, are constructive directions for most speech-language pathology and audiology settings.

The Communications Disorders Family

Providing Services on the Cutting Edge

Excellence through Knowledge, Commitment, and Effort

Quality Training and Service from Those Who Care

Excellence by and for People

Clinical Training and Service-Productivity through People

Quality, Service, Human Dignity

Customer satisfaction is an important value for enhancing organizational effectiveness in all speech-language pathology and audiology settings. In the competitive health care environment, attracting and keeping clientele is critical if an organization is going to survive and flourish. A first step is to determine who the customer is. Recipients of service immediately come to mind. Other customers exist as well. For example, students are customers in academic training, and physicians, support personnel, and funding agencies are customers in health care environments. Drucker (1998) thinks that, in order to thrive, organizations need to be innovative entrepreneurs. This means accurately identifying customers and anticipating their needs. Speech-language pathology and audiology organizations, whether training or health care deliverers, need to give intense thought to the identification of their customers and then actively work to anticipate and meet their needs. In essence, we need to create value for our services in the eyes of the consumer.

Values, once selected, must be communicated to all within the organization. It must be continually modeled by management and rewarded when practiced by supervisees. In particular, the guiding concept needs to be the prime consideration whenever decisions are made. Individual supervisees will also benefit from understanding how their efforts mesh with and contribute to the overall organizational goal.

Under the guise of any of the above ideals, the value-driven environment will view trainees/employees as valuable trustworthy team members who have an intrinsic desire to do well and to contribute to the organization's goals. As a result, these individuals will be treated with consideration and respect, further enhancing their sense of dignity and self-worth. Care will also be taken to ensure that trainees/employees interact with each other and clients in a similar fashion.

In addition, the organization and its members will actively work to remove barriers to successful performance. There will be a bias to move forward with one's best effort with the outcomes analyzed to determine the next step. Risk-taking, entrepreneurship, and enthusiasm will be modeled as well as encouraged and rewarded. There will be an overt reflection of the desire to work in the best interests of the consumer. Finally, evidence of efforts to develop people will be consistently visible.

More specifically, supervisors will be accessible and will listen. They will have respect for those they supervise. They will provide feedback when it is helpful to the supervisee. They will also actively work to assist clinicians in viewing their behavior accurately and in feeling good about themselves.

Continuous Process Improvement

Quality improvement is a fundamental tenet in any setting that is working to achieve its potential. It is also integrally related to the implementation of an organizational value system. Organizations ranging from training programs to service delivery settings benefit from deciding what they want to achieve. This may involve choosing what the goal for a client is today or the image an organization wishes to project. On a day-to-day basis, it is deciding what is to be achieved, how it will be attained, and then analyzing the success of the attempt with an eye to making ongoing improvements.

Organizations that actively implement quality improvement will minimize their errors and are more likely to attain their goals. As a result, they can anticipate and respond to environmental demands, and position the organization for innovation. This becomes increasingly critical in the context of managed care and evidence-based practice (Logemann, 1999).

Critical Thinking

The idea of teaching people to think is most often linked to training at the university level. Thus, is this just an issue relative to students-in-training? Ironically, Perry (1970) finds that the majority of college seniors continue to function at the level of "if there isn't a specific answer, it is just a matter of opinion." This means that the need for fostering critical thinking exists at the college level but it is also likely to be true once people are in the field. This is particularly likely given the diversity of persons providing clinical service. The speech-language pathology assistant and others who have not learned to engage in logical decision making will need assistance from the supervisor. Individuals who have not been taught to build hypotheses, collect data, and analyze outcomes often will not be critical thinkers. As a result, these individuals will not be providing diagnosis or treatment up to their level of potential. They are also unlikely to engage in innovative practices.

If supervisees are making decisions but are unable to verbalize the underlying logic, it will be helpful to assist them in identifying factors that make decision making unclear. Once the source of the ambiguity is identified, the supervisee will be guided to build a logical argument for choices that may be appropriate under the circumstances. Once a decision has been made, data collection should be encouraged to assess the quality of the outcome. The supervisor may need to teach supervisees to collect data and to use it to solve clinical problems because many individuals will not have had exposure to this process. Once logical arguments are being built to support decisions, it is helpful to identify circumstances in which a decision would not be valid or ones that would require a different solution (Dowling & Bruce, 1997). Once this process is underway, supervisees will be more likely to engage in innovative practices as they will have the tools to plan and evaluate outcomes.

In this portion of the chapter, the ideas about motivating others and topics relating to leadership have been applied to the fields of speech-language pathology and audiology. This included the application of how and what motivates, leadership style, value-driven, continuous process improvement, and critical thinking.

Relationship of Creating Productivity and Professional Growth and the Specified Supervision Tasks

As noted at the beginning of the chapter, organizational productivity and professional growth are identified as relevant to seven of the thirteen Supervision Tasks (ASHA, 1985). Establishing and maintaining an effective working relationship, assisting the supervisee in developing and refining assessment skills, assisting the supervisee in developing and refining clinical management skills, assisting the supervisee in observing and analyzing assessment and treatment sessions, and assisting the supervisee in evaluation of clinical performance are at the heart of productivity and professional growth. Indeed, fostering supervisee critical thinking abilities through the use of data collection, directed problem-solving and the building of logical arguments will assist supervisees in accurately identifying the quality of their service delivery and will give them a mental strategy to use in improving their work. The active hypothesis testing in both critical thinking and continuous process improvement will allow the supervisee to accomplish three goals: (1) optimize delivery of services, (2) move toward self-actualization, and (3) become involved in clinical research.

In regard to establishing and maintaining an effective working relationship and the modeling of professional conduct, information about the clinical environment is critical to the successful acculturation of the supervisee. Knowledge of the values that drive a facility focuses the supervisee's efforts and instills a sense of respect for colleagues and those served. In particular, it is important for management to model self-actualizing behavior to ingrain this value. In addition, the Theory Y view that people want to develop as professionals contributes to a constructive work setting. Situational leadership is also relevant. This is particularly true if both a task and person element are reflected in the supervisor's conference style as it shifts along the Anderson continuum from telling to collaborating to consulting. This orientation enhances the impact of the supervisor–supervisee interchange, increases active personnel participation, and maximizes the quality of work output.

In regard to facilitating professional conduct, several of the ideas described above continue to be pertinent. They are: the supervisory style selected, the inclusion of individuals as valued, integral parts of the organization, and the view that people want to develop. Each of these fosters the professional growth of the supervisee. The organization will also actively work to remove barriers impeding the maturation of individuals and capitalize on opportunities to celebrate winning to foster both organizational and self-esteem. The issues regarding how and what motivates that underlie worker productivity then become a consideration. In this regard, goal-setting and the establishment of expectancy and equity are important. In sum, multiple aspects of organizational behavior set the stage for optimal facility performance, personal productivity, and participant satisfaction.

Summary

A variety of topics relating to organizational climate are presented in this chapter. It begins with an overview of the historical development of thought in this area. The issues of "how" and "what" motivates are then considered and are accompanied by examples. These topics are followed by information on leadership, value-driven, continuous process improvement, and critical thinking. The material is then discussed for the purpose of application in speech-language pathology and audiology. Organizational behavior is then linked specifically to the development of seven of the thirteen tasks of supervision. The reader is encouraged to think about and apply the fundamental concepts presented here. Specifically, it is hoped that programs, either related to training or the delivery of services, will (1) become value-driven; (2) make a conscious effort to treat people as respected, valued individuals; (3) assume that people want to self-actualize and feel good about themselves and then act in ways that facilitate this development; (4) serve as a role model by demonstrating efforts toward self-actualization; and (5) celebrate winning whenever it occurs. If these strategies are implemented, clinical services will improve and those in the organization will be more satisfied.

REFERENCES

Alderfer, C. *Existence, Relatedness, and Growth.* New York: Free Press, 1972.

American Speech and Hearing Association. Committee on Supervision in Speech-Language Pathology and Audiology. "Clinical supervision in speech-language pathology and audiology: A position statement." *American Speech Hearing Association, 27* (1985): 57–60.

Anderson, J. *The Supervisory Process in Speech-Language Pathology and Audiology.* Austin, TX: Pro-Ed, 1988.

Barlow, J. "It pays to invest in human assets." *Houston Chronicle,* Feb. 12, 1998.

Barrow, J. "How to motivate without much cash." *Houston Chronicle,* May 11, 1999.

Birnbach, L. "How to work for somebody else and still be yourself." *Parade Magazine,* Oct. 30, 1988: 14.

Bittel, L. *What Every Supervisor Should Know.* (5th ed.). New York: McGraw-Hill, 1985.

Blake, R., and McCanse, A. *The Leadership Grid.* Houston: Gulf Publishing, 1991.

Blake, R., and Mouton, J. "Management by grid principles or situationalism: Which?" *Group & Organization Studies, 6* (4) (1981): 439–455.

Blakeney, R. "Evolution of management theory and thought." In G. Newton, (Ed.), *Certificate in Management Accounting Review: Organization and Behavior, Including Ethical Considerations.* (1983): 1–34.

Bowman, J., and Brady, L. "Dow Chemical, Texas, project makes continuous improvement part of everyone's job." *Industrial Engineering, 20* (1988): 40–45.

Cogan, M. *Clinical Supervision.* Boston: Houghton Mifflin, 1973.

Cohen, S., and Bailey, D. "What makes teams work: Group effectiveness research from the shop floor to the executive suite." *Journal of Management, 23* (3) (1997): 239–290.

Cohen, S., Chang, L., and Ledford, G. "A hierarchical construction of self-management leadership and its relationship to quality of work life and perceived work group effectiveness." *Personnel-Psychology, 50* (2) (1997): 275–308.

Deming, W. *Out of Crisis.* Cambridge, MA: Massachusetts Institute of Technology, Center for Advanced Engineering Study, 1986.

DeShon, R., and Alexander, R. "Goal setting effects on implicit and explicit learning of complex tasks." *Organizational Behavior and Human Decision Processes 65,* (1) (1996): 18–36.

Dowling, S. "Supervisory training, objective setting and grade contingent performance." *Language Speech Hearing Services Schools, 24* (1993): 92–99.

Dowling, S., and Bruce, M. "Improving clinical training through continuous quality improvement and critical thinking." In B. Wagner, (Ed.), *Proceedings: Partnerships in Supervision: Innovative and Effective Practices.* Grand Forks, ND: University of North Dakota, (1996): 66–72.

Dowling, S., and Bruce, M. "Clinical training: Enhancing clinical thought and independence." Seminar presented at the Annual Convention of the American Speech, Language and Hearing Association, Boston, MA, Nov. 1997.

Drucker, P. "Management's new paradigms." *Forbes, 162* (7) (1998): 52–177.

Earley, C., and Kanfer, R. "The influence of component participation and role models on goals acceptance, goal satisfaction and performance." *Organizational Behavior and Human Decision Processes, 36* (1985): 378–390.

Evans, M. "Organizational behavior: The central role of motivation." In J. Hunt & J. Blair (Eds.), *1986 Yearly Review of Management of the Journal of Management, 12* (2) (1986): 203–222.

Fisher, K. "Managing in the high-commitment workplace." *Organizational Dynamics,* Winter (1989): 31–50.

Greenfield, C. "Employer work/life trends: Benefits and beyond." *Compensation and Benefits Management, 13* (4) (1997): 20–30.

Hersey, P., and Blanchard, K. *Management of Organizational Behavior: Utilizing Human Resources.* (4th ed.). Englewood Cliffs, NJ: Prentice-Hall, 1982.

Herzberg, F. *Work and the Nature of Man.* Cleveland: Work Publishing, 1966.

Kotter, J. "Leading by vision and strategy." *Executive Excellence, 14* (10) (1997): 15–16.

Kreitner, R., and Kinicki, A. *Organizational Behavior.* Boston, MA: Richard D. Irwin, 1989.

Leebov, W., and Ersoz, C. *The Health Care Manager's Guide to Continuous Quality Improvement.* Chicago: American Hospital Publishing, 1991.

Levering, R., and Moskowitz, M. "The 100 best companies to work for in America." *Fortune,* Jan. 12, (1998): 84–95.

Lewis, B. "Used strategically, money can really talk to motivate and reward employees." *Infoworld 19,* 41 (1997): 104.

Lieber, R. "Why employees love these companies." *Fortune,* Jan. 12, (1998): 72–74.

Lipton, M. "Demystifying vision." *Executive Excellence, 14* (3) (1997): 5–6.

Locke, E., Shaw, K., Saari, L., and Latham, G. "Goal-setting and task performance." *Psychological Bulletin, 90* (1981): 125–152.

Logemann, J. "The state of our professions." University of Houston, Houston, TX, Jan., 1999.

Maslow, A. *Motivation and Personality.* New York: Harper and Brothers, 1954.

Mawdsley, B., and Scudder, R. "The integrative task-maturity model of supervision." *Language, Speech and Hearing Services in Schools, 20* (3) (1989): 305–315.

McClelland, D. "That urge to achieve." In D. Domm, R. Blakeney, M. Matteson, and R. Scofield (Eds.), *The Individual and the Organization.* New York: Harper and Row, 1973.

McGregor, D. *The Human Side of Enterprise.* New York: McGraw-Hill, 1960.

McGregor, D. "The human side of enterprise." In W. Bennis, D. Benne, and R. Chin (Eds.), *The Planning of Change.* New York: Holt, Rinehart, & Winston, 1961: 422–431.

Moses, N., and Shapiro, D. "A developmental conceptualization of clinical problem solving." *Journal of Communication Disorders, 29* (1996): 199–221.

Murray, H. *Explorations in Personality.* New York: Oxford University Press, 1938.

Nelson, B. "Rewarding employees: Asset appreciation produces best results." *Canadian Manager, 21* (4) (1996): 24.

Nelson, B. "Motivating people." *Executive Excellence, 14* (9) (1997): 16–18.

Nicholls, J. "Congruent leadership." *LODJ,* 7 (1) (1986): 27–31.

Perry, W. G. *Forms of Intellectual and Ethical Development in the College Years: A Scheme.* New York: Holt, Rinehart, & Winston, 1970.

Peters, T., and Waterman, R. *In Search of Excellence: Lessons from America's Best-Run Companies.* New York: Harper and Row, 1982.

Phillips, J., and Gully, S. "Role of goal orientation, ability, need for achievement, and locus of control in the self-efficacy and goal-setting process." *Journal of Applied Psychology, 82* (5) (1997): 792–802.

Popp, G., Davis, H., and Herbert, T. "An international study of intrinsic motivation composition." *Management International Review, 26* (3) (1986): 28–35.

Scherer, J., and Rogers, T. "How to take charge of your professional life in turbulent times." Presented at The Leader's Toolkit, Leadership Conference of the American Speech-Language and Hearing Association, New Orleans, LA, July, 1999.

Shingo, S. *Non-Stock Production.* Cambridge, MA: Productivity Press, 1988.

Shriberg, L., Filley, F., Hayes, D., Kwiatkowski, J. Schatz, J., Simmons, K., and Smith, M. "The Wisconsin Procedure for Appraisal of Clinical Competence: Model and data." *American Speech and Hearing Association, 17* (1975): 158–165.

Skinner, B. *Contingencies of Reinforcement.* New York: Appleton-Century-Crofts, 1969.

Smith, A. *The Wealth of Nations.* New York: Modern Library, 1939.

Spitzer, D. "Supermotivation." New York: AMA-COM, 1995.

Stoffman, D. "Launching a business: The power of positive strokes." *Canadian Business, 60* (1987): 94–95.

Zuber, A. "People—the single point of difference—motivating them." *Nation's Restaurant News, 31* (40) (1997): 114–116.

PART TWO

Developing Tools and Strategies

2 Solving Puzzles: Setting the Stage for Growth

Clinical Supervision Tasks Relevant to Solving Puzzles, Setting Goals, Preparing for Growth

Task 1: Establishing and maintaining an effective working relationship with the supervisee;

Task 2: Assisting the supervisee in developing clinical goals and objectives;

Task 4: Assisting the supervisee in developing and refining management skills;

Task 6: Assisting the supervisee in observing and analyzing assessment and treatment sessions;

Task 8: Interacting with the supervisee in planning, executing, and analyzing supervisory conferences;

Task 9: Assisting the supervisee in evaluation of clinical performance;

Task 12: Modeling and facilitating professional conduct;

Task 13: Demonstrating research skills in the clinical or supervisory process.

Data Collection and Performance Objectives as Supervisory Tools

Two related topics are the focus of this chapter. The first is data collection as a strategy for fostering professional growth. The second topic, a logical outgrowth of the first, is the development of performance objectives. Both are of vital importance to the supervisee and supervisor. Data gathering will be addressed first and then objective setting. These topics will initially be considered in relation to the clinical process followed by the supervisory process.

Clinical Puzzle

Noah, a beginning graduate student clinician, is working with a three-year-old child, Lisa, who has been diagnosed as having Asperger's Syndrome. Lisa does not establish eye contact, engage in parallel play, or converse interactively. Noah feels that he provides good models for the youngster but her meaningful conversation is not improving. Noah thinks that what he is doing is on the right track but doesn't know if change is needed or what to do next.

The situation described in Box 2.1 occurs frequently in treatment and diagnosis. It may occur in relation to any type of disorder and with supervisees at varying levels of professional development. Clinicians have a general sense of the events that are transpiring. They often have a feeling that a procedure is or is not working but they don't know why or what should come next. In most cases, they don't have a mechanism for analyzing the events that occur in a way that allows them to understand the workings of the process or to generate a logical plan of action.

A tool that will help Noah in unraveling this puzzle is data collection. This process allows people to get into the heart of treatment and figure out the "why" of events. Once behaviors are charted, regularities in behavior are noted and then predictions can be made. The information gained from data collection assists clinicians in problem-solving, generating strategies, and testing hypotheses. The understanding of the "whys" of therapy leads to improvements in treatment quality.

Puzzle Solved

Noah and his supervisor discussed the therapy he had been implementing. Together they decided to collect data during his next therapy session. They planned to gather information about the nature of Noah's statements to the child, the length of time between Noah's utterance and the child's response, or Noah's next statement and the length of the child's reply. The collected data appears in Figure 2.1.

Noah had 10 utterances compared to the child's 3. The clinician, on average, paused for 16.8 seconds after he or the child spoke before initiating another response. The range of the clinician's pause time was 5 to 40 seconds before he either spoke again or the child responded. He used 4 questions, 4 prompts, and elaborated on 2 of the child's productions. After considering the data, Noah is concerned about the low number of child responses. He wonders about the types of prompts he was using to stimulate responses from the child and notes the short amounts of time he gave the child to respond. He is pleased he elaborated on two-thirds of the child's utterances.

FIGURE 2.1   **Clinician and Client Responses Speaker Order, Elapsed Time and Length of Client Response.**

Sequential Data Collection

Nature* of Noah's response	Next Speaker		Elapsed Time	Length of Child's Response—# Words
	Noah	*Child*		
Q	>		15"	0
P	>		18"	0
P		>	28"	2
E	>		10"	
Q	>		5"	0
Q		>	32"	1
E	>		5"	
P		>	40"	3
Q	>		5"	0
P	>		10"	0

*Q = question
 P = prompt
 E = elaborated on child's response

After problem-solving with his supervisor, he decides to wait a minimum of 25 seconds after he verbalizes before he says anything else. He hypothesizes that pausing longer will encourage the child to talk more. He plans to test his theory in his next session. Following his next session, he delightedly reports that the frequency of the child's statements doubled. He says he is excited about collecting additional data to look at other aspects of his therapy. He feels he has grasped an important straw in solving the therapy puzzle.

Data Collection

Data collection and analysis in supervision are known to have existed in theory since the early work of Flanders (1970) and Cogan (1973) in the field of education. Flanders discusses interaction analysis systems and Cogan introduces the clinical supervision model that uses a "cycle" of supervision. This cycle begins with establishing the relationship between the supervisor and supervisee and is followed by planning, observing, collecting data, analyzing and conferencing, and then returning once again to the planning stage. Data collection is viewed as the basis for each of the components. Later, in speech-language pathology and audiology, Anderson (1988) parallels and extends the ideas presented by Cogan (1973). She offers a model of supervision that emphasizes data-based collaboration as a primary means to foster the development of the supervisee. Both Cogan and Anderson stress the value of supervising at the supervisee's level of need and incorporating data collection as a critical aspect of supervision. Numerous authors (Anderson [1988], Dowling [1992], Shapiro [1994], Anderson and Frieberg [1995]) talk about the importance of data collection as a tool to foster supervisee growth. Sexton, Whiston, Bleuer, and Walz (1998) view data collection as the basis for effective decision making. Jensen, Parsons, and Reid (1998) report that accurate data collection and feedback regarding teacher assistants' teaching behaviors improves not only the supervisee's performance but also that of the supervising teacher. On a broader scale, clinical data collection is the basis for accountability (Power-deFur, 1999) and the source for the outcome research that will pave the way to identify best practices in treatment (Kreb and Wolf, 1997; Logemann, 1999).

One example of a data collection tool is the Low Inference Self-Assessment Measure (LISAM) developed by Freiberg (1987). It is designed as a mechanism to collect data on a variety of teaching behaviors such as questioning skills, talk time, and wait time between teacher questions and next statement. Later research by Anderson and Freiberg (1995) using the LISAM data collection tool shows that student teachers view the tool as effective for self-assessment. They are surprised by the data, particularly by the discrepancies between what they think is occurring and what actually is. The student teachers also report that the use of data collection gives them the basis for improving specific teaching behaviors.

Data collection is a key to professional development in the context of supervision. The intent of data collection and analysis is to objectify teaching or clinical performance. It does, indeed, objectify behavior and forms a basis for assessing cause and effect. It reduces the level of abstraction when considering a clinical event, facilitates the analysis of a procedure, and makes the testing of assumptions regarding efficacy possible. Most importantly, when actively incorporated into the supervisory process it enhances the clinical problem-solving abilities of both the supervisee and supervisor.

Data Collection Terminology.   An array of terminology relates to data collection. Of particular import are words such as target behavior, baseline, post-test, event versus behavior recording, duration recording, and time sampling. Before data can be collected, the *target behavior* to be recorded must be defined. The description must be precise enough to allow the observer to readily identify it when it occurs. After the data to be collected is defined, a *baseline* is established. The baseline is a premeasure used to assess the occurrence of a behavior in its natural state. Once this information is obtained, attempts to alter it can be implemented. *Post-test* data is then collected to determine the impact of the treatment. In the end, the baseline and the post-test results are compared to determine progress.

Data may be counted in regard to specific *behaviors,* such as making eye contact, or in relation to broader *events,* such as reinforcement strategies. The *duration* may also be of importance. For example, in a clinical session, a record of the instances of clinician versus client talk is important. But this count alone may be misleading if the length of time expended is not shown. To record this data, a mark is made each time a speaker initiates speech and then the actual length of that utterance is timed with a stopwatch. In implementation, the importance of this factor can be illustrated by a session in which the clinician talked 20 times and the client 60. On the surface, this appears to be highly appropriate. When talk time for each participant is considered, however, the clinician verbalized for 30 minutes of the session and the client, only 20. This second piece of information presents a markedly different picture than did the counting alone.

   Time sampling can also be used when gathering information. In this method-ology, a decision is made prior to the observation about the timing of data collec-tion. A supervisor might decide to collect data only on the middle five minutes of a session. Or a tone may be recorded on a tape at specified intervals such as every 5 seconds. During the observation, the supervisor plays the tape and notes the behaviors occurring at the time of the beep only. All other instances are ignored. In time sampling, an assumption is made that the observed behaviors are repre-sentative of the interaction as a whole. The alternative to this approach is contin-uous recording in which specified targets are registered as they occur.

Data Collection Tools.   Actual data collection may take a variety of forms. Casey, Smith, and Ulrich (1988) identify seven types of data collection: verbatim recording, selective verbatim, rating scales, tally, interaction analysis, nonverbal analysis, and those that are individually designed. A *verbatim recording* is one in which a treatment session or conference is written down word for word. *Selective verbatim* (Acheson & Gall, 1992; Reiman & Thies-Sprinthall, 1998) is a similar strategy that focuses on a specific aspect of behavior such as questioning, pupil talk, etc. A literal transcription is then made but is limited to the behaviors spec-ified. *Rating scales,* on the other hand, are less concrete as they classify behaviors on a continuum ranging from low to high or vice versus. A judgment, based on the rater's perception, is made about the frequency, level of occurrence, or qual-ity of a behavior. *Tallies* are simply frequency counts of specified behaviors. In contrast, *interaction analysis systems* are the more structured and complex of the instruments. They are used to chart a variety of observed behaviors and can take the form of a sign, rating scale, or category format. *Sign systems* tally the occur-rence and frequencies of lists of behaviors. These can be as diverse as recording the positions of people in the room to counting actual responses to questions. The *category system*, a more rigorous method, requires the assignment of events to the appropriate classifications. For example, a smile, awarding a sticker, or saying "good" are grouped in the slot designated as reinforcement. The result is a frequency count and, generally, a visual, sequential representation of the events observed. Further, either a sign or category system can be used as an observation-system rating scale by assigning relative judgments of frequency or quality rather than actually recording the objective data. For example, the fre-quency of providing reinforcement may be rated as all of the time or some of the time. The *nonverbal analyses,* as implied, focus on aspects other than what is said during the treatment or supervisory session. Finally, *individually designed systems* are developed by the user as a means to collect specific data. An excellent exam-ple of such an approach is the Kansas Inventory of Self-Supervision (Mawdsley, 1987).

Data Collection Continuum.   In general, data collection systems can be thought of as existing on a continuum from informal to formal, as shown in Figure 2.2. The simplest type is counting or *tallying* the occurrence of a specified behavior. For example, the number of times a clinician uses closure at the end of an activity may be recorded. *Verbatim* and *selected verbatim* are next as the format and content recorded is at the discretion of the collector. It might take the form of a transcription of a supervisee's questions or be a complete record of all verbalizations observed. Shifting still further along the horizontal axis, the *individually designed approaches* appear. The behaviors to be observed are typically preselected and the format for collection predetermined, which gives these methods a more formal air. Two such methods, the profile and sequential methodology, will be discussed extensively in this chapter. *Category observation systems* are the most formal type of data collection tool. These systems allow for extensive data gathering but are less flexible because the categories are predetermined and explicit coding guidelines are provided. Depending on the type of system (sign, rating, or category) selected and the degree of coder training implemented, the collected data from a formal observation system are likely to be more reliable and valid than that gathered through an individually designed system. Finally, the *nonverbal analyses* will vary in formality depending on the strategy selected. They can range from a tally of the frequency of a behavior, such as eye contact or body mirroring, to the use of an observation system to collect nonverbal behavior data.

Formal observation systems mushroomed in the late 1960s and early 1970s in the field of education and continue to emerge in that field today. As an example, O'Connor and Fish (1997) describe the implementation of the Classroom Systems Observation Scale to assess differences between expert and novice teachers. A similar burst in observation systems development occurs in speech-language pathology in the 1970s and early 1980s. The tools that emerge are used primarily to answer specific research questions about the supervisory conference. Representative examples are the work of McCrea (1980), Dowling and Shank (1981), Smith and Anderson (1982), Roberts and Smith (1982), Dowling (1983), Farmer (1984), Dowling (1993), and Shapiro (1994).

Informal ⟵————————————⟶ **Formal**

Tally	Selected Verbatim Verbatim Sign Observation System	Individually designed KISS Profile Sequential	Observation systems 1. Rating Scale 2. Category

Tally ⟵————————————⟶ **Observation
System**

FIGURE 2.2   **Data Collection Continuum.**

Several systems do exist in speech-language pathology for the purpose of analyzing a therapy session: *The Content and Sequence Analysis of Speech and Hearing Therapy,* Boone and Prescott (1972); *Analysis of Behaviors of Clinicians (ABC) System,* Schubert, Miner, and Till (1973); *Therapy Analyzer,* Oratio (1987); *Conover Verbal Analysis System,* Conover (1979); and *The Clinical Interaction Analysis System (CIAS): A system for observational recording of aphasia treatment,* Brookshire, Nicholas, Krueger, and Redmond (1978). Those available to consider the supervisory session are: *Content and Sequence Analyses of the Supervisory Session,* Culatta and Seltzer (1976); *Underwood Category System,* Underwood (1973); *McCrea Adapted Scales for the Assessment of Interpersonal Function in Speech Pathology Supervision Conferences,* McCrea (1980); *A Supervisory Transactional System,* Oratio (1977); and the *Multidimensional Observational System for the Analysis of Interaction in Clinical Supervision (M.O.S.A.I.C.S.),* Weller (1971), a tool for use in education. It is later adapted by Smith (1977) for use in speech-language pathology and audiology. A thorough discussion of these observation systems can be found in Anderson (1988), Casey, Smith, and Ulrich (1988) and Shapiro (1994), who did a comparative study of four of the tools in analyzing the supervisory conference: System for Analyzing Supervisor–Teacher Interaction (Blumberg, 1980); Underwood Category System for Analyzing Supervisor–Clinician Behavior (Underwood, 1973); McCrea Adapted Scales for the Assessment of Interpersonal Function in Speech Pathology Supervision Conferences, McCrea (1980); and Smith's Adaptation of the Multidimensional Observational System for the Analysis of Interactions in Clinical Supervision (Smith, 1977). Shapiro finds that each is a valuable tool for self-study and that the one selected should be based on the types of questions the supervisor and supervisee are interested in answering.

Relative to the formal/informal continuum, the type of data-collection methodology selected will depend on the needs of the user. For research, a category observation system may be most appropriate. It might also be the method of choice for considering the clinical and supervisory process, particularly if completeness of scope is of concern. To answer specific questions and for practical day-to-day applications, tallies and the individually designed strategies may be more useful. It is important to note that these informal systems can also be used for research purposes if they are validated and intercoder agreement is established and monitored.

Data Collection and Its Application to the Clinical Process

Individually Designed Systems

This chapter focuses on the more flexible individually designed approaches, the tally, the profile, and the sequential method. A more thorough discussion of each of the three strategies follows, with examples of their use.

Tally. As stated earlier, the tally is the counting of specific events such as the number of correct responses or the times a clinician uses the discourse filler "ok." It is a quick method of data collection that provides the clinician and supervisor with a simple way of looking at one aspect of performance. It is a means to increase awareness of a particular behavior. Often, realization alone will trigger an increase in a desired behavior or a decrease in one perceived as less effective.

Figure 2.3 reflects the collection and the summary of data for a clinician who was working to reduce her usage of *ok* during treatment. Note that the supervisor tailored the form to meet the need at hand. Thus, as was preplanned, the observer looked at her watch and then made a mark each time she heard *ok* during a five-minute period. During the first observation relevant to this behavior, the clinician said "ok" 12 times in a five-minute period. Subsequently, the clinician was able to eliminate this behavior as continued counting of the behavior allowed her to measure progress toward her goal. Further, as she gained in experience, she was able to record her own behavior within a treatment session or from a videotape.

Profile. A second individually designed method is the profile. It is a more complex version of the simple tally. This approach evolves from work from Dowling and Wall (1988). It simultaneously records more than one or a set of behaviors. Generally, the items collected in this format will be related conceptually. The for-

FIGURE 2.3   Record of the Filler "ok" in a Clinician's Speech During Two Five-Minute Segments of Therapy.

Tally Data Collection

Target Behavior
Number of times clinician says "ok"

Behavior	Time Beginning	End	Date
OK			

(1 recorded for each occurrence)

| 11111111111 | 4:05 P.M. | 4:10 P.M. | April 30. |

Summary of results:

Date: Session 1

NUMBER OF TIMES ___12___ IN A ___5___ MINUTE SEGMENT

Date: Session 5

NUMBER OF TIMES ___0___ IN A ___5___ MINUTE SEGMENT

mat is extremely adaptable and functional. An example of a potential use is to record the variations in verbal/nonverbal reinforcers used during a therapy segment. Another example would be correct and incorrect client responses by task type. The structure for the profile appears in Figure 2.4. The specificity of the labels on the form have been minimized to increase the flexibility of the tool. The user-planned labels might read, clinician–client or clinician–clinician or other persons of interest. It is also set up in multiples of ten for ease of use and to facilitate the calculation of percentages of occurrence. When using the form, a legend will need to be designed and added to identify the behaviors to be recorded. For example, a number might be assigned, such as a 1 or a + (plus) to mean a positive reinforcer, a 2 or a – (minus) to mean a punisher. A space has also been left to identify the activity that is being observed and to pinpoint the relevant time segment as an aid for recall. Areas for comments and notes are also provided.

Date/Time: _____

Clinician/Supervisor: _____

Client/Supervisee: _____

Observation: Treatment/Conference

Goal:

Behaviors to be Charted:

Data Collection: I   II

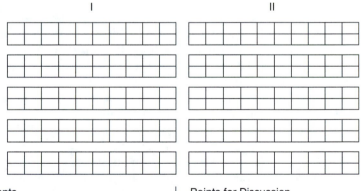

General Comments | Points for Discussion

Observer: _____

FIGURE 2.4   Observation Record

Profile Data Collection

Prompt Array

    1)   Look at me.
    2)   Where are your hands supposed to be?
    3)   Hands on table.
    4)   We can't begin until you look at me.
    5)   Chip placed on clinician's chin to focus attention.
    6)   Clinician touches/turns child's cheek.

Prompt Use

Session 1 (10 minutes)

1	1	1	1	1	1	1	1	1	1
1	1								

Session 6 (10 minutes)

1	2	3	3	1	2	3	1	3	3
1	2	3	1						

Session 10 (10 minutes)

5	2	3	5	5	5	1	3	5	2
5	3	4	5	5					

FIGURE 2.5   Prompts to Promote Attending Behavior.

The first example of a profile relates to a clinician's use of prompts relative to client attending behavior. As seen in Figure 2.5, during 10 minutes of the first session, he uses "look at me" 12 times as a prompt. After reviewing these data, the clinician feels that what he has used was appropriate but hypothesized that more variety in his prompts might be useful. During the sixth session when data are again collected, three different prompts are used: look at me (5), where are your hands supposed to be? (3), and hands on table (6). He has used three variations for a combined total of 13. In considering the results, he is pleased that he has been able to alter his prompts. His next goal is to decrease the volume of verbal prompts and to use ones that he can implement quickly. As a result, he wants to continue to use varied prompts but to incorporate others that may be done swiftly and without clinician talk. During the tenth session, data on types and frequency of prompts are again collected. The following is observed: look at me (1), hands on table (2), we can't begin until you look at me (1), chip on clinician's chin to focus attention (8), and touch/turn child's cheek to focus attention (3). In this latest session, he uses a total of 15 prompts, 4 that are verbal and 11 nonverbal. The clinician, at this point, feels his goals of using varied prompts and increasing efficiency by using a greater proportion of nonverbal are met.

Sequential Data Collection

Instance of Wordfinding difficulty (*)

Client Maladaptive Responses
    a)   stops talking
    b)   closes eyes
    c)   snaps fingers

Client Adaptive Strategies
    S.   Substitutes another word
    D.   Describes the word conversationally
    V.   Produces word after verbal prompt of first letter by clinician

Session 1   Baseline (5 minute segment)

*	*	*	*	*	*	*	*	*	
a,b	a,b	a,b	a,b	a,b	a,b	a,b	a,b	a,b	
c	c	c	c	c	c	c	c	c	

Session 2   (5 minutes)

*	*	*	*	*	*	*	*	*	*
a,b	S	V	a,b	V	D	V	V	S	V
c		a,b	c			a,b	a,b	a	a,b
		c				c	c		c

Session 3   (5 minutes)

*	*	*	*	*	*	*	*	*	
a,b	D	D	S	D	D	D	D	S	
c			a						

FIGURE 2.6   Client Use of Adaptive Strategies When Experiencing Wordfinding Difficulty.

    The second example (see Figure 2.6) using a profile relates to an adult client who exhibits wordfinding difficulties. In conversation, when John is unable to think of a word, he stops, closes his eyes to try to visualize the written word, and snaps his fingers. This method of attempting to recall interrupts the conversation and makes John feel panicky. Because the wordfinding difficulty happens so frequently, he is reluctant to talk to people he does not know well. The clinician is interested in assisting him in developing strategies to use when a word escapes him. The clinician collects a baseline on the client's response to being unable to recall a word. The first time the data is collected for a five-minute period, there are 9 words he has trouble recalling. In each instance, he stops talking, closes his eyes, and snaps his fingers. During the next meeting, session two, the clinician encourages him to use three different strategies to help him recall the word: (1) substitute a different word, (2) describe the word as part of the conversation, and (3) produce the word after the clinician provides a prompt of the first letter of the word. In this session, the client has 10 instances of wordfinding difficulty. In 2 instances, he responds by stopping talking, closing his eyes, and snapping his fingers. In 5 other instances, the clinician provides prompts of the first letter. One works and, in response to the remaining 4, the client responds by stopping talking, closing his eyes, and snapping his fingers. One time, he successfully uses an alternate word and, in another, describes the word as part of the conversation. After thinking about the data and talking with the client about what he perceived to be helpful, they decide that the clinician's provision of a verbal prompt isn't helpful. They note that using another word works sometimes. They decide to focus on using another word and describing a word when it is difficult to recall. Data is collected again 4 weeks later, during session 3. This time there is only one instance when the client stops talking, closes his eyes, and snaps his fingers. He tries to use another word 2 times and is successful once. The remaining 6 times he describes the word he cannot recall but does it within the context of the conversation. As the clinician and client talk about this session, the client feels that he can eliminate the eye closing, stopping, and finger snapping, and he decides that describing the word works best for him. He also reports that he has talked to strangers on four occasions during that week. He says he doesn't panic as often now when he can't think of a word, and he is very pleased with his progress. This sample illustrates a direct translation of data collection and analysis to the improvement of clinical services.

The third example, Figure 2.7 on page 41, using the profile, relates to a clinician's work with a small group of children. The goal for the day is turn-taking and the use of agent–action–object in a child-centered play activity. The children select a shopping basket filled with foods. They are to take turns picking an object and using an agent–action–object sentence to describe it. The speaker then returns the item to the basket or gives it to the next child. The clinician is interested in fostering turn-taking and collects data on this aspect of treatment. A baseline is collected in session 1. Keith is the only child to return the food to the basket after speaking. After considering the data, the clinician decides to verbally praise each turn-taking act. The second time data is collected, all of the children engage in turn-taking on a limited basis: Keith (2), Emir (1), and Ronalese (3). The clinician notes the gains and decides to implement a tangible reinforcer, a star sticker to be put on the child's hand, and data is again collected. This time the frequency of turn-taking increases notably: Keith (5), Emir (6), Ronalese (5). The clinician is very pleased with the results and speculates that once turn-taking becomes more automatic, it may be possible to fade out the tangible reinforcer.

Sequential.   An alternative individually designed data collection approach is a sequential strategy. This is very similar to the profile but has the added feature of maintaining the sequence of events (Dowling and Wall, 1988). Therefore, in regard to plotting client correct/incorrect and self-evaluation accuracy, for exam-

FIGURE 2.7   Frequency of Turn-Taking under Three Conditions.

Profile Data Collection

Baseline—No Specific Intervention

Children	Turn-Taking Acts
Keith	1
Emir	0
Ronalese	0

Time 2—Verbal Praise Condition

Children	Turn-Taking Acts
Keith	2
Emir	1
Ronalese	3

Time 3—Tangible Reinforcer Condition

Children	Turn-Taking Acts
Keith	5
Emir	6
Ronalese	5

ple, it is possible to determine if the correct response is followed by an accurate self-evaluation. Hence, this type of individually designed system maintains the flexibility of the profile but adds information.

The following are three examples using sequential data collection. The particular ones cited reflect recordings at a specific time but the approach can also be used for the gathering of information over an extended time period. The first example, shown in Figure 2.8 on page 42, relates to the ratio of clinician and client talk during one treatment activity. Three categories of clinician talk are recorded: model, reinforcement, and "other" statements. Correct, incorrect, and other responses are also collected for the client but, interestingly enough, "other" responses do not occur for the client. The clinician models 12 times, reinforces in 7 instances, and makes additional comments 32 times for a total of 51 clinician utterances. In contrast, the client has 9 correct responses and 7 incorrect, a total of 16 responses. As part of the analysis, the ratio of clinician to client talk is calculated and is found to be 2.8:1. This number indicates that the clinician is talking too much. It is noted that if the clinician is able to eliminate the "other" comments alone, the level of supervisee to client talk will drop to 1:1. The latter appears to be more appropriate in a therapeutic relationship. As a result of these data, the clinician develops a goal to reduce her talk time in treatment.

In data collection and analysis, there is a tendency to focus on weaknesses. Of equal importance is the identification and monitoring of perceived talents. Borgen and Amundson (1996) refer to this as challenging strengths. The second example, Figure 2.9 on page 43, portrays this strategy. A clinician feels that her reinforcements are strong and that they are carried out in the right sequence. Her clinical

Clinician - Client Talk

Clinician Talk			Client Talk		
Model	Reinforcement	Other	Correct	Incorrect	Other
II	I	IIII	II		
	I	II	I		
I	I	II	I		
II	I	III	I		
			I		
I		I		II	
I	I	II	I		
IIII		II	I	III	
I	I	I	II		
		IIIIIII	I		
	I	IIIIIII		II	
12	7	32	11	7	0

Clinician Talk Total = 51   Client Talk Total = 18

FIGURE 2.8   Record of Clinician/Client Talk during One Therapy Activity.

scheme is to follow each client production with a request for client self-evaluation. After the client has responded, the clinician plans to provide a reinforcer. The supervisee feels she does this successfully but wants to be certain. As can be seen, the client consistently produces the target, is asked to self-evaluate, and is then reinforced, documenting the supervisee's skill in this area.

The third example is a more complex sequential analysis. This is spontaneously collected by the supervisor and is not preplanned. The supervisee is treating a preschool language-impaired child and her goal is for him to use a five-word utterance containing a copula and a preposition. As can be seen in Figure 2.10 on page 44, the clinician models a five-word sentence but the child responds with four words, deleting the copula. The clinician recues the copula and preposition in a three-word fragment, which the child accurately repeats. The identical behaviors occur in the remaining dialogue. The clinician stimulates a five-word utter-

Sequential Data Collection

Order
1–4

Client Production		Clinician Request for Client Self-Evaluation	Client Self-Evaluation		Clinician Reinforcer	
Correct	Incorrect		Correct	Incorrect	Positive	Punishment
1		2	3		4	
	1	2		3		4
1		2	3		4	
1		2	3		4	
1		2	3		4	
1		2	3		4	
1		2	3		4	
1		2	3		4	
1		2	3		4	
1		2	3		4	
1		2	3		4	
	1	2	3		4	

FIGURE 2.9   Sequence of Clinician/Client Talk in Regard to Evaluating Client Productions.

ance using both the copula and preposition. The child deletes the copula producing only four words. The clinician remodels the copula and preposition in a succinct segment, which the child correctly repeats. The clinician is unaware that this pattern has taken place until she examines the data with her supervisor. It rapidly becomes evident that the task is too difficult for the child. A more realistic goal appears to be a four-word sentence with auditory stimulation containing the copula and preposition but not the initial article, or a three-word fragment using the copula, preposition, and noun without auditory stimulation. These data aid the clinician in modifying the procedure.

Summary.   The preceding examples of data collection—tally, profile, sequential—originate from a variety of sources. Some are spontaneously collected, others are preplanned by the supervisor and supervisee. From a collaborative supervision

Sequential Data Collection
Model
*Remodel

	Clinician Model	Client Responds	Used "Is" Correct	Incorrect	Client Response	Number of Words
1.	The dog is in box	1		1	The dog in box	4
	* is in box	1	1		is in box	3
2.	The boy is in school	1		1	The boy in school	4
	* is in school	1	1		is in school	3
3.	The man is in chair	1		1	The man in chair	4
	* is in chair	1	1		is in chair	3
4.	The girl is on chair	1		1	The girl on chair	4
	* is on chair	1	1		is on chair	3
5.	The girl is on bed	1		1	The girl on bed	4
	* is on bed	1	1		is on bed	3

*Goal: 5 Words with Copula and Preposition

FIGURE 2.10   Verbal Behaviors of the Clinician and Client during a Language Stimulation Activity for Standard English.

viewpoint (Anderson, 1988), this process is at its best when the planning, collecting, and analyzing are a product of joint interaction and when both participants are systematically involved. Also, as supervisees move toward self-supervision, they will take increasing responsibility for the process.

To gain insight into the supervisees' perceptions of the value of data collection and analysis, a group of clinicians who have participated in this process during their supervised clinical experience are asked to complete a questionnaire. Their responses are informative. In general, they find the data-collection process helpful and an aid to improving their ability to perform clinically. They also feel that it increases the productivity of the supervisory conference. Most report that it enhances their clinical problem-solving abilities, and a majority indicate that the process is most valuable when both the supervisor and supervisee collect and analyze the data. The supervisees also provided general observations.

"Provides a method to evaluate your therapy";

"It's time-consuming, but worth it";

"The data collected enables me to adjust the ratio of my talking and the client's talking time during the semester";

"Data collection helps me see where changes are needed, where changes are being made, and cause and effect in action";

"It's difficult to chart your own behaviors and sometimes you can get so wrapped up in charting that it can throw you off task"; and

"Data collection makes information about my performance more concrete."

Overall, the reaction to the data collection process from the viewpoint of the supervisee is positive (Dowling & Wall, 1988).

Individuals enrolled in a supervision course also endorse data collection as a tool to enhance treatment quality and to foster professional growth. During the class, the first few times data is gathered relative to videotaped therapy, they feel that the process is difficult. They report that the hardest part is deciding what to observe and how to lay out the format for collecting the information. Once they begin to feel comfortable with the process, they say that they wish they had been exposed to data collection before they began to do therapy and definitely before their externship experiences. At the end of the course, these same class participants were asked to identify aspects of their philosophies about supervision that had changed as a result of the course. Almost half cited issues regarding data collection.

"Effective data collection can enhance self-exploration and improve clinical skill";

"Data collection is the key for change";

Data collection "provides an objective way for us to analyze our behaviors";

Data collection "can be an important tool for measuring outcomes in therapy";

"Data collection is more important for the supervisory process than I realized. It's the main way to objectify comments made";

"Data collection was brand new to me! I am so glad that I learned about it and know that I will use it";

"Data collection takes a lot of the subjectivity out of conferences";

When I begin to supervise "the majority of my conferences with supervisees will revolve around objective data"; and

"Data collection is very important for the supervisor's growth."

In sum, they view data collection and analysis as fundamental tools for enhancing client, supervisee, and supervisor performance.

Supervisee Introduction to Data Collection

Supervisees do need to be trained to engage in data collection and analysis. If the clinicians have not had formal training during previous coursework, a brief exposure to its logic and value is helpful. The examples presented in Figures 2.1–2.10 can be discussed with the supervisee. Individual supervisors may also have collected others from personal experience that can be used to illustrate this process to the supervisee.

The flowchart in Figure 2.11 can also be introduced as it provides a framework for data collection and the analysis process. The initial planning session begins with an exchange of information about professional, clinic, or client goals. It then moves to a discussion of priorities for data sampling, and concludes with a joint supervisor/supervisee decision concerning the area of behavior to be observed and the type of data to be collected. Following this initial interaction, the supervisor will collect and may analyze or assist the supervisee in considering the data. This reflection can precede or be a component of the conference, although opinions, suggestions, and alternate strategies based on the data will likely not emerge until the joint meeting occurs. While the collection and analysis of data begins as a supervisor-guided or joint effort, there should be a progressive shift in emphasis to increased supervisee responsibility and independence. The data accumulated during a term can be helpful during the summary conference in estab-

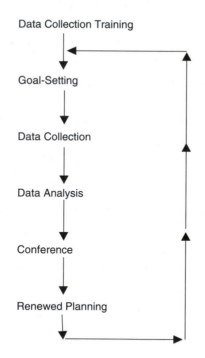

Responsibility shifts with increasing collaboration and self-supervision

Supervisor ───────────▶ Supervisee

FIGURE 2.11   Flowchart: Implementation of Data Collection.

lishing support for evaluations. So, from the initial stages of introduction to the end of the semester or year, when a grade is assigned or a work evaluation is completed, a continuous cycle has taken place. It begins with goal identification, then data collection and analysis, the supervisory conference, and a return to renewed planning as the cycle is reinstituted. The emphasis throughout the series of interactions is the gradual shift of responsibility from the supervisor to the supervisee in the areas of data collection, analysis, and the resulting strategy development (Dowling & Wall, 1988).

Early in the author's interactions with supervisees in training, it became apparent that clinicians need to have at least adequate clinical skills before involving them in extensive self-implemented goal setting, data collection, and analysis procedures. If trainees are struggling to survive, the clinical experience itself is overwhelming. To facilitate performance, a direct, primarily client-focused orientation may be needed. Clinician goals for therapy may include basic ones, for example, keep Johnny in the room, implement an activity appropriate to an objective, and plan sufficient materials and procedures for a whole session. These objectives for supervisee development, framed by the supervisor, should be verbalized to the trainee in a concrete manner. Specific behaviors that must be achieved to attain minimal clinical competence will also be shared. Generally, such goals will probably not emerge from the supervisees' self-reflections. Indeed, Kruger and Dunning (1999) point out that individuals exhibiting low levels of competence are likely to be poor self-evaluators as well. Such people typically see a need for "fixes" for specific events but are unable to view the process as a whole. Further, if they are asked to collect and analyze specific data or plan for their own professional growth, the task is perceived as an addition to an already overwhelming load. They also are not likely to see goal-setting and data collection as assisting them in getting the immediate situation under control.

In these circumstances, data will still be collected by the supervisor and used as the basis for structured, direct feedback to the supervisee. The data may also be used for the purpose of documenting a less than successful experience. The supervisor can even choose to show the data to the clinician as support for specific observations or suggestions. Active supervisee involvement in goal-setting, data collection, and analysis should be minimized until they demonstrate readiness to participate.

Professional Objectives in the Clinical Process

Literature

The setting of objectives is cited repeatedly in the literature as a strategy to enhance personal development and to increase goal attainment. This is true in a variety of settings. For example, Kreitner and Kinicki (1989) endorse a management by objective approach in business and Resick and Bloom (1997) in psychology education. In counselor education, White, Rosenthal, and Fleuridas (1993) view goal-setting and data collection in the context of single-subject research designs as mechanisms to focus learning and objectify aspects of effective clinical behavior. Anderson and Frieberg (1995) report that student teachers using the LISAM data collection tool are more likely to change specific teaching behaviors if a goal is formally written. Jensen and colleagues (1998) find that goal-setting and data collection allow teachers to improve the performance of classroom assistants as well as their own teaching behaviors. Notably, the gains that are made are maintained when assessed seventeen months later. In regard to professional growth, Schmoker (1996) notes that improvement is unlikely without specific goals.

According to Evans (1986), objectives stimulate and guide behavior. They help supervisees focus on the relevant aspects of the task and encourage persistence in goal attainment. Locke, Shaw, Saari, and Latham (1981) indicate that acceptance of a target triggers four related events: (1) increases attention to the relevant aspects of the task, (2) stimulates effort, (3) encourages persistence in behavior, and (4) fosters the emergence of strategies for effective performance. Joyce and Showers (1988) contend that to be effective targets selected must mirror one's stage of development. Anderson (1988) states that goals are of little value unless they are at the participant's level of readiness. Objectives that are slightly out of reach are thought to encourage individuals to stretch toward improvement. Successful completion also makes individuals feel competent (Locke, Frederick, Lee, and Bobko, 1984; Dowling, 1993; 1994). In addition, the recipients state that the process is helpful, it contributes to job satisfaction (Daley, 1985), and facilitates learning (Dixon, 1988).

Thus, once data collection is underway, a logical extension is to develop professional objectives. This is true for both the supervisee and supervisor. The following section addresses the former and the latter will be considered separately. Therefore, in regard to the supervisee, two aspects of objective setting will be presented. First, the identification of goals will be discussed and then their selection. Examples chosen by previous supervisees will also be incorporated.

The Clinical Process

Identification.   When working with supervisees, the concepts of determining professional objectives and monitoring growth have immediate credibility and typically generate an eager response. The development of goals, however, is easier said than done. Often supervisees will say, "I tried but I couldn't think of any" or state objectives that are superficial or minimally appropriate. The strategy that follows is often helpful.

After approximately three weeks of therapy with a given set of clients, supervisees may be asked to make a list of their own professional strengths and weaknesses. In essence, this is a listing of the things they perceive they do well and those that are difficult for them. To assist supervisees in this process, it can be helpful to provide a clinical evaluation sheet, or a list of competencies or key aspects of diagnosis or treatment for them to consider in regard to their own performance. The supervisor can also make a similar list based on observations of treatment and interactions with these individuals. Rockman (1977) suggests this as a strategy to diagnose the supervisee and to open lines of communication between the participants. Then, during the subsequent supervisory conference, the lists are shared and discussed. The supervisor adds information or an alternate viewpoint when appropriate.

It is important that strengths as well as weaknesses be discussed as there is a general tendency to overlook what one does well and to dwell only on aspects perceived as less strong. In rare cases, the supervisee may have an overly inflated view of self and not be aware of serious areas of weakness that need to be identified. Kruger and Dunning (1999) note that the same skills underlying competence are also necessary to recognize levels of competence. Thus, poor performers may not be aware of the quality of their work. An important supervisory role, then, is to assist supervisees in accurately viewing their professional self. Therefore, if the supervisee's strength list is short or missing key behaviors that have been observed, the list can be lengthened as the supervisee and supervisor talk.

Selection. Once the strength and weakness list has been discussed, a joint supervisor–supervisee prioritization is helpful. Items that will have the greatest impact and/or importance and those appearing to be realistically achievable may be identified. Then, it is relatively easy to translate assets and deficits into goals for growth. Borgen and Amundson (1996) suggest increasing the number and variety of circumstances in which an identified strength is implemented. In weak areas, for example, if a supervisee rarely provides positive reinforcement, an appropriate target would be to increase the frequency of this behavior. After the initial identification of objectives, it is important to review those selected to ensure that a balance between enhancing the supervisee's strengths and alleviating weaknesses has been achieved. Indeed, for some clinicians who have great difficulty acknowledging their own skill, an appropriate objective may be to increase the length of the asset inventory during the term.

Examples. For a supervisor or supervisee who wants to write goals but has never done so, it is sometimes difficult to imagine the nature of professional objectives. The examples that follow, although not written in a formal behavioral format, are those identified by and for previous supervisees.

Clinician 1   *Therapy*
                Be more assertive; end conversations as needed
                Delay clinician evaluation until client self-evaluates
                Eliminate fillers in own speech

                Conference
                Come to the meeting with at least two agenda items
                Identify two aspects of therapy that went well and two that did not

Clinician 2   *Therapy*
Increase problem-solving abilities
Refine target word selection
Decrease clinician verbalizations
Improve clinician listening skills for judging articulation productions
Learn to give negative feedback

Conference
Analyze a two-minute segment of therapy for clinician–client talk time before each conference

Clinician 3   *Diagnostics*
Increase pace of interaction
Enhance adaptability to deal with the unexpected
Monitor voice volume
Improve analytic ability to adjust as needed rather than after the fact
Augment frequency of follow-up questions when appropriate in the interview

Conference
Increase personal comfort in expressing own viewpoints during the conference

It is important to note that although the majority of objective setting occurs at specific times, the process is continuous and ongoing. As skills are learned, new targets evolve. To demonstrate this progression, Figures 2.12 and 2.13 show the objectives for two clinicians over a two-semester period. Note that some of the items are identified and achieved in the same term while others continue across both and, in one instance, are not completed by the end of the second semester. For each clinician, new goals emerge during term two that were not previously recognized. As expected in a growth process, achievement of individual skills does set the foundation for attempting those behaviors previously out of reach.

The focus of this chapter up to this point has been the supervisee's clinical and professional growth. An area that has only been alluded to, but one that is a key aspect of development, is the supervisee's participation in the supervisory conference. It is highly appropriate to target active involvement in the conference as a supervisee objective. This is particularly true in the areas of data analysis, problem-solving, and responsibility for the conference agenda. In summary, clinician professional development is diverse in nature. Clinical skill development, personal growth, as well as taking an appropriate amount of responsibility for the outcomes of the supervisory process are all suitable components.

FIGURE 2.12   A Clinician's Professional Objectives for Two Consecutive Terms.

Clinician 1

Objectives Selected > Objectives Achieved *	Semester 1	Semester 2
1. Build clinician self-confidence	>*	
2. Catch client errors and incorporate into current activity	>*	
3. Give clear directions	>	>*
4. Provide closure at the end of the activity	>	>*
5. Increase clinician eye contact/verbal responsiveness	>*	
6. Control task difficulty	>*	
7. Teach client to self-evaluate	>	>*
8. Vary tasks/procedures	.	>*
9. Reinforce more often and in correct sequence	.	>*

FIGURE 2.13   Another Clinician's Professional Objectives for Two Consecutive Terms.

Clinician 2

Objectives Selected > Objectives Achieved *	Semester 1	Semester 2
1. Decrease clinician talk	>	>
2. Respond to client self-evaluation in an unbiased manner	>*	
3. Improve charting during treatment	>*	
4. Increase creativity of activities	>*	
5. Refine target work selection	>*	
6. Label phonological processes accurately	>*	
7. Note client errors outside of structured activities	>*	
8. Increase client response rate		>
9. Increase clinician problem-solving ability		>*

Data Collection: Its Application in the Supervisory Process

Supervisory Puzzle

Martha has been supervising for five years in a professional work setting. She observes staff members a minimum of two times a year and then has conferences with them. Tom has been on staff for three years. Martha feels Tom's performance has plateaued. He continues to have significant difficulties managing client behavior but is excellent in planning sessions and implementing them in an organized manner. Tom is pleasant during conferences but seems to think everything is fine, with no need for change. Two individuals complain to Martha that Tom has "snapped" at their family members. They also state that Tom isn't helpful to them in figuring out how to control aggressive behaviors demonstrated by the family member in treatment. Martha is feeling frustrated. Tom's behavior needs to change but she is not sure what she can do to bring this about.

As we will see, data collection, analysis, and objective setting also underlie quality supervision and foster the ongoing professional growth of the supervisor. An examination of the supervisory conference is suggested by several authors, including Anderson (1988), Farmer and Farmer (1989), and Dowling (1992), as a means to provide a foundation for improving the quality and outcomes of supervision. Dowling (1993) shows that objective setting as a part of supervisory training results in supervisors modifying targeted conference talk behaviors. It makes sense that if a supervisor is unaware (other than on a subjective level) of what is occurring in the interaction, there is little basis for growth. As in the clinical process, data needs to be collected and used for problem-solving. As in the clinical process, objectives are set. Progress toward goals is then guided and documented through the use of objective data. In Martha's case, we will see how she uses data to adapt her supervisory style to encourage change in the supervisee's performance.

Puzzle Solved

As Martha reflects on her concerns about Tom, she begins to think about her conferences with him. Her supervisory philosophy (in relation to the Anderson Continuum) is to use as much collaboration as possible. She likes to see supervisees functioning independently. She concludes she needs to look at her next conference with Tom and collect data to see if she can figure out why Tom has stopped growing professionally. Is it something in the way she confers with him? She decides to collect several pieces of data in relation to the conference to get a picture of her supervisory style. She wants to know the number and types of questions used in the conference and who asks them, how much each participant talks, who is problem-solving and developing strategies, whether data is used in the conference, and who initiates or changes topics.

A summary of the data from her audiotaped conference with Tom appears in Figure 2.14. Martha notes several points in examining this information. Tom dominates talk time almost 6 to 1 and initiates 22 topics during the conference in contrast to the 2 she introduces. She notes that questions are limited in the conference but that she uses almost twice as many open-ended questions as closed ones. In considering just these behaviors, Martha concludes that this is consistent with her philosophy of encouraging the supervisee to be an active participant in the conference, placing this conference well within the collaborative stage of the Anderson model (1988). She is concerned that very little problem-solving occurred in the conference and, when it did occur, she did it. In addition, data as the basis for problem-solving and strategy development is only introduced once. Lots of strategies are suggested by the supervisee. In reflecting on this component of the data, she feels that her conference wasn't truly collaborative. She also thinks about the content of the conference. Tom did talk a lot about therapy but any time behavior was broached, he changed the topic. Tom shared his ideas about therapy and had lots of ideas about what to do next, but engaged in no actual problem-solving.

After reviewing and thinking about this information, Martha reaches several conclusions. First, she questions the general conference style she is using with Tom. Because the behavior management issue isn't improving and Tom appears to avoid the topic in the conference, she feels she needs to shift to a more direct, telling style with him. She also thinks she needs to become more focused on collecting data when she observes. She will then use this data in the conference with a particular focus on addressing behavior management. Tom may not be able to accurately self-evaluate and the data should help. She also needs to more actively control topic initiation to foster problem-solving and strategy development in relation to those issues problem-solved. Goal setting for professional growth also needs to be incorporated. With these thoughts in mind, she feels she has an action plan and is confident in her ability to assist Tom in improving his performance.

FIGURE 2.14   Summary Analysis of Supervisory Conference.

Profile Data Collection

Supervisor	Supervisee
Number of Talks	Number of Talks
50	299
Number of Times Uses Data	Number of Times Uses Data
1	0
Number of Problem-Solves	Number of Problem-Solves
2	0
Number of Strategies	Number of Strategies
0	21
Number/Type of Questions	Number/Type of Questions
Open Closed	Open Closed
13 6	0 6
Initiator of Topics	Initiator of Topics
2	22

In the example in Figure 2.14, Martha uses data collection and goal-setting as tools to improve her supervision and to increase the supervisee's effectiveness. The strategy of collecting data and setting objectives is as important in the supervisory process as it is in the clinical process. The continuing growth of the supervisor and the enhancement of the provision of supervision is the goal. As with the supervisee, after data is gathered about their supervision, supervisors benefit from making a list of their own strengths and liabilities. Input from supervisees is also helpful. The supervisor will, then, set goals and collect data to facilitate and monitor their growth processes. In the material that follows, general background information regarding data collection in the supervisory process will first be presented. Examples of data collection as it relates to specific objectives will follow. Finally, potential supervisor goals will be discussed.

Data Collection Strategies

As previously mentioned, several category observation systems exist for the analysis of the supervisory conference. Informal systems may also be used for data collection. The strategy selected is best determined by the nature of the question posed. For an overview of the conference or to answer research queries, a category observation system or a validated, reliable, individually developed method may be the technique of choice. On the other hand, a personally designed approach may be tailored to analyze specific issues of interest and may, on a day-to-day basis, be more efficient. The material that follows will focus on the informal tools. Some of the examples fit the previously described tally and profile formats while others do not. The data collection strategy being implemented will be identified prior to the illustration.

Implementation

Tally.   After reflecting on the collaborative portion of the Anderson Continuum of Supervision, a supervisor decides to assess her conference style. She decides to begin by looking at talk time in the conference, that of both the supervisor and the supervisee. She plans to audiotape her conference and then select a five-minute segment in the middle of the conference for analysis. She is going to tally each utterance made by the participants. She wants to know if her talk time is consistent with the collaborative phase of the Anderson model. After collecting the data on this session, the supervisor is startled because her talk time is much greater than she expected. She finds she talks more than two talks for each supervisee. This is not consistent with her view of collaboration. As a result, the supervisor sets a goal of reducing her talk time by 10 percent. She again collects data during conference 4 and is pleased to see that she has met her goal. She has reduced her talk time from 57 to 48 in a five-minute period exceeding her goal of 10 percent. She is also pleased to see that the incident of supervisee talks has increased from 25 to 32. After reviewing the data, she observes that she is still talking more (1 and ½ talks) than the supervisee (1 talk). The supervisor feels that this doesn't reflect the degree of collaboration she would like to attain. Her new goal is to increase the equality of their talk time by reducing her talk time while increasing that of the supervisee. She collects data during conference 10. Equality of talk time is nearly achieved with 45 for the supervisor and 42 for the supervisee. She is satisfied with her efforts and plans to work to maintain this level of talk time with the supervisee in future conferences.

Profile. Now that talk time is consistent with her view of collaborative supervision, this supervisor wants to monitor other aspects of her conference. She decides to look at two related issues, problem-solving and strategy development. She wants to know if either is occurring in her conferences and who is doing it, the supervisor or supervisee. She selects the profile format to record the data summarized in Figure 2.15 on page 56. The supervisory conference is first audiotaped and the supervisor and supervisee's instances of problem-solving and strategy development are recorded. The intent is to establish a baseline for these behaviors. On examination of the first exchange, it is noted that the supervisor solves two problems and provides six strategies, but the supervisee does no problem-solving or strategy development. In reviewing this data, the supervisor reflects on the goal of collaboration, which is to assist the supervisee in becoming more independent and active in analyzing therapy and in planning for future sessions. She feels that she is taking too much responsibility in the conference and wants to begin to shift it to the supervisee.

The data in Figure 2.16 on page 57 reflects a change in that direction as time progresses. When data is again gathered, during conference 5, the supervisee problem-solves three times and generates two strategies for the next session. The supervisor solves two problems and provides one strategy. A picture of equality emerges. After thinking about the findings and the growth of the supervisee, the supervisor feels that it is time to increase the supervisee's independence. This will be reflected by the latter doing more of the problem-solving and strategy development. The supervisor and supervisee are both delighted when the analysis of conference 10 shows growth in this area. The supervisee solves five problems and provides six strategies for possible implementation as compared to two problem-solves by the supervisor. In addition, the supervisee expresses confidence in her abilities and feels she is well on her way toward self-supervision, the goal of the Anderson Continuum of Supervision.

Individually Designed. Another supervisor, a firm believer in the Anderson collaborative model of supervision, makes a commitment to data collection and analysis in theory but finds it hard to implement. She notes that her previous data collection attempts have been predominantly tallies of the occurrence of specific behaviors or the use of formal observation systems such as the *Content and Sequence Analysis of Speech and Hearing Therapy* (Boone-Prescott [1972]). To obtain a baseline on the frequency of the data she has previously collected, she reviews the observation records for three clinician–client pairs from a previous semester. Over the term, she finds that their data was gathered only 20 percent of the time

Tally Profile Data Collection

<u>TARGET BEHAVIOR</u>
Participant talk time during the supervisory conference
(5-minute segments from middle of conference)

Conference 1—Baseline

	Supervisor	Supervisee
Utterances	57	25

Conference 4

	Supervisor	Supervisee
Utterances	48	32

Conference 10

	Supervisor	Supervisee
Utterances	45	42

FIGURE 2.15   Summary of Data Collected during Three Conferences Assessing Supervisor and Supervisee Talk Time.

for clinician–client pairs one and two and 38 percent for pair three. The overall average is 26 percent.

Following examination of this information, the supervisor establishes the goal of increasing the frequency of data collection during clinical observations. At the end of that semester, observation records are again reviewed to see if the objective was achieved. The records indicate that data has been collected for

Profile Data Collection

TARGET BEHAVIOR

Participant problem-solving and strategy development during the supervisor conference
(5-minute segments from middle of conference)

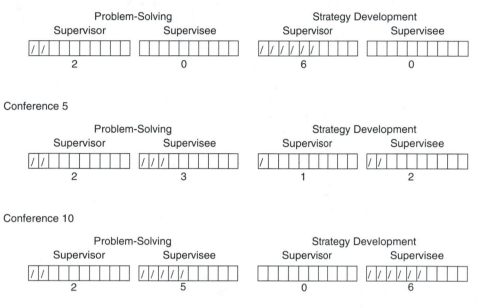

FIGURE 2.16 **Summary of Data Collected during Three Conferences Measuring Supervisor and Supervisee Problem-Solving and Strategy Development.**

clinician–client pair one 60 percent of the time, for pair two, 38 percent, and for three, 66 percent, with an average of 54.66 percent. The supervisor feels she has successfully met her objective of increasing the frequency of the data she collected during observations.

In considering the data further, two new concerns emerge. First, the supervisor notes that, although the total amount of data collected has improved, the volume per observation now appears to be erratic. For clinician–client pair one, the number of areas for which data is collected per observation varies from two to four, while for pair two either one or two target areas are observed and for pair three it varies from one to six. The supervisor speculates that the collection of data in only one area per observation may be insufficient, while collecting six different types of information during one observation may be overwhelming to the clinician. Secondly, in reviewing the data, the lack of organization in the way it is collected and summarized becomes apparent. For example, data is gathered in areas other than those targeted as objectives for the clinician. It is also difficult to determine, from the way the data are gathered and recorded, whether objectives are being met and if appropriate closure is being made.

As a result, the supervisor's new goal is to limit data collection to no more than four areas per observation and to collect data in a more organized manner. The supervisor quickly discovers that the task is more difficult than she expected. Limiting areas to be observed to four is not difficult, but gathering only data pertinent to individual clinician objectives is more so. A need to streamline the process quickly becomes apparent. The form that appears in Figure 2.17 is designed to make the task more manageable.

Procedurally, the clinicians' perceptions of their strengths and the areas in which they need growth, as well as their objectives, are transferred to this form. To make it possible to track progress, the date is recorded when a goal is selected, data are collected in regard to that objective, and the goal is achieved. A quick glance at the sheet enables the supervisor to identify the objectives in progress and those achieved.

To further make the task manageable, the following procedure is suggested. A folder, containing the above form for all supervisees being observed by the supervisor, is taken to each observation so that individual clinicians' objectives are readily available. In addition, the observation record, previously discussed and presented in Figure 2.4, is used for preplanning. During each conference, each clinician is asked to select the type(s) of data to be collected during the supervisor's next observation. The requests are recorded on the top of the observation form. This is then attached to the clinician's objectives. At the start of the observation, the observation form specifying the data to be collected and the attached objectives are pulled out as an organizational aid for gathering data. At the end of the observation, the date, the type of data gathered, and percentages of accuracy for those objectives observed are recorded on the summary form shown in Figure 2.17.

The supervisor will discover that with a concerted effort and the forms discussed above, the objective of keeping data in a more organized, functional manner is achievable. It is important to note that, with the use of the forms and procedures described above, the time demands relating to data collection are slightly more or no different than supervising without a formal data-collection strategy. In addition, this process assists both at midterm and at the end of the semester in summarizing the clinician's professional growth.

Profile.   A third supervisor is also actively involved in furthering his own professional growth. After viewing videotapes of his conferences and informally recording data, he analyzes the content. He feels that numerous positive behaviors are occurring. He observes that he is an active listener, gives positive feedback, and frequently asks for the supervisees' opinions, thoughts, and strategies. In response, the supervisees are involved in the conference and frequently engage in problem-solving. In the negative domain, relating to a more superficial aspect of conferencing, he finds that he uses an excessive number of verbal greasers/encouragers to let the supervisee know he is listening and to stimulate

Perceived Strengths   Perceived Areas for Growth

Objectives

1.
2.
3.
4.
5.
6.

Objective 1.

Date Identified   Observation Date(s) Data Collected   % Achieved

Date Achieved

Objective 2.

Date Identified

Date Achieved

Objective 3.

Date Identified

Date Achieved

Objective 4.

Date Identified

Date Achieved

FIGURE 2.17   Observation Summary Form.

further clinician talk. The supervisor notes that in one five-minute segment, he uses 18 "uh huh, ok, all right" filler statements. A goal is then set to reduce the number of verbal encouragers per conference and to collect data regarding this behavior. He chooses to count the occurrence of the fillers during the conference across supervisees. Therefore, as the supervisor participates in a conference, he makes a mark each time he uses a verbal facilitator.

Figure 2.18 documents the progress the supervisor makes in pursuing this goal. Note that the baseline is a five-minute segment while the collected tallies reflect entire conferences. Awareness of the behavior allows the supervisor to rapidly alter this behavior. In the first set of conferences, the highest incidence is 16 per 30-minute interaction as compared to 18 per five minutes in the baseline condition. By the sixth week of conferencing, the supervisor feels that he has achieved his goal by reducing filler usage to an acceptable level.

Undocumented Objective.   In another instance, a supervisor who regularly targets and achieves goals by setting objectives and collecting related data listens to her audiotaped conferences. She finds that she is often straining to make out her own words but has no problem hearing the clinician. As a result, she sets a goal of increased vocal volume but feels she can improve this behavior through conscious effort without formally collecting data to monitor change. At the end of the term, she again listens to her conferences on audiotape but discovers that she is still very difficult to hear. She subsequently reaches the conclusion that good intention alone is insufficient to alter behavior. She verbalizes that collecting and reviewing data has been instrumental in her previous achievement of objectives. Consequently, she writes a new plan for growth and incorporates a data-collection strategy for increased vocal volume during conferences.

Objectives.   In the preceding examples, several supervisory goals are considered: (1) adjusting talk time in the conference, (2) increasing problem-solving and strategy development, (3) implementing a higher instance of supervisor data collection, (4) gathering data consistently and in a volume tolerable to the supervisee, (5) reducing excessive encouragers for supervisee communication during the conference, and (6) augmenting vocal volume during meetings with the supervisee.

FIGURE 2.18   Record of Verbal Encouragers Used by One Supervisor during One Semester.

Tally Data Collection

	Supervisor/Supervisee Conference Pair			
Conference	A	B	C	D
1	10	4	3	16
2	6	1	4	4
3	1	1	2	3
4	4	6	4	4
5	1	3	1	2
6	0	2	0	3

Baseline: 18 verbal facilitators per 5-minute conference segment

The following are additional examples of supervisors and the objectives they set.

Supervisor 1

After diagnosing supervisees, adjust conference style to their levels of need

Increase active listening by paraphrasing, restating, and summarizing

Supervisor 2

Decrease supervisor talk time in the conference

Increase the use of open-ended questions in the conference

Use a minimum of three pieces of data for problem-solving in the conference

Supervisor 3

Reduce total number of supervisor questions in the conference

Allow the supervisee 30 seconds to respond before the supervisor makes another statement or asks a question

Mirror supervisee nonverbal behavior in conference at least six times to increase rapport

Data Collection and Goal-Setting Options

The types of data collected and the questions to be asked in regard to the supervisory process are limited only by the individual's imagination. Supervisory models or an individual's perception of needs may be used to prioritize potential objectives. For example, if one is interested in the interpersonal tone of the conference, several behaviors can be monitored. The supervisor's use of verbal or nonverbal encouragers for the supervisee to keep talking will be worth analyzing. It may also be helpful to consider the room arrangement and the flow of the verbal interaction to determine if the tone of the exchange is superior–subordinate, a factor likely to interfere with open discussion. Noting the use of active listening and restating for clarification purposes is also a good idea. Or, an assessment to ascertain if the supervisor exhibits facilitative genuineness and positive regard might be undertaken. The data collection strategy for considering the interpersonal domain may vary in sophistication from the simple tally to the use of a formal observation system such as the McCrea Adapted Scales (McCrea, 1980).

Supervisor and supervisee conference talk behaviors will often be a key focus for the analysis. Issues such as participant talk time, questioning and answering behaviors, verbalizations reflecting data analysis, problem-solving, and strategy development are at the heart of effective conferencing. Of key importance is who is doing it and how much. The amount of positive and punishing feedback is also worth monitoring, as is evidence of agenda setting and preconference preparation. Data-collection strategies in this area may also vary from the tally to the individually designed system or the use of a formal observation system.

As stated earlier, the aspects of the conference or supervisory interaction that can be studied are limitless. The supervisor may begin by completing a global analysis of the conference and then identifying a specific area for change, recalling that the enhancement of strengths may be as beneficial as the modification of weaknesses. Initially, the supervisor may want to select areas for growth that are readily attainable or those that will significantly improve supervisory skills. As an individual's confidence grows and commitment to self-improvement increases, more complex or challenging objectives can be targeted. Each effort will contribute to the goal of lifelong learning and the maintenance of competence (Kamhi, 1995).

Relationship of the Specified Supervision Tasks to Solving Puzzles, Setting Goals, Preparing for Growth

Eight tasks of supervision are identified at the outset of this chapter as pertinent to the topic of solving puzzles and setting the stage for growth. Data collection, analysis, and objective setting underlie the establishment and maintenance of an effective working relationship. Data collection removes subjectivity and makes it clear that the supervisory relationship is devoted to the improvement of both clinical and supervisory performance. Goal-setting gives supervisees the vision and the tool to move toward clinical independence. The application of these same strategies to client performance allows supervisees to set realistic treatment goals. Once goals are in place, data-gathering and analysis of this information will allow supervisees to continually refine their clinical management skills and to assess treatment outcomes. Through this process, supervisees will also be able to realistically assess the quality of their clinical performance because they have the tools to determine if procedures are working. Once clinical process data collection and analysis is underway, application of the same strategies may be applied to the supervisory process to foster supervisor growth, but also to increase supervisee participation in the conference. Through active involvement, supervisees learn to take charge of their growth by requesting supervisor behaviors that meet their needs. Supervisors and supervisees who engage in joint data collection and analysis are also exhibiting objective problem-solving behavior characteristic of a professional. In addition, they are practicing basic research skills in the assessment of efficacy. In sum, data collection and objective setting are key factors in the implementation of eight of the tasks underlying effective supervision.

Summary

This chapter begins with a puzzle demonstrating the value of data collection as a clinical tool. A continuum of data collection strategies is presented with the major emphasis on the individually designed approaches. Several examples are provided relating to specific questions supervisee and supervisors might ask regarding issues in the clinical process. The idea of objective setting is discussed and followed by a strategy for doing so with clinicians. Several examples are provided. Next, attention is directed to the supervisory process. The purpose here is supervisor growth through data collection and goal-setting. Following a supervisory process puzzle, several questions that might be asked and the related collected data follow. This chapter ends with a discussion of the role of data collection and objective setting regarding the eight supervision tasks listed at the outset. In addition, a therapy and conference script is provided in the appendices to give the reader an opportunity to practice data collection and analysis.

REFERENCES

Acheson, K., and Gall, M. *Techniques in the Clinical Supervision of Teachers: Preservice and Inservice Applications.* (3rd ed.). New York: Longman, 1992.

American Speech-Language-Hearing Association. Committee on Supervision in Speech-Language Pathology and Audiology. "Clinical supervision in speech-language pathology and audiology: A position statement." *American Speech Hearing Association, 27* (1985): 57–60.

Anderson, J. *The Supervisory Process in Speech-Language Pathology and Audiology.* Austin, TX: Pro-Ed, 1988.

Anderson, J., and Freiberg, J. "Using self-assessment as a reflective tool to enhance the student teaching experience." *Teacher Education Quarterly,* Winter (1995): 77–91

Blumberg, A. "A system for analyzing supervisor-teacher interaction." In A. Blumberg, (Ed.), *Supervisors and teachers: A private cold war* (2nd ed.) Berkeley, CA: McCutchan, 1980: pp. 99–101.

Boone, D., and Prescott, T. "Content and sequence analyses of speech and hearing therapy." *American Speech and Hearing Association, 14* (1972): 58–62.

Borgen, W., and Amundson, N. "Strength challenge as a process for supervision." *Counselor Education and Supervision, 36* (1996): 159–169.

Brookshire, R., Nicholas, L., Krueger, K., and Redmond, K. "The clinical interaction analysis system: A system for observational recording of aphasia treatment." *Journal of Speech and Hearing Disorders, 43* (1978): 437–447.

Casey, P., Smith, K., and Ulrich, S. *Self-Supervision: A Career Tool for Audiologists and Speech-Language Pathologists.* Rockville, MD: National Student Speech Language Hearing Association, 1988.

Cogan, M. *Clinical Supervision.* Boston, MA: Houghton Mifflin, 1973.

Conover, H. "Conover verbal analysis system." Unpublished manuscript. Athens, OH: Ohio University, 1979.

Culatta, R., and Seltzer, H. "Content and sequence analyses of the supervisory session." *American Speech Hearing Association, 18* (1976): 8–12.

Daley, D. "An examination of the MBO/performance standards approach to employee evaluation: Attitudes toward performance appraisal in Iowa." *Review of Public Personnel Administration, 6* (1) (1985): 11–28.

Dixon, G., "MBO: Tried and true management tool on a new setting." *Nonprofit World 6* (4) (1998): 26–28.

Dowling, S. "Teaching clinic conference participant interaction." *Journal of Communication Disorders, 16* (1983): 385–397.

Dowling, S. *Implementing the supervisory process: theory and practice.* Englewood Cliffs, NJ: Prentice-Hall, 1992.

Dowling, S. "Supervisory training, objective setting, and grade-contingent performance. *Language, Speech, and Hearing Services in Schools, 24* (2) (1993): 92–99.

Dowling, S. "Supervisory training: Comparison of grade contingent/non-contingent objective setting." In M. Bruce, (Ed.), *Proceedings: International and Interdisciplinary Conference on Clinical Supervision: Toward the 21st Century.* Burlington, VT: University of Vermont, (1994):180–183.

Dowling, S., and Shank, K. "A comparison of the effects of two supervisory styles, conventional and teaching clinic, in the training of speech and language pathologists." *Journal of Communication Disorders, 14* (1981): 51–58.

Dowling, S., and Wall, B. "Data collection: Analysis application to the clinical and supervisory process." Miniseminar presented at the Annual Convention of the American Speech-Language and Hearing Association, Boston, Nov., 1988.

Evans, M. "Organizational behavior: The central role of motivation." In J. Hunt & J. Blair (Eds.), *1986 Yearly Review of Management of the Journal of Management, Vol 12* (2) (1986): 203–222.

Farmer, S. "Supervisory conferences in communicative disorders: Verbal and non-verbal interpersonal communication pacing." (Doctoral dissertation, University of Colorado, 1983). *Dissertation Abstracts International, 44* (1984): 2715 B. (University Microfilms No. 84-00, 891.)

Farmer, S., and Farmer, J. *Supervision in Communication Disorders,* Columbus, OH: Merrill, 1989.

Flanders, N. *Analyzing Teaching Behavior.* Reading, MA: Addison-Wesley, 1970.

Freiberg, J. "Teacher self-evaluation and principal supervision." *NASSP Bulletin, 71* (498) (1987): 85–92.

Jensen, J., Parsons, M., and Reid, D. "Supervisory training for teachers: Multiple, long-term effects in an education program for adults with severe disabilities." *Research in Developmental Disabilities, 19* (6) (1998): 449–463.

Joyce, B., and Showers, B. *Student Achievement through Staff Development.* New York: Longman, 1988.

Kamhi, A. "Research to practice: Defining, developing and maintaining clinical expertise." *Language, Speech and Hearing Services in Schools, 26* (4) (1995):353–356.

Kreb, R., and Wolf, K. *Successful operations in the treatment-outcomes-driven world of managed care.* Rockville Pike, MD: National Student Speech Language Hearing Association, 1997.

Kreitner, R., and Kinicki, A. "Motivation through equity, expectancy and goal-setting." *Organizational Behavior.* Boston, MA: Richard D. Irwin, 1989: 174–208.

Kruger, J., and Dunning, D. "Unskilled and unaware of it: How difficulties in recognizing one's own incompetence lead to inflated self-assessments." *Journal of Personality and Psychology, 77* (6) (1999).

Locke, E., Frederick, E., Lee, C., and Bobko, P. "Effect of self, self-efficacy goals, and task strategies on task performance."*Journal of Applied Psychology, 69* (1984): 241–251.

Locke, E., Shaw, K., Saari, L., and Latham, G. "Goal-setting and task performance." *Psychological Bulletin, 90* (1981): 125–152.

Logemann, J. "The state of the profession." Presentation at the University of Houston Department of Communication Disorders. Houston, TX, Jan., 1999.

Mawdsley, B. "Kansas inventory of self-supervision." In S. Farmer, (Ed.), *Clinical Supervision: A Coming of Age.* Proceedings of a national conference on supervision held at Jekyll Island, GA: Las Cruces, New Mexico State University, 1987.

McCrea, E. "Supervisee ability to self-explore and four facilitative dimensions of supervisor behavior in individual conferences in speech-language pathology." Doctoral dissertation, Indiana University. *Dissertation Abstracts International, 41* (1980): 2134 B.(University Microfilms No. 80-29, 239).

O'Connor, E., and Fish, M. "Differences between the classrooms of expert and novice teachers on the dimensions of the 'Classroom Systems Observation Scale.'" Paper presented at the Annual Meeting of the New England Educational Research Organization, Portsmouth, NH, April, 1997.

Oratio, A. "A supervisory transactional system." In A. Oratio (Ed.). *Supervision in Speech Pathology: A Handbook for Supervisors and Clinicians.* Baltimore, MD: University Park Press, 1977.

Oratio, A. *Therapy Analyzer.* Ridgewood, NJ: Ridgewood Center for Communication Disorders, 1987.

Power-deFur, L. "Predicting the future of speech-language pathology in public schools." In S. Cornett (Ed.), *Clinical Practice Management for Speech-Language Pathologists.* Gaithersburg, MD: Aspen Publishers, (1999):243–257.

Reiman, A., and Thies-Sprinthall, L. *Mentoring and supervision for teacher development.* New York: Addison-Wesley-Longman, 1998.

Resick, C., and Bloom, A. "Effects of goal setting on goal commitment, team processes, and performance." *Psychology: A Journal of Human Behavior, 34* (3–4) (1997):2–8.

Roberts, J., and Smith, K. "Supervisor-supervisee role differences and consistency of behavior in supervisory conferences."*Journal of Speech and Hearing Research, 25* (1982): 428–434.

Rockman, B. "Supervisor as clinician: A point of view." Paper read at Annual Convention of the American Speech and Hearing Association, Chicago, 1977.

Schmoker, M. "Results: The key to continuous school improvement." Alexandria, VA: Association for Supervision and Curriculum Development, 1996.

Schubert, G., Miner, A., and Till, J. "The analysis of behavior in clinicians (ABC) system." Unpublished manuscript, University of North Dakota, Grand Forks, 1973.

Sexton, T., Whiston, S., Bleuer, J., and Walz, G. *Integrating Outcome Research into Counseling Practice and Training.* Alexandria, VA: American Counseling Association, 1998.

Shapiro, D. "Interaction analysis and self-study: A single-case comparison of four methods of analyzing supervisory conferences. *Language, Speech, and Hearing Services in Schools, 25* (1994): 67–75.

Smith, K. "Identification of perceived effectiveness components in the individual supervisory conference in speech pathology and an evaluation of the relationship between ratings and content in the conference." (Doctoral dissertation, Indiana University, 1977). *Dissertation Abstracts International, 39* 680B. (University Microfilms No. 78-13, 175).

Smith, K., and Anderson, J. "Relationship of perceived effectiveness to content in supervisory conferences in speech-language pathology." *Journal of Speech and Hearing Research, 25* (1982): 243–251.

Underwood, J. "Interaction analysis between the supervisor and the speech and hearing clinician." (Doctoral dissertation, University of Denver, 1973). *Dissertation Abstracts International, 34* (1973): 2995B. (University Microfilms No. 73-29, 608).

Weller, R. *Verbal Communication in Instructional Supervision.* New York: Teachers College Press, Columbia University, 1971.

White, L., Rosenthal, D., and Fleuridas, C. "Accountable supervision through systematic data collection: Using single-case designs." *Counselor Education and Supervision, 33* (1993): 32–46.

Clinical Data Collection Challenge

A sample therapy script follows. Using a profile format, the accuracy of the client's responses may be charted. If the reader wishes to do a more complex analysis, a sequential pattern may be used to assess the relationship between the clinician's verbal behaviors and the client's responses. After completing and interpreting the scoring, one may wish to consider two possible solutions suggested by the author.

Observation: Treatment

Goal: To increase correct production of /s/ marker.

Behaviors to be charted:

Clinician
M = Model
R+ = Positive Reinforcer
P = Punishment
O = Other

Client
+ = Correct Production
- = Incorrect Production
T = Off-Task Response

Clinician	**Client**
1. Say dog jumps.	Dog jump.
2. No. You need to say *jumps*.	Jumps.
3. Good. Try again.	Jump.
4. Dog. . .	Jump.
5. Say *dog jumps.*	Dog jumps.
6. Now, say it three times.	Dog jump. Dog jump. Dog jump.
7. No, *dog jumps.*	This is too hard. I don't want to do this.
8. If you say two more, you'll get a star.	Dog jump.
9. Say *dog jumps.*	Dog jumps.
10. That's good. Say one more.	Dog jump.

Data collection:

Clinician				Client		
M	R+	P	O	+	-	T

Clinician				Client		

FIGURE 2A.1   Treatment Observation

Sample Solution

Goal: To increase correct production of the /s/ maker.

Behaviors to be charted
1.   Client's correct responses
2.   Client's incorrect responses

Data collection:

I   II

Client

M	R+	P	O		+	-	T
						-	
					+		
						-	
						-	
					+		
						-	
						-	
						-	
						-	
					+		

Client
+   =   Correct Productions
            (27%)

-   =   Incorrect Productions
            (73%)

					-	

Possible Interpretation:
       The task appears to be too difficult for the client.

FIGURE 2A.2   Possible Solution to Figure 2A.1

Alternate Solution

Observation: Treatment

Goal: Correct production of the /s/ maker.

Behaviors to be charted:
1.   Client responses: correct, incorrect, off-task
2.   Supervisor verbalization: models, positive reinforcement, punishment

Data collection:

Clinician

M   =   Model
R+   =   Positive Reinforcer
P   =   Punishment
O   =   Other

Client

+   =   Correct Production
-   =   Incorrect Production
T   =   Off-Task Response

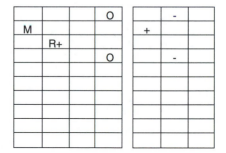

Clinician				Client		
M	R+	P	O	+	-	T
M					-	
		P				
M				+		
	R+					
			O		-	
			O		-	
M				+		
			O		- - -	
		P				
M						TT
			O		-	
M				+		
	R+					
			O		-	

Possible Interpretation:
   An increased number of clinician models would enhance the client's success rate, as the correct responses that did occur followed a model.

FIGURE 2A.3   Alternate Solution

A P P E N D I X   2 - B

Supervisory Data Collection Challenge

A sample conference script follows. A profile format can be used to record the questions and answers used by the supervisor and supervisee to identify the volume of questions and answers produced by each participant. A more extensive sequential analysis will allow one to assess the relationship between question type and response complexity. After completing and interpreting the scoring, one may wish to compare the results to two possible solutions.

FIGURE 2B.1   Conference Script

Supervisor	Clinician
Did your session go well today?	I thought so.
What was Tommy's behavior like today?	Much better.
You mentioned that you were going to increase the number of activities. Is that what helped?	Definitely.
Did you alter any other aspect of therapy that may have had an impact?	Not really.
Now that you have his behavior under control, have you given thought to your own professional goals?	Yes.
What have you considered?	Well, there are still several areas giving me problems. I don't have enough confidence in my own judgment.
I don't understand.	I thought Tommy was bored and needed more variety, but I was afraid to try it until we talked.
So you are saying that you have good ideas but don't feel confident in trusting your own instincts.	That's right.
What do you plan to do about that?	Well, I think one of my goals should be to develop strategies and write my lesson plan without discussing everything with you first. Then, I'll get your feedback, but I will be less dependent.
That's a good idea. I often sense you are on the right track, but feel you are reluctant to go out on a limb. So, one goal for you will be to become more independent and to increase your own abilities. Right?	Yes.

Sample Solution

Observation: Conference

Behaviors to be charted:
Pattern of Questions and Answers/Statements

Data collection:

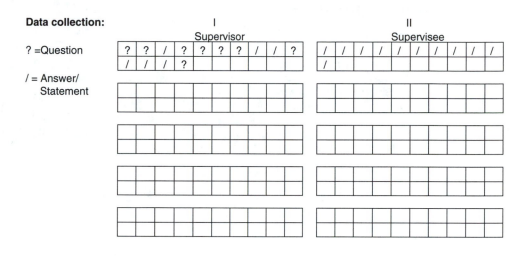

% of Questions Asked
  1. 100%–Supervisor
  2.   0%–Supervisee

Possible Interpretation:
  The supervisor needs to encourage the supervisee to participate in questioning.
  Supervisor may also wish to decrease his or her number of questions.

FIGURE 2B.2   Sample Solution

Alternate Solution

Sequential Method

Observation: Conference

Behaviors to be charted:

Types of questions and answers

Data collection:

C = Closed-ended questions
O = Open-ended questions
S = Simple response (yes, no)
E = Elaborated response

Supervisor					Clinician				
C					S				
C					S				
C					S				
C					S				
C					S				
O					E				
O					E				
C					S				

Possible Interpretation:
     Open-ended questions are more likely to elicit
     elaborated responses from the supervisee.

FIGURE 2B.3   Alternate Solution

3 Maximizing Feedback in the Supervisory Process

Clinical Supervision Tasks Relevant to Maximizing Feedback in the Supervisory Process

Task 1: Establishing and maintaining an effective working relationship with the supervisee;

Task 2: Assisting the supervisee in developing clinical goals and objectives;

Task 3: Assisting the supervisee in developing and refining assessment skills;

Task 4: Assisting the supervisee in developing and refining clinical management skills;

Task 6: Assisting the supervisee in observing and analyzing assessment and treatment sessions;

Task 7: Assisting the supervisee in the development and maintenance of clinical and supervisory records;

Task 9: Assisting the supervisee in the evaluation of clinical performance;

Task 10: Assisting the supervisee in developing skills of verbal reporting, writing, and editing;

Task 12: Modeling and facilitating professional conduct.

Literature

The previous chapter on data collection provides a strong foundation for the provision of objective information to supervisees. In a clinical (Cogan, 1973), cognitive coaching (Costa and Garmston, 1994), or collaborative (Anderson, 1988) model of supervision, the majority of verbal and written input will be in this domain. Supervisees will be guided to analyze the information and arrive at a valuative conclusion alone or in conjunction with the supervisor. At times, though, direct praise or criticism from the supervisor or supervisee is appropriate. Thus, this chapter will explore varying types of feedback, their effects, and strategies for implementation. Feedback as it relates to the thirteen tasks of supervision will also be considered.

Nature and Effects

Feedback, whether valuative or not, is perceived as an integral part of the supervisory relationship. It is generally viewed as having a twofold purpose: to foster supervisee development and to form the basis for evaluation. Typically, superiors, peers, individuals, and the task itself are the sources of such information. But feedback may also come from others interacting with the supervisee if a strategy such as 360 evaluation is used (Manatt, 1997). In that case, recipients of service become an important source of information.

According to Bandura and Cervone (1983), two factors determine reactions to feedback: an internal system in which individuals compare actual performance with their own goals or standards, and a consideration of one's capabilities to achieve or perform. In general, individuals feel fulfilled by positive feedback and tend to view it as accurate. In contrast, those receiving negative input are less satisfied and often perceive it as incorrect (Taylor, Fisher, and Ilgen, 1984; Stone and Stone, 1985, Kruger and Dunning, 1999). In fact, negative feedback is even recalled less accurately and is more likely to be rejected. This is particularly true when the supervisee has a view of performance differing from that of a given supervisor (Bernstein and Lecomte, 1979). Others feel that criticism may have a generally positive effect when it is timely, constructive, and specific (Abbott and Lyter, 1998). Another factor is the sex of the supervisor. Male supervisors tend to give negative feedback more frequently than do female supervisors, an area of specific gender difference (Brewer, Socha, and Potter, 1996).

Stone and Stone (1985) find that subjects with high levels of self-esteem have elevated self-perceptions of their task competence independent of how they have actually performed. Second, perceptions of their ability to accomplish an assignment are enhanced by successful performance. Third, consistent feedback from two evaluators has a greater impact on their perception of self-competence than does inconsistent information. Finally, when variable ratings are given by different judges, the provider of the more positive component is perceived as the more credible.

Contingent positive reinforcement is linked to increases in motivation and the enhancement of subsequent job performance (Podsakoff, Todor, Grover, and Huber, 1984) as is objective, meaningful feedback (Sama, Kopelman, and Manning, 1994). Leaders who use contingent positive reinforcement reward subordinates through praise, acknowledgment, and commendation. Conversely, contingent punishment takes the form of a reprimand when workers fail or, in general, exhibit low productivity. Of the two types of reinforcement, contingent positive feedback is found to be the most effective in changing behavior and enhancing job satisfaction (Podsakoff et al., 1984; Sama et al., 1994).

A supervisor's decision to provide feedback is often tempered by specific conditions. It is more likely to be given if the observed event or behavior is perceived as important by the supervisor, and if supervisee performance is directly linked to the supervisor's achievement and job evaluation (Evans, 1986). The supervisor's attributions regarding performance also are a factor in determining whether to react to an employee's behavior. If the supervisee is not perceived as responsible due to luck or task difficulty, comments often are not made. Conversely, events attributable to supervisee responsibility and effort typically are noted and shared during the conference or on a written evaluation. McCready, Roberts, Bengala, Harris, Kingsley, and Krikorian (1996) also find supervisors' attributions are a factor in selecting a strategy for managing supervisee noncompliance. If the reason for nonperformance is beyond the supervisee's control, the supervisor will react less negatively than if it is a controllable situation.

In speech-language pathology, Kennedy (1981) determines that the supervisor's provision of written subjective versus objective verbatim data differentially impacts both supervisor and supervisee talk in subsequent conferences. Cimorell-Strong and Ensley (1982) also examine conferences under two conditions. Following each meeting, one group of subjects provides written remarks to the supervisor regarding the latter's performance in that interaction. The others do not. The absence or presence of this feedback has no impact on the talk behaviors in the conference, although the researchers report a tendency for supervisors in the nonfeedback mode to provide the highest frequency of negative information. Dowling and Wittkopp (1982) further find that supervisees want valuative comments, in either written or checklist form, following an observation. These supervisees indicate a desire for information regarding both the positive and negative aspects of their performance. In addition, Brown and Block (1975) report that student teachers did not perceive supervisors as helpful unless they provided specific observations about performance.

In sum, there is a diversity of viewpoints about the effects, nature, and content of feedback. As noted, feedback may be verbal or written. In addition, certain other factors affect a supervisor's decision to provide feedback and the strategies to be used.

Effective Feedback Criteria

According to Pfeiffer and Jones (1972) effective feedback has the following characteristics: (1) descriptive, (2) specific, (3) responsive to the needs of the system, (4) oriented to modifiable behavior, (5) solicited rather than imposed, (6) well-timed, and (7) validated with the receiver. They elaborate by noting that evaluation typically reflects the supervisor's "should," which is likely to trigger defensiveness in others, and, for this reason, they emphasize the importance of objective rather than valuative data. Further, global information is often not meaningful as the supervisee remains unclear as to what is to be changed. Typically, the greater the specificity, the more helpful the input. The readiness and willingness of the recipient is also cited as a key consideration. Feedback in areas beyond the individual's current ability to modify behaviors is without value. Similarly, requested feedback is more likely to be viewed as acceptable than that determined solely and/or is imposed by the supervisor. Timing is critical in that immediate, rather than delayed, input is seen as more efficient (Reid & Parsons, 1996). Finally, the importance of validating feedback to check perceptions and to be sure the message is received and interpreted as intended is underscored. Views parallel to these regarding the provision of information to supervisees are voiced by Crago (1987) in speech-language pathology.

Sama, Kopelman, and Manning (1994) agree that feedback enhances job performance if it is relevant and meaningful. Abbott and Lyter (1998) stress the importance of being consistent and systematic. Systematicity is also echoed by Freeman (1985), who notes that effective feedback must be "systematic, timely, clearly understood, acceptable and reciprocal." According to her, systematic input is objective, accurate, and consistent. Thus, it is data-based and verifiable rather than being rooted in subjective impressions. In addition, consistency in the information provided over a period of time is thought to assist the supervisee in modifying behavior. Timeliness is related to the provision of data in close proximity to the occurrence of the event. In order to be clearly understood the information must be lucid, specific, and accompanied by explicit expectations or guides for modification. Acceptability is related to the balance of positive and negative information provided to the supervisee. Freeman stresses the importance of supervisor judgment in equalizing information so that the supervisee is neither overwhelmed nor allowed to become complacent about performance. She further states that the mixture of feedback selected will depend on the training the supervisee has had in data collection and analysis, the level of that individual's personal self-esteem, and the quality of the supervisory relationship. The final criterion discussed by Freeman is reciprocity, mutuality between the supervisor and supervisee. This factor influences the supervisee's willingness to ask for elaboration and question input, and the supervisor's acceptance of feedback from the supervisee. Finally, Wilkins-Canter (1997) notes that competent feedback is frequent, specific, continuous, relevant to the supervisee's needs, and delivered by someone trained in providing feedback.

According to Latting (1992), in order to give effective feedback, decisions must be made in four areas: (1) whether to give feedback, (2) what to say, (3) how and when to give the feedback, and (4) how to handle the recipient's responses. In addition, Cousins (1995) says that all feedback needs to foster supervisee growth. Therefore, appraisal should be a growth-oriented process. Thus, supervisors benefit from reflection on the characteristics of effective feedback and the intended outcomes for supervisees.

Supervisee Experiences

A discussion between two clinicians highlights concerns when feedback is not helpful.

PAIGE: That wasn't very helpful! She kept saying that there is a problem, there is a problem. When I asked what it was, she said it's the way you organize your session. I asked what she meant. She went on some more about how I organize procedures and my session. I asked for an example. She got annoyed and said she shouldn't have to hold my hand. Something is obviously wrong but I don't know what it is.

BRANDON: Wow, that's frustrating.

PAIGE: It is and I still don't have an idea of what's really wrong or how to fix it.

In this situation, the supervisor is either unaware of the criteria for effective feedback or is choosing not to provide it. In particular, the input is not systematic because it is neither objective nor specific. It is obvious that it is not clearly understood by the supervisee and the reciprocity aspect is being ignored. In addition, the feedback is all negative, which, in this case, may affect the supervisee's perception of her ability to modify her therapy strategies.

A different perception of feedback follows. Again, two clinicians are talking.

LAURA: Getting feedback is hard sometimes. I do appreciate my supervisor though. She always asks me what I think before she gives me her view. She always has something concrete to back up what she is saying. I like that.

TILLY: That's interesting. Ms. White doesn't give me feedback—you know—saying it's good or bad. We collect data and figure out what happened together. I often change things I do but I never feel I've been told if it's good or bad. I've had other supervisors tell me what they liked and didn't like. I hadn't thought about it being so different this time.

These supervisees are more satisfied with the feedback they are receiving. It is systematic, specific, and reciprocal. Their supervisors are incorporating a number of effective feedback strategies. In addition, Tilly's supervisor is encouraging her to self-evaluate, a feedback tactic to be discussed later in this chapter.

Feedback and Direct Observation

Feedback prepared during or in conjunction with direct observation may take a variety of forms. The method and format used may vary markedly from one supervisor to another and across facilities. Students at the end of their training have provided the following observations about clinical performance and the related valuative information. First, supervisees appreciate clear expectations for performance. They value helpful suggestions, prompt feedback, honest and specific input, praise, being respected, and being encouraged to self-evaluate before the supervisor does so. They do not like an absence of feedback, that which is predominantly negative, reactions given in a cutting, domineering, or sarcastic manner, nasty written notes, discrepant evaluations between supervisors, or a supervisor's refusal to discuss assigned ratings (Dowling, 1999). The impressions of these clinicians are important to keep in mind as the feedback process is further explored.

Four commonly used types of feedback will now be discussed: written narratives, valuative checklists, objective data, and competency-based assessment. Recall that Freeman's (1985) criteria for effective feedback include: systematicity, timeliness, understandability, acceptability, and reciprocity. The implementation of these criteria will be considered in relation to each of the four types of feedback.

Narrative Feedback

Narrative Description.   A narrative strategy, which Anderson (1998) refers to as "field notes," can take a variety of forms. Some supervisors describe the events that take place by writing a sequential account of behaviors or making a transcription of the entire session. A variation on this idea is selected verbatim (Acheson & Gall, 1992). In implementation, specific aspects of diagnosis or treatment are recorded, such as directions or reinforcement. The latter strategy is more focused and generally more helpful than a complete transcription.

When using a narrative format, supervisors usually describe isolated behaviors and record related impressions. While Wilkins-Canter (1997) reports that supervisors are actually reluctant to give written feedback, it is the preferred style of others. When narratives are used, positive and negative comments, as well as suggestions for altering or refining behaviors, are interspersed among the descriptions. Jans, Hagler, McFarlane, McCrea, and Casey (1994) find that the absence or presence of narrative notes has no impact on the amount of evaluation that occurs in the subsequent supervisory conference. One variation of a narrative strategy used by some individuals is to write a list of questions intended to stimulate supervisee reflection on the diagnosis or treatment session. In another situation, at the supervisee's request, a supervisor made a list of events representing strengths and those reflecting weaknesses during each observation. In sum, the content and form of written feedback may be highly diverse and reflective of individual differences among supervisors, supervisees, and the perceived needs of the participants. As is typically true, it is most effective when it is a jointly preplanned event.

Effective Narrative Usage.   It is helpful to use Freeman's five criteria, mentioned previously, to insure effective narrative usage. Systematicity may be somewhat difficult using the narrative approach because a specified structure is not used to guide the observation. Instead, the supervisor reacts to what is seen. Inconsistency from observation to observation may occur in terms of volume and the aspects of behavior singled out for comment. To deal with this issue, professional objectives for the supervisee, requests for specific types of feedback from the supervisee, and preselection of a specific goal for observation will help structure the narrative. The supervisor will then approach the observation with a mental picture of the types of notations desired by the supervisee. Consequently, the narrative will have a consistent, meaningful focus over time. The issue of timeliness is readily met using this style as long as the supervisor makes a concerted effort to deliver the narrative to the supervisee as soon as possible after the session. The concepts of clarity and reciprocity are closely linked in narrative usage. The supervisor needs to take care that the content conveys what is intended. The information and observations must be sufficiently complete and coherent to be accurately interpreted by the reader. On receipt, supervisees may wish to restate their impressions to confirm the accurate delivery of the intended message. In this same vein, supervisees benefit from being encouraged to give the supervisor feedback in regard to the helpfulness of the information being provided. The final criterion of acceptableness can easily be addressed in this methodology. For example, the supervisor must take care to limit the volume of issues addressed during each observation to avoid overwhelming the supervisee. In addition, a conscious effort to balance the tone of the feedback is likely to increase the level of acceptability to the supervisee.

One final observation with reference to narratives is worthy of consideration. If the supervisor opts to use a strategy such as listing a number of questions for the supervisee, the type and quantity used warrants thought. Conferences in which the supervisor uses numerous questions are considered direct in style (Smith, 1979). Typically, these questions set the tone for a supervisor-dominated interaction in which the supervisee functions as a passive participant (Roberts and Smith, 1982). Care must be taken that a list of questions to the supervisee, resulting from the observation, does not have the same impact on the subsequent supervisory conference. In particular, the supervisor must guard against dominating topic selection and talk time during the exchange. It is also important to note that people often react defensively to "why" questions (Flynn, 1978). Thus, if the strategy of listing questions is used, the supervisor must take extreme care in regard to the type and quantity used.

Rating Scale Feedback

Rating Scale Description.   Rating scales are widely used during clinical observations for the purpose of evaluation. They are noted for their efficiency and effectiveness (Anderson, 1998). These instruments vary in two primary ways: the number of items included and the continuum used for scoring each entry. Some facilities use a tool with as few as ten items spanning the breadth of clinical work. Thus, each individual element is broad in scope. An example might be "Clinical management was proficient." Other rating scales might have as many as thirty to forty entries. Here the items are more finite, such as "Closure was provided at the end of each procedure." A general rule is that increasing the level of specificity of an item results in a higher level of concreteness. Indeed, variability is minimized by selecting scale items that are as concrete as possible.

Checklist-type rating tools also differ due to the continuum range used to evaluate behavior. That is, an entry such as "Behavior management is implemented appropriately" is rated qualitatively on a defined scale. A varying number of distinctions may be found on those tools that are or have been in actual use. Some have as few as two descriptors while others extend to as many as ten ratings. A common example is one that uses a one-to-seven scaling with the lowest number representing an exceptional rating and the highest, seven, considered unacceptable. Table 3.1 reflects instruments that range from five to ten evaluative categories.

TABLE 3.1 Continuums and Descriptors for Rating Scale Instruments.

5-Item Range
(Lougeay-Mottinger, Harris, Perlstein-Kaplan, and Felicitti, 1984)

(5) Good, (4) Adequate, (3) Developing, (2) Inadequate, (1) Skill not evident. Each rating is further operationalized for four levels of clinical development: entry, primary, intermediate, and advanced. Level 3 (developing) is described as follows in regard to "Accurately records responses":

Entry

Has difficulty with qualitative description of behavior; needs supervisor's assistance and rarely charts behavior.

Primary

Does little or no charting within session but relies on tape recorder. Progress notes indicate good qualitative and quantitative description of behaviors.

Intermediate

Attempts to implement recording system and, as evidenced by progress notes, has good qualitative and quantitative description of behavior.

Advanced

Attempts to determine recording system and has good quantitative and qualitative description of behaviors.

James Madison University (Runyan and Seal, 1996)
- 1 = Unacceptable
- 2 = Acceptable
- 3 = Approaching competency
- 4 = Competent
- 5 = Outstanding

6-Item Range
Wayne State University, 1974
Communication Disorders and Sciences

5   (Outstanding clinical skills: able to operate independently);
4   (Appropriate clinical skills: able to operate with minimal supervision);
3   (Acceptable clinical skills: needs guidance);
2   (Unable to determine appropriate or specific procedures);
1   (Behavior absent);
       (Not applicable).

7-Item Range
Dowling & Bliss (1984)

1–2 (Inferior), 3–5 (Average), 6–7 (Outstanding)

10-Item Range
(Shriberg et al. [1974])

1   (Specific direction from supervisor does not alter unsatisfactory performance and inability to make changes);

TABLE 3.1   *(Continued)*

2–4	(Needs specific direction and/or demonstration from supervisor to perform effectively);
5–7	(Needs general direction from supervisor to perform effectively);
8–10	(Demonstrated independence by taking initiative; makes changes when appropriate, and is effective).
Note:	The clinician's level of development is factored in with the above ratings for the evaluation of performance.

Flahive (1996)

0	Does not apply
1	Not acceptable at any level of training
2, 3, 4	These values represent increasing skill shown by the student but with constant or very specific input from the supervisor necessary.
5, 6	These values represent adequate or good performance shown by the student with general or broad guidance necessary from the supervisor.
7, 8, 9	These values would be applied when the student functions with minimal specific instruction from the supervisor. Here the student is demonstrating initiative and is to a large extent self-directed in terms of preparation, carrying out, and reporting therapeutic sessions. The different values in this range (7, 8, 9) allow for discrimination between adequate (7) and truly outstanding (9) clinicians, keeping in mind that these values would be applied only when the faculty member feels that the student can function independently.

An issue that is frequently raised in the use of evaluation rating scales is the criteria against which the supervisee is to be judged. Some supervisors feel that the standard should be the proficient professional. Others state that the comparison should be limited to those at a similar level of development. For example, the beginning clinician, when observed, is to be compared to those with less than 50 clock hours or a new employee considered relative to those with experience of less than a year. The criterion used, without question, influences the range of ratings individuals at various levels receive. If proficiency is the gauge, beginning clinicians may expect to be rated at the lower end of the continuum, indicating room for growth. To minimize inconsistency in ratings, supervisors within a facility need to discuss the meaning and use of items on the scale relative to supervisees with varying levels of experience.

A limited number of tools designed for summative evaluation in training do adjust for varying levels of experience and/or presenting skills. Note that they are not intended for the day-to-day observation of therapy. The W-PACC (Shriberg, Filley, Hayes, Kwiatkowski, Schatz, Simmons, and Smith, 1974) and the UTD Competency Based Evaluation System (Lougeay-Mottinger et al., 1984) are illustrations of such methods. In all other cases, individual supervisors must make the adjustments in their own minds at the time rating-scale numbers are used for the purposes of summarizing performance.

Romero (2000) presents a rating scale strategy adaptable to the level of supervisee skill and experience. She suggests developing a tool to allow supervisees to rate themselves on skills needed in a particular time frame or setting. The intent is for supervisees to rate themselves as a basis for setting professional goals. Romero provides an example of such an instrument for the assessment process (see Appendix A).

Research and Rating Scale Objectivity.   Several studies address the issue of subjectivity in the use of rating-scale evaluation tools. Schalk and Peroff (1972) compare the findings of twenty supervisors, representing four universities, who observe the same videotape of therapy on two occasions. After observing it a first time, they see it again four weeks later. Following each viewing, they complete a checklist on which they judge each behavior on a seven-point scale. Marked inconsistency is found among the supervisors as each interpreted various points along the scale differently. Some people consistently rate high while others rate low. Interrater variability is extensive, but internal consistency is found to be high as individual supervisors' assessments are similar on both ratings.

The subjectivity of ratings is further highlighted by the work of Andersen (1981). She assesses the impact of supervisor bias and the subsequent evaluation of a supervisee's therapy. Prior to viewing a videotape of treatment, supervisors are randomly given varying information about the supervisee's grade-point average, clock hours accrued, and a summary of the quality of previous therapy and conference behavior, either acceptable or outstanding. Even though all supervisors view the same tape, the evaluations vary significantly. Grade-point average and information regarding previous performance bias the supervisors' judgments regarding the quality of the therapy session.

Acknowledging the inherent variability among supervisors' evaluations, three researchers have attempted to reduce such variance in degree. First, Hagler and Fahey (1982) provide supervisors with information about expected supervisee performance by reporting average W-PACC (Wisconsin Procedure for the Analysis of Clinical Competence)(Shriberg et al., 1974) scores earned by previous supervisees. The hypothesis is that knowledge of average or typical performance will reduce variability; supervisors will be more likely to rate supervisees much as they have been evaluated in the past. The information has no impact on the ratings given by supervisors as the spread in scores is not reduced. Second, Sbaschnig (1987), in a clinical training program, set specific guidelines for supervision. For example, all supervisors are required to complete a rating scale evaluation form five times per term per supervisee and to conference with each individual weekly. In addition, the supervisors meet in a group to view and rate three videotapes of therapy per term with the goal of a mean variation of less than .5 on the observation checklist. Discrepant views are then discussed after each viewing. During the third term, consistency among the ratings is achieved by the supervisors. In a follow-up study, the same procedure is used at externship sites. Consistency among supervisory ratings is not accomplished in these environments. Sbaschnig (1987) reports, in accounting for this finding, that the supervisors at externship sites exhibited less commitment to the goal than did in-house supervisors. Third, Balloun (1996) describes efforts to reduce grade inflation and variability among supervisors. The staff first modifies a published evaluation form to increase its specificity and then standardizes the procedure for grade calculation. Doing so does not reduce grade inflation though. The supervisors then meet to discuss and generate a consensus about clinician characteristics representing various grade levels. As a result, the criteria for evaluating are interpreted more stringently. Improvements are noted in the ratings of those supervisors who strongly agreed with the grading standards but less so in others.

These studies (Schalk and Peroff, 1972; Andersen, 1981; Hagler and Fahey, 1982; Sbaschnig, 1987; Balloun, 1996) underscore the seriousness of the issue of consistency in supervisor's evaluations of supervisees. The Sbaschnig and Balloun information provides encouragement. It appears that consistency is attainable with sufficient commitment and effort directed to that end. These same studies also highlight the concentrated focus required to achieve such a goal because others have had little success in increasing the congruity of ratings.

Due to the apparent variability attributable to checklist rating scales, the user of this type of tool must make every effort to minimize subjectivity. Rating scales that operationalize the meaning of the numbers on the continuum have a greater chance of reducing the variation due to supervisor interpretation. Thus, in selecting a tool for a facility, thought needs to be given not only to the range or number of items on the rating continuum but also to the degree of specificity defined for those points.

Effective Rating Scale Usage.   The Freeman (1985) effective feedback criteria of systematicity, timeliness, clarity, acceptability, and reciprocity are also applicable to the use of rating scales. Systematicity is easily met with this type of instrument because the same tool is used throughout an interaction. Thus, the supervisee will receive information in similar areas after each observation. Likewise, the goal of timeliness is addressed by delivering the completed form to the supervisee soon after the observation. The concept of clarity requires a mutual understanding of the intent of individual items on the scale. Written comments in addition to a number rating will help clarify the intended meaning. The reciprocal aspect is also important here. The supervisor and supervisee benefit from actively working to insure that both individuals interpret items similarly. In addition, they may need to negotiate the relative importance attached to given behaviors by each member of the team. Reciprocity will also be enhanced if the supervisee conveys information regarding the helpfulness of the feedback to the supervisor. Also, the acceptability of information from rating scales may be increased by the supervisor who actively looks for positive attributes and insures a balance between negative and affirming impressions recorded on the form.

A practical issue often emerges in relation to the use of rating scales. Multi-item instruments are usually subdivided into areas such as preparation for therapy, implementation, client behavior, and personal/professional behavior. If an overall average is calculated across all items at the end of the observation, a supervisee may interpret the score erroneously. Often, the tools have a number of items relating to preparation, material/equipment usage, and the personal/professional domain. These areas are critical in some cases. But, for most clinicians, the execution of these related components is well within an acceptable range. For these people, these significant but peripheral components are less important than skillfully implementing therapy. Thus, an average computed across all items may skew the overall picture because all areas are treated as equal in weight. To deal with this concern, a supervisor may choose to rate individual behaviors but not calculate a summative average. Or, the supervisor may provide an overall rating for the session but use only those behaviors reflecting actual therapy performance. A final strategy is to identify the factor(s) of prime importance during that observation and give a specific, separate rating for that subset. Therefore, if a supervisee is having difficulty in an area, such as the interpersonal domain or actual therapy implementation, the relevant segment can be isolated for the purpose of feedback.

In summary, the most helpful rating scales for supervisees will be those with specific items that are easily related to performance. Operationalized definitions for the points along the rating continuum will also identify the level of behaviors the supervisee needs to exhibit to demonstrate improvement. Thus, the more precise the items and the clearer the criteria for evaluation, the more likely the supervisee is to perceive the use of the tool as constructive.

Objective Feedback

Objective Feedback Description.   Objective feedback, by definition, is not valuative or judgmental (Wilkins-Canter, 1997), and its use enhances job performance on a continuous basis (Sama, Kopelman, & Manning, 1994). Information regarding this strategy is discussed extensively in the chapter on data collection. Recall that it may range from the use of formal observation systems to informal strategies such as simply counting behaviors to the previously described profile and sequential strategies. The nonvaluative aspect is a prime characteristic and advantage of this approach. It affords supervisees the opportunity to analyze the collected data, problem-solve, and arrive at their own decisions. Supervisees also accept this data as a valid representation of the occurring behaviors (Wilkins-Canter, 1997) This is particularly true if supervisees request the types and quantities of data to be gathered.

Effective Objective Data Usage.   The Freeman (1985) criteria—systematicity, timeliness, clarity, acceptability, and reciprocity—for effective feedback are also applicable to objective data. To be *systematic,* a supervisor must make a conscious effort to collect relevant, specified information on an ongoing basis. If this is not done, the supervisor may document widely diverse areas; as a result, the evaluation will lack an integrated focus. In general, the orderliness and value of objective data will be enhanced by using the supervisee's professional objectives and related requests for data collection as a guide to determining targets for observation. The goal of timeliness is met by insuring the delivery of the recordings to the supervisee in close proximity to the session observed. Clarity is addressed by collecting data in a manner that facilitates interpretation. For example, when the sequence of events during reinforcement are recorded, a notation that this was the purpose guides the clinician in considering the information. Similarly, legends that identify the intent of markings are also important. In regard to the issue of acceptability, collected data are likely to be more so if they are limited to those areas requested by the supervisee and specified in the clinician's objectives. Further, the collection of data reflecting a balance of strengths and weaknesses increases the supervisee's comfort in interpreting the findings. Reciprocity is achieved by encouraging the supervisee to question, ask for clarification, compare analyses of the data, and to provide feedback to the supervisor regarding the helpfulness of the information.

If the supervisor's primary mode of feedback is collected data, a word of caution is in order. The exclusive use of objective data may distort supervisees' perceptions of their level of competence. Theoretically, they should "know" how they are performing because they are being guided to identify the presence or absence of success in goal attainment. In practice, supervisees are not always able to do this. They may recognize the parts but not accurately perceive the whole. As a result, periodic valuative information from the supervisor may be necessary to assist the supervisee in developing a well-balanced view of self. If both types of information are provided, performance evaluations, such as grades or job reviews, are more likely to be consistent with the supervisees' self-perceptions of performance, although poor performers often have difficulty self-evaluating accurately (Kruger & Dunning, 1999).

Competency-Based Assessment

Runyan and Seal (1996) describe competency-based assessment in a clinical training program. Competencies in four areas are defined: (1) diagnostic evaluation, (2) treatment process, (3) personal and interpersonal behaviors, and (4) other areas of clinical training available at a field placement. Supervisees are given a dichotomous rating of pass/fail for each skill. A percentage of competency achievement is then calculated. The percents achieved may also be placed in a hierarchical order for evaluation purposes. More importantly, the competencies are a template for supervisee growth as the behaviors underlying clinical effectiveness are stated. Perkins and Mercaitis (1995) also use a competency-based system to aid novice clinicians in developing clinical skills. The behaviors identified as keys to successful performance, at various points in the treatment process, are used to structure clinician performance and are the focal point of weekly conferences. The Perkins and Mercaitus competencies and guides for weekly implementation appear in Appendix B.

Relative to Freeman's five requirements for effective feedback, competency-based assessment easily meets the systematicity requirement. The behaviors to be obtained are clearly stated and readily available to supervisees. Timeliness is also achievable although its definition may vary according to the defined use of a particular system. For example, Runyan and Seal (1996) use the competencies for the summative conference, meaning that they are reviewed only once a term. Perkins and Mercaitis (1995) use competencies on a weekly basis and highlight those to be achieved in a given week. Thus, depending on the intent and frequency of use, the timeliness will vary. Because the competencies to be achieved are specifically stated they are easily and clearly understood, and they are acceptable because they are the targets for the development of clinical excellence. Competency assessment is reciprocal as long as supervisors request supervisee input into their definitions and feedback about the competencies when applied. Supervisees may also give supervisors information about ways to enhance the clinicians' growth.

Supervisee Feedback Involvement

The importance of incorporating the supervisee in the feedback process cannot be overemphasized. Self-supervision skills are widely recognized as critical to the development of a competent professional (Anderson, 1988; Anderson and Freiberg, 1995; Dowling, 1998), so self-reflection is a fundamental goal of clinical education (Taylor and Horney, 1997). McBride and Skau (1995) note that, in an effort to foster self-reflection, supervisees must feel safe, supported, and respected by their supervisor. McLeod (1997) views self-evaluation as the basis for goal-setting and supervisor/supervisee discussion. Ironically, Wilkins-Canter (1997) finds that student teachers are often not given the objective data needed for reflection on their own performance, undermining the idea of collaborative supervision.

Of the four global approaches—narrative, rating scale, objective data, and competency-based assessment—the narrative strategy may be the most difficult for supervisees to self-apply. Typically, supervisees have difficulty observing themselves in a manner similar to that of a supervisor or other observers. Of course, the exception to this rule is when they have the opportunity to view themselves on videotape. Even then, however, they have not had broad experience in observing therapy, and thus may have difficulty pinpointing their areas of strength and weakness. One strategy used to assist supervisees in implementing narrative recordings in regard to themselves is to have them watch a tape of their own work and write comments that seem pertinent to them. A priori, joint discussion with the supervisor about critical aspects of performance may help structure this task. Similarly, the Crago (1987) strategy of having clinicians identify three aspects of therapy—one that was successful, one that was unsuccessful, and another that was surprising—provides a format for organizing the task. Also, encouraging the supervisees to comment in areas relevant to their professional objectives serves a similar purpose. Still another way to use a self-narrative, on a smaller scale, is for the supervisor to ask the supervisees to make notations about specific aspects of a session.

In contrast, rating-scale checklists are much easier for the supervisee to use for the purpose of self-feedback. Following the session, the supervisee completes an observation checklist. This guides the supervisee toward reflection on the events that take place. In using this strategy, the supervisee might think about the criteria for performance for specific behaviors and focus on executing them during the session. Following the session, the supervisee then rates the quality of completion in that area. The supervisee and supervisor might then compare impressions when both have evaluated the same session. This would increase the reciprocal aspect of the relationship. In addition, Donnelly and Glaser (1992) note that opportunities for supervisees to use and receive feedback when using an evaluative checklist increases the accuracy of their self-evaluation.

Objective data collection can also be used by the supervisee. Initially, clinicians may need to collect data from a videotape of therapy. But, as they grow in skill, they will be able to collect specified aspects of performance data regarding their own behavior during clinical sessions. As discussed in the previous chapter, supervisee involvement in the process will gradually increase in degree.

Competency-based assessment is of particular value as a basis for supervisee self-evaluation. The behaviors to be exhibited are specifically stated, which clarifies the expectations for their performance. These competencies also reflect the values of a profession (Taylor and Horney, 1997), something that will aid clinicians in incorporating them into their professional repertoires. Supervisees may also use competency-based tools to assess their acquisition of targeted skills and to plan strategies for continuing development. Two examples of competency-based assessment appear in Appendices C and D. The first is intended for use with student teachers (Glaser, Prudhomme, and Rogero, 2000) and the second for practicum experiences during clinical training (Runyan and Seal, 1996).

Supervisee self-evaluation fosters the development of clinical competence and a sense of professional self. Kamhi (1995) notes that beginning clinicians see their personal self as distinct from their developing professional self. As supervisees gain in competence, their views of personal and professional selves merge. The use of the four feedback strategies, *narrative, rating scale, objective data,* and *competency-based,* as tools for feedback, will hasten this process.

Feedback Strategies

Feedback Techniques

A variety of techniques other than written approaches for the delivery of feedback are cited in the literature or are observed in practice. Some enjoy more widespread use than others. Examples that will be discussed are the "bug-in-the ear," induction loops, audiotape and videotape, and audiotaped and written journals.

Terrio and Magee-Bender (1984) and Hagler (1986) describe the "bug-in-the-ear" strategy, and Wilson, Welch, and Welling (1996) present the interactive supervision system (ISS), a more mobile "bug-in-the-ear." Supervisees wear a hearing aid receiver in concert with a sound transmission system or a treatment room wired with a loop induction system. A supervisor in the observation room is then able to speak directly to the clinician during therapy. For example, the supervisor might evaluate client sound productions simultaneously with the supervisee as a means to develop listening skills. The timing of reinforcement might also be prompted. This same idea is used with diagnostic teams in other facilities. It provides immediate feedback to supervisees so that they can optimize the diagnostic session. For example, the supervisor might initially demonstrate an evaluation modeling the "bug-in-the-ear" strategy, and the supervisees can ask specific questions during the actual testing session through the sound system. For example, a supervisee might ask why testing is stopped at a certain point. The supervisor who is wearing the hearing aid receiver responds verbally, indicating that a test ceiling has been attained. Once this exchange is accepted as a natural component of the interaction, the supervisees feel comfortable receiving similar queries as they conduct the testing. Rooms equipped for free-field sound are also in use. In this circumstance, the feedback is delivered directly to the room rather than through an earpiece. Again, the supervisor can provide direct, specific feedback to the clinician during the treatment or diagnostic session.

Tape recordings are also in use in some settings. A tape recorder is placed in the observation corridor during therapy, and the supervisor then makes comments that are recorded simultaneously with the events as they occur during treatment. The supervisee can then listen to the tape later. The advantage is that the event precipitating the comment is readily identifiable by the supervisee. The disadvantage is the need to listen to the entire session to gather the feedback from the supervisor. An alternative is to record only the significant segments of therapy relating to issues for discussion. The latter significantly reduces the supervisee's listening time.

Videotape is widely used as a feedback mechanism. As a function of viewing their own tapes, supervisees often are able to step outside themselves and view their behaviors more objectively, and can frequently identify their own strengths and weaknesses without input from the supervisor. Videotape also has another advantage in that the need to recall events is reduced. Therefore, the conferences in which videotapes are used may shift from the supervisee's description of events to discussions of cause and effect and problem-solving. This is particularly true when data-collection strategies are used in conjunction with the viewing.

Crago (1987) uses videotape to actively teach both supervisees and supervisors to self-explore. Indeed, she states that it is "central to Student–Supervisor Interactional Self-Exploratory Training." Clinicians learn this skill by taping their sessions and coding them with a variety of observation tools such as The Content and Sequence Analysis of Speech and Hearing Therapy (Boone and Prescott, 1972) and the McGill Guidelines for Tape Analysis (Crago, 1983), and then present the tape segments to class members using the Teaching Clinic format (Dowling, 1992), which will be discussed at length in a later chapter. As a result, supervisees learn to analyze their tapes and actively seek feedback from their supervisors and peers. Crago uses a similar strategy with supervisors in training.

Audiotape journaling as a feedback strategy is described by Schill and Swanson (1993) as a supplement to traditional observation and conferencing. Once a week, supervisees make entries into an audio journal concerning self-reflections, comments about events in treatment, and areas in which the supervisee desires feedback. The supervisor listens to the journal and responds to the supervisee's concerns. Using this method, supervisees say that they receive more feedback than is typical of written responses, it increases the level of their own self-reflection, and they obtain the feedback requested. Drawbacks to the approach are tape recorder availability, the added time for the process, and the necessity for the dialogue to be continuous if it is to be meaningful.

Written journals can also be incorporated into the supervisory process. Supervisees use entries to describe and reflect on their experiences, then their supervisors review these writings and provide feedback as needed. Pickering (1989–1990) uses journals to aid supervisees in developing self-reflection skills and to increase the effectiveness of the interpersonal relationship between the supervisor and supervisee. Anderson (1998) finds such journals particularly helpful in circumstances such as field placements in which direct observation is less frequent.

Supervisee Observations

The effect of implementing the various feedback strategies is being discussed by two friends in the workplace, Pat and Bobbie. Note that in these instances, feedback is viewed as a constructive, helpful process.

> **PAT:** I'm really glad JoAnn decided to take Lee Ann's position. I like that she observes once in a while. I like that she collects data. It's been fun to get someone else's perspective. Even when we disagree on a certain procedure, I've felt good about the process. She is so positive. I like her a lot. It is sure different than when Lee Ann was here. I dreaded being observed then.
>
> **BOBBIE:** I like her too. I've really gotten into the competencies and self-reflection. We are lucky to have her.
>
> Near the end of a term in a university setting, two clinicians, Joel and Barbara, are eating lunch and talking about their training experiences.
>
> **JOEL:** I think I'm going to make it. Only two more treatment sessions.
>
> **BARBARA:** Me too. This has been a challenging term. I've grown so much. I was lucky to work with Ms. Hoff, although I wouldn't have admitted it earlier. I've never had a supervisor who wanted me to take so much responsibility.
>
> **JOEL:** She has been good. At first I didn't know what to think of the journals we had to keep. It's really made me think about the way I do therapy.
>
> **BARBARA:** The data has been good too.

> **JOEL:**   And the competencies. I've had more of a sense of where I'm going than ever before.
>
> **BARBARA:**   The other thing I like is that she always treats me with respect. She is honest with me so it hasn't always been roses. But I feel valued.
>
> **JOEL:**   Yeah.

These supervisors have incorporated numerous strategies to involve supervisees in self-reflection and the analysis of the clinical process: data collection, competencies, and journals. The supervisors' interpersonal styles are also effective. As a result, the supervisees have grown and are satisfied with the process.

Verbal Feedback Strategies

Ideas for giving verbal feedback abound. For example, Crago (1987) indicates a need for a balance between positive and negative input during the conference. Anderson (1988), too, feels that both positive and negative are appropriate, as do Abbott and Lyter (1998). Cogan (1978) stresses the need for positive comments only to avoid having supervisees reject the supervisor's input altogether. Borgen and Admundson (1996) suggest focusing on supervisee strengths, and Juhnke (1996) says that it is more effective to stress solutions rather than problems. Jans and associates (1994) note that, in general, supervisors are reluctant to provide verbal valuative comments, and Wilkins-Canter (1997) report the same observation in regard to negative written commentary. In contrast, Costa and Garmston (1989) indicate that direct suggestions should not be used at all. Instead, the supervisee should be guided through the processes of problem-solving and discussion to arrive at his or her own conclusions. Some supervisees prefer receiving all the negative and then all of positive comments, or vice versa. Some supervisors suggest sandwiching or alternating positive and negative comments (Abbott and Lyter, 1998). In sum, views on the nature of feedback and strategies for implementation do vary. In general, though, it is safe to say that most people believe that supervisees should leave the interaction on a positive note.

As a supervisor, the strategy of downplaying the negative aspects of supervisees' performance or alternating positive and negative feels like gameplaying. One does this and then that. Yet, managing feedback is a fundamental issue in building constructive supervisory relationships. The important idea to remember, regardless of the strategy selected, is that supervisees are people. They have feelings and need to feel good about themselves personally and professionally. They may also have varying levels of tolerance for certain types of information, so a supervisor must show sensitivity to that individual and temper his or her feedback accordingly.

Contingent positive and negative reinforcement is identified in business management and psychology as essential to the modification of performance. Reid and Parsons (1996) note that immediate input is preferred to delayed, while Pfeiffer and Jones (1972) speak of the importance of specific feedback addressed only to those behaviors perceived by the supervisor as modifiable. Similarly, Sama and associates (1994) state that feedback must be both relevant and meaningful if it is to enhance the supervisee's performance. Crago (1987) further states that input is best when it is descriptive and behaviorally oriented rather than judgmental. Pfeiffer and Jones (1972) say that it's most effective when comments are solicited, not imposed. The importance of shared opportunities to discuss and compare perceptions of given feedback is highlighted by both Freeman (1985) and Crago (1987). Finally, the quantity of feedback at any one time must be adjusted to the level of supervisee need.

Feedback Timing

Three issues in regard to the timing of feedback continually recur. The first two relate to the frequency and synchrony of providing information and the other to the scheduling of conferences. The question on a day-to-day basis is whether objective and/or valuative input should be provided after each observation. Individual supervisors may choose to do so. Others will alternate between collected data, no information, and valuative scoresheets. Research shows that supervisees in training programs object to observations for which they receive no feedback (Dowling and Wittkopp, 1982). On the other hand, a continuous flow of valuative data may interfere with supervisee learning. Wilson (1967) points out that learning a skill requires time. To maximize self-learning, supervisees need the opportunity to attempt, reflect, and reorganize their thoughts without interference from the supervisor. To avoid this problem, objective data may be provided when valuative data seems inappropriate. In fact, if supervisors want to implement a collaborative (Anderson, 1988) model of supervision, their input will be predominantly data-based.

Timing also relates to the actual delivery of information to the supervisee. Learning theory states that the closer the reinforcer follows the event, the more effective it is in modifying behavior. Reid and Parsons (1996) report that professionals prefer immediate to delayed feedback, yet Wilson (1967), cited earlier, indicates that immediate feedback may actually interfere with learning. In addition, Crago (1987) states that, before the supervisor provides feedback, the supervisee needs to have the opportunity to discuss the behaviors that occurred as well as the related feelings. Thus, in some circumstances, the supervisee benefits from receiving the data or evaluation tool as they leave the treatment room. In others, effectiveness is increased by allowing the supervisee to reflect on his or her own data and perceptions prior to input from the supervisor. In the latter, the supervisor may choose to hold the written input until either the next day or the next conference.

Frequency and type of feedback is best determined jointly by the supervisor and supervisee. Optimally, the supervisor will share his or her philosophy regarding the provision of valuative feedback, collected data, and instances when direct input will not be given. In turn, the supervisee will reflect on his or her own needs and the likelihood that the supervisor's strategy will address those concerns. If the two participants are not in agreement, a compromise solution is necessary to enhance the working relationship.

The actual scheduling of meetings is the final issue in regard to the timing of feedback. Trainees need regularly scheduled conferences. In training settings, these meetings are most beneficial when they occur prior to the submission of weekly lesson plans but after at least one scheduled treatment session per week. Conferences scheduled within two or three hours preceding the actual session often are difficult for the clinician, because alternate strategies, techniques, data collection approaches, and/or a need for additional information are likely to be discussed during these meetings. Usually the supervisee will make an attempt to follow through with the decisions made. However, if the individual has not had time to think through modifications, implementation may be inefficient or disorganized. Thus, if conferences are not optimally scheduled, agreed-on changes that were determined the day of the therapy session are best delayed until a session held on a successive day.

In contrast, for those more skilled, such as the working professional, conferences are likely to occur less often. Yet, they too benefit from having regularly scheduled meetings. These may follow observations or be set to discuss progress toward professional goals.

Feedback on Written Material

The development of the supervisee's professional writing skills is an important aspect of the supervisory process. This is almost always true for the individual in training, but it can also relate to the employed professional. For those in the latter group, accommodation to the unique requirements of a facility will be the focus. Some people have difficulty with writing well into their professional career. Because reports sent to others are viewed as a reflection of an individual's competence, this aspect of clinical performance is very important in all settings.

To begin the writing process, Rassi (1990) suggests orienting supervisees to the types of material typically found in professional reports, and advises following this information with completed examples. She also recommends guidebooks such as *Report Writing in Audiology* (Billings and Schmitz, 1980), *Report Writing in the Field of Communication Disorders* (Knepflar and May, 1989), and Meyer (1998) *Survival Guide for Beginning Clinicians,* which provide strategies for the novice writer. Rassi indicates that, in some instances, supervisees may need to be gradually taught the process by a supervisor who co-writes varying amounts of the final product.

Farmer (1989a) suggests an alternate strategy. For supervisees who have significant writing difficulties, she suggests introducing formula writing. In this approach, a skeletal format is given to the supervisee. The form may range from the element formula, which prescribes only the sequence for organizing the information, to a slot-filler formula. The latter contains complete sentences and the supervisee only has to fill in the blanks. Farmer also describes a nine-step strategy to teach formula writing.

In the more typical case, feedback takes the form of editing and narrative suggestions on lesson plans, reports, and other written materials. Supervisees, in training, often express concern about the time devoted to report writing and the number of rewrites requested (Baxley & Bowers, 1991–1992). The comments from the supervisor may relate to the appearance of the document, or its content, style, organization, grammar, wording, and spelling. Given this variety, there are at least three helpful things that supervisors can do, other than providing technical information, to help trainees develop their writing skills. First, the supervisor should make a conscious effort to identify writing strengths as well as areas that need revision, an approach that makes the information more palatable. Second, consistent input from the supervisor aids learning. The changes requested for rewrites should be similar to those made on the original submission. Smith (1990) suggests having supervisees submit all of their drafts with the revised reports to facilitate the consistency of feedback. The exception to this is when there are so many suggested revisions that they need to be dealt with in layers. As the major writing problems are resolved, attention can then be focused on specifics. In this latter case, the supervisee may feel that the supervisor's comments have been contradictory because some parts of a report were acceptable at one stage but unacceptable at the next. An explanation to the supervisee often satisfies this concern. Third, remarks are most beneficial when they are specific and helpful. In that regard, general valuative notes are of minimal value. Rather, precise guides or directives assist the completion of the task. In view of the above, the supervisor would be wise, after editing a document, to review the written comments, ensuring that they are a mix of positive and negative, if appropriate, consistent, specific, and helpful.

If the goal is to truly teach writing skills, open communication about the process needs to take place. In the interest of saving time, some supervisees rotely make alterations requested by the supervisor. In these cases, little or no effort is made to understand why the proposed changes enhance the quality of the final document. To avoid this situation and to maximize learning, it may be best to establish an environment in which the supervisee is encouraged to question the supervisor's comments and understand the reasoning behind specific editorial notations. Farmer (1989a) suggests that, when the supervisor and supervisee's styles differ, the differences and the related underlying rationales are an important topic for the conference.

Another comment in regard to feedback on written materials is in order. Clinicians frequently are heard to comment "My report bled to death." Supervisees often attach negative connotations to the color red from previous school experiences. Indeed, they may react more to the color and quantity of notations than to the comments themselves. Although it clearly is a superficial aspect of supervision, supervisors may want to consider the use of a pencil or different pen color when editing the written work of supervisees in order to minimize this affective reaction.

Electronic editing of written work (Densmore, Runyan, and Hagler, 1990) assists in the teaching of professional writing. It also increases the efficiency from the viewpoint of both the supervisor and supervisee. If both people are on a computer network, they can call up the document for editing without ever having to print a hard copy. If not, and both members have access to compatible software and hardware, the supervisee may submit a disc and the file name to the supervisor. In both of these circumstances, the supervisor may use an editing software feature to insert comments or highlight aspects in need of revision. Smith (1990) suggests an additional strategy. She encourages supervisees to save each draft of a document under a different file name. Then, if either the supervisor or supervisee wants to look at an earlier version, it is readily available.

Similarly, to reduce the stress attached to professional writing, the volume of material required at each point and the scheduling of due dates may be considered. For example, instead of having the complete case report submitted at the end of a term, it might be broken into successive segments spaced out over the term. For example, the assessment, analysis, and objectives might be due early and be followed by the first half of the entire report. At the end, all of the earlier components would have been revised and accepted so that only the results and recommendations are open to review at the last interval. The distribution of the quantity of writing due, at any point in time, makes the process more manageable and probably a better learning experience for the supervisee.

Work environments may have more flexibility in varying completion dates. For example, if case reports are due on dismissal or at the end of a specified number of sessions, patient data may be segmented so that a manageable number of reports are due at a time. This would avoid having the majority of the writing turned in at once. Continuous case notations rather than lengthy reports can also reduce demands in this area.

In work settings, the nature and formality of report writing varies. In general, it is usually shorter, more structured, and to the point. The reporting requirements in a given facility are responsive to reimbursement requirements, the readers of the report, federal stipulations, and, in the schools, state mandates. Thus, supervisees transitioning from one type of facility to another will need assistance in adjusting to the differences in documentation and reporting.

Grades and Salary Increment Determination

Various strategies are used to translate feedback about clinical behavior into grades or salary increases. There is not a best method nor is there one that satisfies all of the participants. Several options exist: subjective impression, rating scales, published criteria, performance contracting, and competency-based evaluation. The first is a subjective impression of an individual's performance expressed as "He is an 'A' clinician," "I feel he is the most effective clinician this term," or "He is the best person on my staff." Most people vigorously object to this type of system because of its lack of objectivity and the inherent potential for bias. A behaviorally based observation scale or other documentable approach is generally seen as more fair. One alternative is to take the formal valuative system used in a facility, rate each person, and then rank-order people on the basis of performance. Rodgers (1990) suggests a pair-by-pair comparison of people within a category, identifying in each case the better performer. After completing such a process, those in the top echelon earn the highest grade or increment, the next group receives less but more than those ranked lower. The ordering may also be done by supervisee category such as beginning clinician, working professional with more than five years of experience, and so on. This sets the stage for comparing individuals with others who have a similar background and level of experience. A second approach for using a given valuative tool in a facility is to establish consistent criteria for each grade or salary increment. A specific level of performance then earns a stated amount of reward independently of how others performed, and the criteria can be adjusted to reflect the experience level of the supervisee. A third option is to contract with supervisees. To earn a given rating, they agree to a target level of performance. The level achieved then translates directly into a specified grade or salary adjustment. Competency-based evaluation is a fourth, but somewhat similar, strategy. The skills to be acquired and the expected levels of performance are specified. Supervisees are then evaluated in relation to their success in demonstrating behaviors reflected by the competencies. Concerning the method of evaluation selected, recall the variability that has been documented among supervisors when judging supervisees. A strategy to deal with this issue will need to be incorporated when a system is placed in use or the ratings are likely to be skewed.

Relationship of Maximizing Feedback in the Supervisory Process to the Specified Tasks of Supervision

Feedback is identified at the outset of this chapter as relevant to nine of the thirteen tasks of supervision. Clearly, it relates to the establishment and maintenance of an effective working relationship. Indeed, feedback is instrumental to the growth of the relationship. This is particularly true when the flow of information is bidirectional. That is, not only does the supervisee receive feedback but the supervisor does as well. Input from a supervisor is often critical to the development of effective client goals. At times, data may be missing or overlooked. In other circumstances, an alternate point of view stimulates thought, discussion, and the identification of optimal objectives. Others of the specified tasks relate to the development and refinement of assessment and treatment skills as well as those linked to the observation and analysis of client and clinician performance. These competencies tend to evolve only in the presence of feedback. Of course, data-based and valuative information may emerge from oneself, the supervisor, or peers. But whatever the source, it is the foundation for maintaining and modifying behavior. The task of developing observation and analysis skills is basic to super-visee self-evaluation and growth of independence in the clinical process. To change behavior, one must first be able to recognize it and acknowledge its rele-vance to cause and effect. Feedback assists the supervisee in accurate identifica-tion, analysis, and problem-solving. Another task, the improvement of writing skills through feedback, is directly addressed in this chapter. The last task, model-ing and facilitating professional conduct, is also enhanced through the feedback process. This is particularly true if supervisors model these behaviors. They thereby demonstrate the relevance of data-based and/or valuative information to one's ongoing professional growth. Also, the fact that the supervisor engages in the gathering of data and problem-solving relative to both the clinical and super-visory process demonstrates the appropriateness of using evidence-based practice (Logemann, 2000) as a basis for growth. It also shows the value of openly study-ing behavior. In sum, feedback underlies effective implementation of nine of the thirteen tasks of supervision.

Summary

This chapter covers an array of topics in regard to feedback. First, the relevant literature is considered. Criteria for effective feedback are presented as are four strategies for implementation: narrative, rating scale, objective data, and competency-based. The importance of involving the supervisee in this process is stressed throughout. Alternative techniques for providing information, such as the "bug-in-the-ear," induction loops, audiotape and videotape, and written journals are presented. Then, tactics for providing input during the conference are discussed as is the issue of timing. This is followed by a section on providing constructive comments in the area of professional writing. Finally, how perfor-mance information is translated into a grade or salary increment is considered, and the last section explores the relevance of feedback to nine of the thirteen tasks of supervision.

REFERENCES

Abbott, A., and Lyter, S. "The use of constructive criticism in field supervision." *The Clinical Supervisor, 17* (2) (1998): 43–57.

Acheson, K., and Gall, M. *Techniques in the Clinical Supervision of Teachers.* (3rd ed.) New York: Longman, 1992.

Andersen, C. *The effect of supervisor bias on the evaluation of student clinicians in speech/language pathology and audiology.* (Doctoral dissertation, Indiana University, 1981.) *Dissertation Abstracts Interna-tional, 41,* 4479B. (University Microfilms No. 81-12, 499.)

Anderson, J. *The Supervisory Process in Speech-Language Pathology and Audiology.* Austin, TX: Pro-Ed, 1988.

Anderson, J., and Freiberg, J. "Using self-assessment as a reflective tool to enhance the student teaching experience." *Teacher Education Quar-terly, 22* (1) (1995): 77–91.

Anderson, N. "Providing feedback to preservice teachers of reading in field settings." *Reading Research and Instruction, 37* (2) (1998): 123–136.

American Speech and Hearing Association. Com-mittee on Supervision in Speech-Language

Pathology and Audiology. "Clinical supervision in speech-language pathology and audiology: A position statement." *American Speech Hearing Association, 27* (1985): 57–60.

Balloun, L. "Grading student clinicians effectively: A case study." In B. Wagner (Ed.), *Proceedings: Partnerships in Supervision: Innovative and Effective Practices.* Grand Forks, ND: University of North Dakota, 1996: 178–182.

Bandura, A., and Cervone, D. "Self-evaluative and self-efficacy mechanisms governing the motivational effects of goal systems." *Journal of Personality and Social Psychology, 45* (1983): 1017–1028.

Baxley, B., and Bowers, L. "Clinical report writing: The perceptions of supervisors and supervisees." *National Student Speech Language Hearing Association Journal, 19* (1991–1992): 35–40.

Bernstein, B., and Lecomte, C. "Supervisory-type feedback effects: Feedback discrepancy level, trainee psychological differentiation, and immediate responses." *Journal of Counseling Psychology, 26* (4) (1979): 295–303.

Billings, B., and Schmitz, H. *Report Writing in Audiology: A Handbook for Students and Clinicians.* Danville, IL: Interstate Publishers, 1980.

Boone, D., and Prescott, T. "Content and sequence analysis of speech and hearing therapy." *American Speech Hearing Association, 14* (1972): 58–62.

Borgen, W., and Amundson, N. "Strength challenge as a process for supervision." *Counselor Education and Supervision, 36* (1996): 159–169.

Brewer, N., Socha, L., and Potter, R. "Gender differences in supervisors' use of performance feedback." *Journal of Applied Social Psychology, 26* (9) (1996): 786–803.

Brown, E., and Block, F. "Evaluating supervision." Paper presented at the Annual Convention of the American Speech-Language and Hearing Association. Washington, D.C., 1975.

Cimorell-Strong, J., and Ensley, K. "Effects of student clinician feedback on the supervisory conference." *American Speech Hearing Association, 24* (1982): 23–29.

Cogan, M. *Clinical Supervision.* Boston, MA: Houghton Mifflin, 1973.

Cogan, M. "Clinical supervision and exploration." Paper presented in the conference Supervision of Students in Communication Disorders. University of Wisconsin, Madison, WI, 1978.

Costa, A., and Garmston, R. "The art of cognitive coaching: Supervision for intelligent teaching." Workshop presented at the conference, "Supervision: Innovations" of the Council of Supervisors in Speech Pathology and Audiology. Sonoma Co., CA, 1989.

Costa, A., and Garmston, R. *Cognitive coaching: A foundation for renaissance schools.* Norwood, MA: Christopher Gordon Publishers, 1994.

Cousins, J. "Using collaborative performance appraisal to enhance teachers' professional growth: A review of what we know." *Journal of Personnel Evaluation in Education, 9* (1995): 199–222.

Crago, M. "Student supervisor interactional self-exploratory training: A description and model." Short course presented at the Annual Convention of the American Speech-Language and Hearing Association. Cincinnati, OH, 1983.

Crago, M. "Supervision and self-exploration." In M. Crago and M. Pickering, (Eds.), *Supervision in Human Communication Disorders: Perspectives on a Process.* San Diego, CA: Singular Publishing Group, 1987: 137–167.

Densmore, A., Runyan, S., and Hagler, P. "What are supervisors doing with computers?" Paper presented at the Annual Meeting of the Council of Supervisors in Speech-Language Pathology and Audiology (CSSPA). Seattle, WA, 1990.

Donnelly, C., and Glaser, A. Training in self-supervision skills. *The Clinical Supervisor, 10* (2) (1992): 85–96.

Dowling, S. *Implementing the Supervisory Process: Theory and Practice.* Englewood Cliffs, NJ: Prentice-Hall, 1992.

Dowling, S. Facilitating Clinical Training: Issues for Supervisees and their Supervisors. *Contemporary Issues in Communication Science and Disorders 25* (1998): 5–11.

Dowling, S. "Students' perceptions of supervision at the end of clinical training." Unpublished, 1999.

Dowling, S., and Bliss, L. "Cognitive complexity, rhetorical sensitivity: Contributing factors in clinical skill?" *Journal of Communication Disorders, 7* (1984): 9–17.

Dowling, S., and Wittkopp, J. "Students' perceived supervisory needs." *Journal of Communication Disorders, 15* (1982): 319–328.

Evans, M. "Organizational behavior: The central role of motivation." *Journal of Management, 12* (2) (1986): 203–222.

Farmer, J. "Clinical literacy." In S. Farmer and J. Farmer (Eds.), *Supervision in Communication*

Disorders. Columbus, OH: Merrill Publishing Company, 1989a: 229–249.

Farmer, S. "Assessment in supervision." In S. Farmer and J. Farmer, (Eds.), *Supervision in Communication Disorders.* Columbus, OH: Merrill, 1989b.

Flahive, L. "Coming into the '90s: Revising an evaluation of practicum performance form. In Wagner, B., (Ed.), *Proceedings: Partnerships in Supervision: Innovative and Effective Practices.* Grand Forks, ND: University of North Dakota, 1996: 190–195.

Flynn, P. "Effective clinical interviewing." *Language Speech Hearing Services in the Schools, 9* (1978): 265–271.

Freeman, E. "The importance of feedback in clinical supervision: Implications for direct practice." *The Clinical Supervisor, 3* (1) (1985): 5–26.

Glaser, A., Prudhomme, M., and Rogero, E. Competency based objectives for student teaching in speech-language pathology and audiology. Miama, OH: Miami University of Ohio, 2000.

Hagler, P., and Fahey, R. "Effects of providing supervisors with normative statistics before student evaluation." Paper presented at the Annual Convention of the American Speech-Language and Hearing Association Convention, Toronto, Canada, 1982.

Hagler, P. *Effects of verbal directives, data, and contingent social praise on amount of supervisory talk during speech-language pathology supervision conferencing.* Doctoral dissertation: Bloomington, IN, 1986.

Jans, L., Hagler, P., McFarlane, L., McCrea, E., and Casey, P. "Effects of supervisors' written session comments on their verbal feedback during supervisory conference." In M. Bruce, (Ed.), *Proceedings of the 1994 International and Interdisciplinary Conference on Clinical Supervision.* Burlington, VT: University of Vermont, 1994: 107–110.

Juhnke, G. "Solution-focused supervision: Promoting supervisee skills and confidence through successful solutions." *Counselor Education and Supervision, 36* (1996): 48–57.

Kamhi, A. "Research to Practice: Defining, developing and maintaining clinical expertise." *Language, Speech and Hearing Services in Schools, 26* (4) (1995): 353–356.

Kennedy, K. *The effect of two methods of supervisor preconference written feedback on the verbal behavior of participants in individual speech pathology supervisory conferences.* (Doctoral dissertation, University of Oregon, 1981). *Dissertation Abstracts International, 42,* 2071A. (University Microfilms No. 81-23, 492).

Knepflar, L., and May, A. *Report Writing in the Field of Communication Disorders: A Handbook for Students and Clinicians.* Danville, IL: Interstate Publishers, 1989.

Kruger, J., and Dunning, D. "Unskilled and unaware of it: How difficulties in recognizing one's own incompetence lead to inflated self-assessments." *Journal of Personality and Psychology, 77* (6) (1999): 1121–1134.

Latting, J. "Giving corrective feedback: A decisional analysis." *Social Work, 37* (5) (1992): 424–430.

Logemann, J. "What is evidence-based practice and why should we care?" *ASHA Leader, 5* (5) (2000):3.

Lougeay-Mottinger, J., Harris, M., Perlstein-Kaplan, K., and Felicetti, T. "UTD Competency based evaluation system." *American Speech Hearing Association, 26* (1984): 39–43.

Manatt, R. "Feedback from 360 degrees: Client-driven evaluation of school personnel." *The School Administrator, 54* (3) (1997): 8–13.

McBride, M., and Skau, K. "Trust, empowerment, and reflection: Essentials of supervision." *Journal of Curriculum and Supervision, 10* (3) (1995): 262–277.

McCready, V., Roberts, J., Bengala, D., Harris, H., Kingsley, G., and Krikorian, C. "A comparison of conflict tactics in the supervisory process." *Journal of Speech and Hearing Research, 39* (1996): 191–199.

McLeod, S. "Student self-appraisal: Facilitating mutual planning in clinical education." *The Clinical Supervisor, 15* (1) (1997): 87–101.

Meyer, S. *Survival Guide for the Beginning Speech-Language Clinician.* Gaithersburg, MD: Aspen Publishers, 1998.

Perkins, J., and Mercaitis, P. "A guide for supervisors and students in clinical practicum." *The Clinical Supervisor, 13* (2) (1995): 67–78.

Pfeiffer, J., and Jones, J. "Openness, collusion and feedback." *The 1972 annual handbook of group facilitators.* University Associates, 1972: 197–201.

Pickering, M. "The supervisory process: An experience of interpersonal relationships and personal growth." *National Student Speech Language Hearing Association Journal, 17* (1989–1990): 17–28.

Podsakoff, P., Todor, W., Grover, R., and Huber, V. "Situational moderators of leader reward and punishment behaviors: Fact or fiction?" *Orga-*

nizational Behavior and Human Performance, 34 (1984): 21–63.

Rassi, J. "Verbal and written reports." In American Speech-Language-Hearing Association (Ed.), *Clinical Supervision across Settings: Communication and Collaboration.* Rockville, MD: ASHA, 1990.

Reid, D., and Parsons, M. "A comparison of staff acceptability of immediate versus delayed verbal feedback in staff training." *Journal of Organizational Behavior Management, 16* (2) (1996): 35–47.

Roberts, J., and Smith, K. "Supervisor–supervisee role differences and consistency of behavior in supervisory conferences." *Journal of Speech and Hearing Research, 25* (1982): 428–434.

Rodgers, T. "No excuses management." *Harvard Business Review, 68* (4) (1990): 84–98.

Romero, D. Goal-setting self-assessment tool. 2000.

Runyan, S., and Seal, B. "Competency-based Assessments of Supervisee Performance." In B. Wagner, (Ed.), *Proceedings: Partnerships in Supervision: Innovative and Effective Practices.* Grand Forks, ND: University of North Dakota, 1996: 57–61.

Sama, L., Kopelman, R., and Manning, R. "In search of a ceiling 'effect' on work motivation: Can Kaizen keep performance 'risin'?" *Journal of Social Behavior and Personality, 9* (2) (1994): 231–237.

Sbaschnig, K. "Accountability in supervision: The reliability audit." In S. Farmer, (Ed.), *Proceedings: Clinical Supervision: A Coming of Age.* A national conference on supervision, Jekyll Island, GA: Las Cruces, NM, New Mexico State University, 1987: 199–203.

Schalk, M., and Peroff, L. "Consistency and reliability of supervisory evaluations at university training centers." Paper presented at the Annual Convention of the American Speech-Language and Hearing Association. San Francisco, CA, 1972.

Schill, M., and Swanson, D. "Use of an audiotaped dialogue journal in the supervisory process: A case study." *The Supervisors' Forum, 1* (1993): 33–35.

Shriberg, L., Filley, F., Hayes, D., Kwiatkowski, J., Schatz, J., Simmons, K., and Smith, M. *The Wisconsin Procedure for Appraisal of Clinical Competence (W-PACC).* Madison, WI: Department of Communicative Disorders, University of Wisconsin-Madison, 1974.

Smith, K. "Supervisory conference questions: Who asks them and who answers them." Paper presented at the Annual Convention of the American Speech and Hearing Association, Atlanta GA, 1979.

Smith, K. Personal communication, 1990.

Stone, D., and Stone, E. "The effects of feedback consistency and feedback favorability on self-perceived task competence and perceived feedback accuracy." *Organizational Behavior and Human Decision Processes, 36* (1985): 167–185.

Taylor, C., and Horney, M. "A phenomenographic investigation of students' approaches to self-evaluation of their clinical practice." *The Clinical Supervisor, 16* (2) (1997): 105–123.

Taylor, M., Fisher, C., and Ilgen, D. "Individuals' reactions to performance feedback in organizations: A control theory perspective." In K. Rowland, and G. Ferris, (Eds.), *Research in Personnel and Human Resources Management* (Vol. 2). Greenwich, CT: JAI Press, 1984: 81–124. Wayne State University. Communication Disorders and Sciences' Clinical evaluation form. Unpublished. 1974.

Terrio, L., and Magee-Bender, L. "Supervising in a loop." *American Speech Language Hearing Association, 26* (1984).

Wilkins-Canter, E. "The nature and effectiveness of feedback given by cooperating teachers to student teachers." *Teacher Educator, 32* (4) (1997): 235–250.

Wilson, B. "Learning theory applied to the therapy process." In D. Kirtley, (Ed.), *Proceedings: Institute on Supervision of Student Teaching in Speech and Hearing Therapy.* Series #2. Indiana Department of Public Instruction, Division of Special Education, West Lafayette, IN, 1967.

Wilson, J., Welch, N., and Welling, R. "Interactive supervision system: A tool for clinical teaching." In Wagner, B., (Ed.), *Proceedings: Partnerships in Supervision: Innovative and Effective Practices.* Grand Forks, ND: University of North Dakota, 1996: 196–198.

A P P E N D I X   3 - A

Goal-Setting Criteria for the Student Clinician

Interval rating scale for select tasks of the clinical supervisee

Read the following descriptors carefully, then rate the statements below.

7 strongest   I have acquired a professional level of knowledge and expertise on this task through study and experience and have had multiple opportunities to apply this knowledge skillfully and independently.

6 strong   I have acquired a high level of knowledge and expertise on this task through study and experience and have had many opportunities to apply this knowledge with some supervision.

5 emerging   I have acquired a level of knowledge on this task through study and some experience; I have had some opportunities to apply this knowledge under direct supervision.

4 untested   While I have some knowledge of this task acquired through study, I have not had the opportunity to apply this knowledge clinically.

3 weak   I have adequate knowledge of the task acquired through study but relevant opportunities to apply it clinically have not been provided for me.

2 weaker   I have insufficient knowledge of the task required and would perform inadequately if called upon to perform this task.

1 weakest   I have no knowledge of this task.

II. Assessment Tasks

1. I can gather case history information as part of the assessment process.

7	6	5	4	3	2	1
STRONGEST	STRONG	EMERGING	UNTESTED	WEAK	WEAKER	WEAKEST

2. I can interpret case history information accurately in making a diagnosis.

7	6	5	4	3	2	1
STRONGEST	STRONG	EMERGING	UNTESTED	WEAK	WEAKER	WEAKEST

3. I accurately interpret medical information in the case history to help make a diagnosis.

7	6	5	4	3	2	1
STRONGEST	STRONG	EMERGING	UNTESTED	WEAK	WEAKER	WEAKEST

4. I interpret personal information in the case history to help make a diagnosis.

7	6	5	4	3	2	1
STRONGEST	STRONG	EMERGING	UNTESTED	WEAK	WEAKER	WEAKEST

5. I interpret educational information in the case history to help make a diagnosis.

7	6	5	4	3	2	1
STRONGEST	STRONG	EMERGING	UNTESTED	WEAK	WEAKER	WEAKEST

Romero, D. Goal-setting self-assessment tool. Reprinted with the permission of the author. 2000.

6. I administer standardized tests reliably.

7	6	5	4	3	2	1
STRONGEST	STRONG	EMERGING	UNTESTED	WEAK	WEAKER	WEAKEST

7. I choose specific tests to answer the referral question.

7	6	5	4	3	2	1
STRONGEST	STRONG	EMERGING	UNTESTED	WEAK	WEAKER	WEAKEST

8. I apply normative data to help answer the referral question.

7	6	5	4	3	2	1
STRONGEST	STRONG	EMERGING	UNTESTED	WEAK	WEAKER	WEAKEST

9. I interpret standardized scores to answer referral questions.

7	6	5	4	3	2	1
STRONGEST	STRONG	EMERGING	UNTESTED	WEAK	WEAKER	WEAKEST

10. I take speech/language samples as part of assessment.

7	6	5	4	3	2	1
STRONGEST	STRONG	EMERGING	UNTESTED	WEAK	WEAKER	WEAKEST

11. I use instrumentation as part of assessment.

7	6	5	4	3	2	1
STRONGEST	STRONG	EMERGING	UNTESTED	WEAK	WEAKER	WEAKEST

12. I integrate all assessment information to make a diagnosis.

7	6	5	4	3	2	1
STRONGEST	STRONG	EMERGING	UNTESTED	WEAK	WEAKER	WEAKEST

Based on your self-ratings related to assessment tasks, write a goal or goals which you would like to accomplish this semester with help from your clinical supervisor and/or other members of the faculty and staff. Then write some steps you feel are necessary to accomplish the goal. An example is listed below:

Example: "My goal is to move from **4** to **5** in administering standardized tests reliably. I feel I need to observe reliable administration of standardized tests, video tape the administration of two or three commonly used instruments by a mentor or supervisor, then administer these instruments under the guidance of my supervisor."

Or

"My goal is to move from a **5** to a **6** in administering standardized tests reliably. To accomplish this goal I feel that I need multiple opportunities to administer a core battery of standardized tests. I would like to be video-taped three times during the semester with follow-up conferences and feedback from my supervisor."

My goal(s) for assessment tasks this semester are:

1. _____

    _____

    _____

_____

_____

_____

_____

_____

2. _____

_____

_____

_____

_____

_____

_____

_____

3. _____

_____

_____

_____

_____

_____

_____

APPENDIX 3 - B

A Guide for Clinical Practicum and Instructions for Implementation

Instructions for the Use of the Clinical Practicum Guide

Supervisor Copy

1. The purpose of the guide.
   a. Help the clinician plan in advance for the upcoming week.
   b. Provide specific feedback to the clinician each week to allow her to know how she is doing in specific areas.
   c. Structure feedback from observations.
   d. Structure supervisory conferences.
   e. Allow for easier grading at the midterm and final point in the semester.

2. The clinician plans each week in advance according to the guide.
   a. The clinician is provided with a copy of the guide.
   b. You will have a master copy.
   c. Each week the clinician will prepare for supervisory conferences and interpret observation feedback according to the week designated on the guide.

3. Provide specific feedback to the clinician each week on level of performance.
   a. The clinician will hand in a copy of her guide each week with her lesson plan and log.
   b. On your master copy, you will have rated the student (1–7) in all possible areas on that week of the guide.
   c. You will transfer those numbers to the student's copy and return it with the lesson plan and log each week.

4. Structure feedback from observations according to the guide.
   a. Each week's focus will be designated by the guide.
   b. While observing therapy, write comments in outline form on your observation sheet following the outline of that week on the guide.
   c. Some areas may not be observable; write n/a.
   d. Feel free to write about additional areas as well, as long as you have remarked on the areas designated on the guide.
   e. Some weeks will focus on therapy observations more than others.

5. Structuring conferences.
   a. Prior to each conference the student will prepare questions and comments about areas that are designated on the guide that were also observed.
   b. The student will come to the conference and it will be structured according to the guide.

Perkins, J., and Mercaitis, P. A Guide for Clinical Practicum and Instructions for Implementation. Related to the article "A guide for supervisors and students in clinical practicum." *The Clinical Supervisor, 13* (2) (1995): 67–78. Reprinted with permission of the authors.

   c. Feel free to discuss additional areas as well as long as you have discussed the areas
      that were targeted on the guide.

6. Ease of grading at midterm and final point in the semester.
   a. At the end of each week you will assign a rating to each area on your master copy
      (rating 1–7).
   b. Transfer this information to the student copy and return it to the student.
   c. At the midterm and final point in the semester, transfer the ratings to the clinic
      grade sheet.

Student Copy

1. Purpose of the guide.
   a. Help the clinician to plan in advance for the upcoming week.
   b. Structure feedback from supervisor observations of therapy sessions.
   c. Structure supervisory conferences.
   d. Provide specific feedback to the clinician each week on level
      of performance
   e. Allow for student to know how they are performing up to the midterm
      and final point in the semester.

2. The clinician plans each week in advance according to the guide.
   a. The clinician is provided with a copy of the guide.
   b. Each week the clinician will prepare for sessions, supervisory conferences,
      and interpret observation feedback according to the week designated
      on the guide.

3. Structure feedback from the supervisor observations of therapy sessions
   by following the guide.
   a. Each week's focus will be designated by the guide.
   b. While observing therapy the supervisor will write comments in outline
      form on your observation sheet following the outline of that week
      on the guide.
   c. Some areas may not be observable; the supervisor will write n/a.
   d. Other areas may be commented upon in addition to the designated issues outlined
      in the guide.
   e. Some weeks of the guide will focus on therapy observations more than others.

4. Structuring conferences.
   a. Prior to each conference the student will prepare questions and comments about
      areas that are designated on the guide for that week.
   b. The student will use the guide to prepare for the conference, which will be
      structured according to the guide.
   c. Additional areas may be discussed as long as you have targeted the areas on the
      guide.

5. Provide specific feedback to the clinician each week on level of performance.
   a. The clinician will hand in a copy of her guide each week with her lesson plan and
      log.

b. The supervisor will have rated her (1–7) in all possible areas on that week of the guide.

c. The supervisor will transfer those numbers to the clinician's copy and return the student copy along with the lesson plan and log each week.

6. Allow students to know in advance how they are performing at the mid and final point in the semester.
   a. At the end of each week the supervisor will assign a rating to each designated area on the guide (rating 1–7).
   b. At the midterm and final point in the semester, the supervisor will transfer this information to the clinic grade sheet.
   c. The student will be assigned mid and final ratings according to the weekly ratings that were provided throughout the semester.

A Guide for Clinical Practicum

Judy M. Perkins and Patricia A. Mercaltis

Week I: Professional Skills/Obtaining a History

1. Review ASHA Code of Ethics and state/federal regulations.
2. Abstract relevant information from the chart (e.g., medical, personal).
3. Develop a problem statement based on information obtained from the chart and your theoretical knowledge.
4. Develop relevant interview questions to clarify vague background information.
5. Select tests that address all suspected problem areas (if formal testing was recently conducted you may elect to obtain informal baseline measures).
6. Have the above mentioned prepared for our first supervisory meeting.

Week II: Execution of Diagnostic/Baseline Collection

1. Read manual and practice administration of all tests (or if applicable baseline measurements) prior to the session.
2. Prepare a checklist of the logical sequence you will follow to administer the tests and budget your time accordingly.
3. Establish rapport with the client.
   a. introduce yourself.
   b. explain procedure to the client.
   c. dress and act professionally.
   d. respond to client feedback.
4. Obtain information from the client during the interview
   a. ask only relevant questions.
   b. use open ended questions that are not leading the client.
   c. use appropriate follow up questions for clarification.
5. Administer all tests/baselines according to appropriate procedures.

Week III: Development of Goals

1. Score all tests/baselines.
2. Interpret and integrate all raw data to formulate a specific diagnostic/level of functioning.

3. Determine if the client will benefit from treatment.
4. Identify specific levels at which the client has difficulty and is successful.
5. Determine a realistic long term goal based on: current level of functioning, premorbid level of functioning, your theoretical knowledge of the deficit, and the client's expectations.
6. Develop short term goals and objectives following a logical sequence of difficulty from current level of functioning to projected long term goal.
7. Within short term goals and objectives, determine criteria to be met to enable the client to progress to the next level of difficulty.

Week IV: Lesson Plan & Report Writing

1. Writing lesson plans
    a. correctly write objectives to meet short term goals.
    b. write specific tasks to accomplish these objectives.
    c. write specific reinforcement techniques.
    d. specify criteria to be met.
    e. report responses and consequences in the log.
2. Write the projected treatment plan
    a. follow the report format in the clinic manual.
    b. summarize the relevant background information.
    c. report raw data, interpret and explain results.
    d. sequence goals and objectives in an organized manner.
    e. use correct spelling, grammar and terminology.
    f. include criteria, method of data collection, schedule of reinforcement, and home programs.
3. Explain to the client the testing/baseline results, long and short term goals, and objectives to achieve them.

Week V: Organization of Sessions & Data Collection

1. Pre-plan all sessions to maximize use of time during the session
    a. pace sessions to allow sufficient time for responses.
2. Tasks should be structured using a stimulus, response, reinforcement paradigm and be clear to the client to maximize participation.
3. Determine what specific response you will measure.
4. Determine how you will measure it.
5. Determine when you will take measurements.
6. Establish a method for recording the information.
7. Refer to the previous criteria to determine when to move the client to the next level.
8. Mid semester supervisory conference to discuss performance to date.

APPENDIX 3-C

Competency Based Objectives for Student Teaching in Speech-Language Pathology and Audiology

[ ] Midterm   [ ] Final

Student's Name: _____

Cooperating Therapist: _____

School District: _____

Semester: _____

Competencies student teachers will demonstrate by the end of student teaching:

Rating Key:

  C = Competent: Is proficient for level of training

  E = Emerging: Making appropriate progress

 NI = Needs improvement

 NE = Not showing effort

NA = Not applicable

Professionalism.   Demonstrates a professional attitude and work ethic by:

C	E	NI	NE	NA	
C	E	NI	NE	NA	1. Effectively balancing work and personal responsibilities
C	E	NI	NE	NA	2. Attending professional meetings
C	E	NI	NE	NA	3. Exhibiting interest and enthusiasm about his/her work
C	E	NI	NE	NA	4. Interacting appropriately with cooperating therapist
C	E	NI	NE	NA	5. Arriving at school on time
C	E	NI	NE	NA	6. Regular attendance
C	E	NI	NE	NA	7. Showing initiative
C	E	NI	NE	NA	8. Being dependable
C	E	NI	NE	NA	9. Dressing appropriately
C	E	NI	NE	NA	10. Utilizing appropriate vocal quality, rate and intonation

Laws and Standards

C   E   NI   NE   NA   1. Explain IDEA (Individual with Disabilities Education Act)

C   E   NI   NE   NA   2. Participate in Intervention Assistance Team (IAT)

C   E   NI   NE   NA   3. Participate in MFE/IEP Team/Annual Review

C   E   NI   NE   NA   4. Prepare Individualized Education Plans (IEP)

C   E   NI   NE   NA   • Utilize diagnostic information to determine present levels of performance

C   E   NI   NE   NA   • Utilize diagnostic information to determine annual goals

C   E   NI   NE   NA   • Utilize diagnostic information to write measurable objectives

Daily Planning Procedures

C   E   NI   NE   NA   1. Write lesson plans in advance

2. Write plans to meet IEP objectives for:

C   E   NI   NE   NA   • individual/small group

C   E   NI   NE   NA   • classroom

C   E   NI   NE   NA   3. Plan therapy that addresses multiple goals in a session

C   E   NI   NE   NA   4. Collaborate effectively with other school personnel

C   E   NI   NE   NA   5. Use information and evaluations from previous therapy sessions

C   E   NI   NE   NA   6. Utilize a variety of materials appropriate to client's interests, abilities, age level, and curriculum

C   E   NI   NE   NA   7. Manipulate equipment and materials before therapy sessions

Diagnosis

C   E   NI   NE   NA   1. Informally assess the need for further testing

C   E   NI   NE   NA   2. Select appropriate diagnostic instruments and procedures

3. Effectively complete:

C   E   NI   NE   NA   a. an oral–facial examination

C   E   NI   NE   NA   b. diagnostic tests for articulation/phonology

C   E   NI   NE   NA   c. diagnostic tests for language

C   E   NI   NE   NA   d. a spontaneous language sample analysis

C   E   NI   NE   NA   e. a diagnostic assessment for voice

C   E   NI   NE   NA   f. a diagnostic assessment for fluency

C   E   NI   NE   NA   g. hearing screening/thresholds

C   E   NI   NE   NA   h. classroom observation/teacher consultation

C   E   NI   NE   NA   i. a parent checklist or interview

C   E   NI   NE   NA   j. other _____

4. Interpret and communicate diagnostic results:

C E NI NE NA   • verbal

C E NI NE NA   • written

Scheduling

C E NI NE NA   1. Select caseload based upon eligibility criteria established by school district

C E NI NE NA   2. Schedule therapy program in relation to total school schedule

C E NI NE NA   3. Communicate with parents and school personnel about therapy schedule

Therapy

C E NI NE NA   1. Establish and maintain good rapport with client

C E NI NE NA   2. Provide the rationale for selection of specific therapy techniques

3. Employ therapy procedures appropriate to child's:

C E NI NE NA   • age level

C E NI NE NA   • ability level

C E NI NE NA   • curriculum

4. Give directions clearly to

C E NI NE NA   • individual/small group

C E NI NE NA   • classroom

5. Handle child's behavior effectively in

C E NI NE NA   • individual/small group

C E NI NE NA   • classroom

C E NI NE NA   6. Begin and end therapy on time

C E NI NE NA   7. Provide for carry-over to classroom and home

C E NI NE NA   8. Communicate goals, therapy techniques and progress to parents

C E NI NE NA   9. Communicate goals, therapy techniques and progress to teacher

Articulation Therapy

C E NI NE NA   1. Conduct articulation/phonology therapy techniques appropriate to child's needs.

C E NI NE NA   2. Conduct therapy consistent with goals

C E NI NE NA   3. Discriminate correct/incorrect sound production with 85% agreement with cooperating therapist

C E NI NE NA   4. Provide appropriate type and level of cue

C E NI NE NA   5. Implement oral motor exercises

C   E   NI   NE   NA   6. Obtain maximum number of responses per therapy session

C   E   NI   NE   NA   7. Provide appropriate reinforcement

C   E   NI   NE   NA   8. Be flexible in therapy situations

C   E   NI   NE   NA   9. Evaluate the pupil's performance with respect to moving on to the next therapy step

C   E   NI   NE   NA   10. Record progress on a consistent basis for a specific goal

Language Therapy

C   E   NI   NE   NA   1. Conduct language therapy techniques appropriate to child's needs

C   E   NI   NE   NA   2. Recognize correct/incorrect language productions with 85% agreement with the cooperating therapist

C   E   NI   NE   NA   3. Provide appropriate level of models and prompts

C   E   NI   NE   NA   4. Obtain appropriate number of responses per therapy session

C   E   NI   NE   NA   5. Utilize a variety of appropriate activities

C   E   NI   NE   NA   6. Record progress on a consistent basis for a specific goal

Fluency Therapy

C   E   NI   NE   NA   1. Provide information and consultation to teachers and parents

C   E   NI   NE   NA   2. Conduct fluency therapy appropriate to child's needs

C   E   NI   NE   NA   3. Be flexible in therapy situations

C   E   NI   NE   NA   4. Record progress on a consistent basis for a specific goal

Voice Therapy

C   E   NI   NE   NA   1. Conduct appropriate therapy techniques

C   E   NI   NE   NA   2. Conduct therapy consistent with goals

C   E   NI   NE   NA   3. Counsel pupils/parents/teacher about vocal hygiene

C   E   NI   NE   NA   4. Discriminate appropriate voice production

C   E   NI   NE   NA   5. Be flexible in therapy situations

C   E   NI   NE   NA   6. Provide appropriate reinforcement

C   E   NI   NE   NA   7. Provide student with self-evaluation and self-management techniques for appropriate vocal behavior

C   E   NI   NE   NA   8. Explain the steps of making a medical referral

C   E   NI   NE   NA   9. Record progress on consistent basis on a specific goal

Self-Evaluation

C   E   NI   NE   NA   1. Evaluate therapy through audio/videotapes or reflective journals

C   E   NI   NE   NA   2. Follow through on suggestions from the cooperating therapist

C   E   NI   NE   NA   3. Set personal objectives for change as a result of self-evaluation

Augmentative/Alternative Communication Systems

C   E   NI   NE   NA   1. Identify a variety of systems (sign, communication board, electronic device, hearing aids, etc.)

C   E   NI   NE   NA   2. Collaborate with students, peers, teachers/family in order to select vocabulary

C   E   NI   NE   NA   3. Prepare and/or program systems appropriate to child's level of functioning

C   E   NI   NE   NA   4. Train student, teacher, family in use of communication systems

Feeding/Oral Motor Therapy

C   E   NI   NE   NA   1. Collaborate with support personnel on diagnostic results and intervention strategies

C   E   NI   NE   NA   2. Implement strategies (positioning, textures, cues and safety precautions)

C   E   NI   NE   NA   3. Implement oral motor exercises

C   E   NI   NE   NA   4. Record progress and adopt plans as needed

Observation

C   E   NI   NE   NA   1. Gain knowledge about a range of disabilities by working with or observing students with a variety of speech/language disorders.

C   E   NI   NE   NA   2. Gain knowledge about a range of related professions by working with or observing professionals in related fields

Comments

A P P E N D I X   3 - D

James Madison University Department of Communication Sciences and Disorders Clinical Competency Record and Student Evaluation Form

Student's Name _____   Date_____

Placement_____   Date Degree Expected _____

Semester Hours Toward Degree _____   Clock Hours Accumulated to Date _____

Number of Diagnostics _____ of 80   Number of Therapy Hours _____ of 80

Number of Audiology Hours _____ of 15   Number of A. R. hours _____ of 15

Rating Legend:

Graded Practicum Scale: 1 to 5	**(Field Placements and Externships) Credit/No Credit Key:**
1 = Unacceptable	+ = Skill present
2 = Acceptable	− = Skill not present
3 = Approaching competency	+ = Skill emerging
4 = Competent	
5 = Outstanding	

Area I. Diagnostic Evaluation:

Total number of complete evaluations supervised at JMU SHC: _____

Types of Evaluations	*Number in each category*	*Supervisor*	*Scale*
_____	_____	_____	_____
_____	_____	_____	_____
_____	_____	_____	_____

Preparation:

_____ 1. Extracts and accurately summarizes pertinent information from client's medical and referral information

_____ 2. Suggests appropriate evaluation procedures and interview questions based on client information and knowledge of communication problem

James Madison University Department of Communication Sciences and Disorders Clinical Competency Record and Student Evaluation Form from Runyan, S., and Seal, B. "Competency-based Assessments of Supervisee Performance." In Wagner, B., (Ed.), *Proceedings: Partnerships in Supervision: Innovative and Effective Practices.* Grand Forks, ND: University of North Dakota, 1996: 57–61. Reprinted with permission of the authors.

_____ 3. Explains rationale for tests and procedures taking into account the following factors:
- evaluation procedures specific to problems
- validity and reliability of standardized tests
- developmental age appropriateness
- interest level of materials
- formal versus informal procedures
- test is suitable in view of other handicapping conditions
- knows when alternate form of test should be given

_____ 4. Adequately prepares physical setting including:
- environment free from distracting objects
- materials and tests are available and organized
- audio-taping set up
- video-taping set up
- specialized equipment

_____ 5. Other_____

Diagnostic:

_____ 6. Establishes professional atmosphere with client and family
- clinician introduces self and supervisor
- clinician provides a brief overview of evaluation format

_____ 7. Begins and ends interview smoothly

_____ 8. Extracts pertinent and accurate information from the interview

_____ 9. Formulates follow-up questions appropriately

_____ 10. Sequences and switches topics smoothly

_____ 11. Uses an interview style which encourages free expression (e.g., open ended questions)

_____ 12. Redirects informant skillfully

_____ 13. Recognizes inconsistent responses from informant

_____ 14. Reacts appropriately to informant's expressions of emotion

_____ 15. Administers and scores tests accurately

_____ 16. Understands the limitations, utility, and interpretations of test instrument

_____ 17. Obtains information via formal and informal observation

_____ 18. Makes effective use of time

_____ 19. Shows flexibility (i.e., recognizes need to depart from pre-arranged plan when necessary)

_____ 20. Demonstrates skills necessary to maintain client's on-task behavior

_____ 21. Shows resourcefulness in obtaining information specific to the problem

_____ 22. Obtains information about client's response to instruction (i.e., stimulability)

_____ 23. Gives appropriate feedback during testing procedure

_____ 24. Organizes and uses materials efficiently

_____ 25. Demonstrates familiarity with motor and speech-language developmental norms

_____ 26. Other_____

Wrap-Up:

_____ 27. Accurately interprets results obtained from formal and informal probes

_____ 28. Shows independence in formulating a statement about nature and extent of problem

_____ 29. Makes an insightful prognostic statement using pertinent history, client's response to teaching, and test results

_____ 30. Makes appropriate recommendations for management

_____ 31. Other_____

Parent, Client, and Family Counseling:

_____ 32. Recognizes potential need for additional interview data

_____ 33. Reviews and interprets the evaluation in a clear and concise way

_____ 34. Gives parent or client opportunity to ask questions and express concern

_____ 35. Responds to parent's or client's questions and reacts appropriately

_____ 36. Consults supervisor if needed

_____ 37. Other_____

Report Writing and Documentation:

_____ 38. Includes all pertinent information

_____ 39. Shows ability to prioritize information obtained from evaluation

_____ 40. Meets deadlines for reports

_____ 41. Reports information accurately

_____ 42. Uses professional terminology

_____ 43. Uses objective rather than subjective statements

_____ 44. Uses appropriate mechanical writing skills (spelling, grammar, organization, etc.)

_____ 45. Observes time lines to submit drafts

_____ 46. Proofreads for spelling, grammar, and format

_____ 47. Other_____

Area II. Treatment Process:

Types of Disorders assigned	Number in each category	Supervisor	Scale
_____	_____	_____	_____
_____	_____	_____	_____
_____	_____	_____	_____

Programming:

_____ 1. Treatment was appropriate to the disorder

_____ 2. Treatment was aimed at the appropriate level for the client

_____ 3. Clinician sequentialized learning steps

_____ 4. Clinician demonstrated ability to branch within a session appropriately and quickly

_____ 5. Clinician achieved programming independently

_____ 6. Clinician cued client appropriately

_____ 7. Clinician used effective instruction and modeling (data confirms effectiveness)

_____ 8. Clinician adapted materials and techniques to fit the client's needs and abilities

Properties of Reinforcement:

_____ 9. Was consistently administered
_____ 10. Was of the appropriate type for client
_____ 11. Was administered on an appropriate schedule
_____ 12. Was administered clearly

Data Collection:

_____ 13. Was consistently taken
_____ 14. Was accurate and reliable
_____ 15. Was collected quickly and discreetly

Interactions in the Session and with the Client:

_____ 16. Clinician recognized need for behavior controls
_____ 17. Clinician set limits clearly
_____ 18. Clinician used techniques effectively to maximize client cooperation and motivation
_____ 19. Behavior controls employed were appropriate for client's level, age, etc. (control of session)
_____ 20. Clinician's pace of session allowed for maximum use of time
_____ 21. Clinician counseled client quickly and efficiently; returned to remedial activity quickly
_____ 22. Clinician conducted session in an organized manner

Organization of the Session:

_____ 23. Clinician prioritized remediation so that client's primary needs were taken into account; sequenced session appropriately

Report Writing and Documentation:

_____ 24. Includes all pertinent information
_____ 25. Shows ability to prioritize information obtained from evaluation
_____ 26. Meets deadlines for reports
_____ 27. Reports information accurately
_____ 28. Uses professional terminology
_____ 29. Uses objective rather than subjective statements
_____ 30. Uses appropriate mechanical writing skills (spelling, grammar, organization, etc.)
_____ 31. Observes time lines to submit drafts
_____ 32. Proofreads
_____ 33. Other_____

Area III. Personal and Interpersonal Behaviors:

_____ 1. Demonstrates warmth, appropriate eye contact, ease and sensitivity to the client's or family's feelings
_____ 2. Reduces anxiety in client and family
_____ 3. Interacts with client in a way appropriate to age and abilities
_____ 4. Sets and enforces limits

_____ 5. Motivates client to perform

_____ 6. Demonstrates independence

_____ 7. Demonstrates initiative

_____ 8. Demonstrates willingness to assume responsibility

_____ 9. Accepts criticism appropriately

_____ 10. Assesses own strengths and areas which need improvement

_____ 11. Suggests ways to improve performance through self-supervisory analysis

_____ 12. Demonstrates cooperation and teamwork

_____ 13. Keeps verbal commitments

_____ 14. Never has an unexcused absence

_____ 15. Adheres to legal mandates

_____ 16. Other_____

_____ 17. Offered empathetic understanding, warmth, and respect to client and family

_____ 18. Enabled problem solving and encouraged client and family responsibility in management

_____ 19. Responses reflected awareness of the client's needs expressed or implied by feelings or performance (clinician sensitivity)

_____ 20. Dealt tactfully with client's frustration in a session

_____ 21. Appeared confident about own performance and remedial activities employed

_____ 22. Consistently utilized positive clinical interactions

_____ 23. Dealt successfully with own frustration in the session

_____ 24. Dealt with client resistance as a part of the remedial management

_____ 25. Was punctual in starting and ending sessions

Demonstrates Developing Attitudes of Professional Behavior:

_____ 26. Observes clinic policies of confidentiality

_____ 27. Dresses for clinic activities with respect for observers, clients, and the professional setting

_____ 28. Nonverbal behaviors positively influence communication

_____ 29. Communicates directly with supervisor for any absences from client assignments, clinic meetings, or supervisor's conferences

_____ 30. Considers supervisory suggestions and openly discusses differences in ideas and evaluations of clinical situations

_____ 31. Respects the privacy of daily clinical operations and all personnel assigned to the Speech and Hearing Center

_____ 32. Demonstrates reflective practice and growing independence for self-supervision

_____ 33. Prepares for conferences and engages in problem-solving

Health Precautions:

_____ 34. Demonstrates care and concern for client's well being

_____ 35. Adheres to standards of health practices for clinic materials

_____ 36. Adheres to standards of sanitary conditions for room space and equipment

_____ 37. Understands and signs the health precautions information provided by the setting

_____ 38. Other (specialized emergency medical knowledge or skills)

Area IV. Other Areas of Clinical Training Available at This Field Placement:
Competencies demonstrated included:
(please attach list)

Area V.
Primary Supervisor: _____   Asha CCC Number: _____

Address: _____   Telephone Number: _____

Recommended use: Areas I & III or II & III or Both + added list of specialized competencies

4 Structuring Effective Supervisory Conferences

Clinical Supervision Tasks Relevant to Structuring Effective Supervisory Conferences

Task 1: Establishing and maintaining an effective working relationship with the supervisee;

Task 2: Assisting the supervisee in developing clinical goals and objectives;

Task 3: Assisting the supervisee in developing and refining assessment skills;

Task 4: Assisting the supervisee in developing and refining clinical management skills;

Task 6: Assisting the supervisee in observing and analyzing assessment and treatment sessions;

Task 7: Assisting the supervisee in the development and maintenance of clinical and supervisory records;

Task 8: Interacting with the supervisee in planning, executing, and analyzing supervisory conferences;

Task 9: Assisting the supervisee in evaluation of clinical performance;

Task 10: Assisting the supervisee in developing skills of verbal reporting, writing, and editing;

Task 11: Sharing information regarding ethical, legal, regulatory, and reimbursement aspects of professional practice;

Task 12: Modeling and facilitating professional conduct;

Task 13: Demonstrating research skills in the clinical or supervisory process.

The conference is at the heart of the supervisory process. It will be considered in this chapter from a variety of perspectives. As will be seen, many writers, in describing the conference, emphasize the feedback aspect. Because this topic is discussed at length in the previous chapter, it will only be touched on here. The context of conferencing will be the primary focus of this section, including factors ranging from supervisee expectations to behaviors that facilitate interactions. The content of meetings and the relationship of effective conferencing to the realization of the thirteen tasks of supervision will also be explored.

Literature

The supervisory conference, although widely discussed, varies in description. According to Anderson (1988):

> Traditionally, the conference is seen as a time when the supervisor provides feedback to the supervisee about the observation. This feedback has been perceived to be something of a one-way street—from supervisor to supervisee. The supervisor talks; the supervisee listens.

Anderson further elaborates:

> For the Collaborative or Consultative styles, the broader term of integrating seems more appropriate than feedback in describing the interaction that takes place when the supervisor and supervisee meet . . . It is here where the components of *Understanding, Planning, Observing* and *Analyzing* will merge . . . The conference will also include discussion of procedural topics such as administrative issues or report writing, the supervisory process, professional issues, personal concerns, and general information relevant to the development of all the participants.

More specifically, in the area of audiology, Rassi suggests that, when there is ample time, the following topics should be considered: the test findings and their implications; the decision making that took place throughout the evaluation (what steps were taken and why?); the patient and his or her reactions to the evaluation, and how they affected the clinical decision-making process; possible alternative actions (what could have been done differently?) (Rassi, 1978). Finally, it is Cogan's (1973) opinion that the supervisory conference cannot be separated for independent definition because "The clinical conference defines itself in its context. It is an integral part of the process in the cycle of supervision."

The thirteen tasks of supervision further provide a framework for considering the conference as many of those tasks are achieved in the context of supervisor–supervisee meetings. In addition, common threads connect the varying descriptions of conferences. For example, the supervisor and supervisee are meeting face-to-face. They are communicating about events that have occurred and are developing strategies to enhance the quality and productivity of future therapy/teaching. Data collection and analysis are stressed. Feedback is viewed as an integral part of this discussion and supervisee involvement in data-based analysis and problem-solving is emphasized. The key elements of the conference are thus defined, with one exception: The importance of discussing the supervisory process itself as an integral part of the process. The remainder of this chapter, then, will be devoted to thoughts and strategies that can be used to structure effective supervisory conferences.

Conference Reflections

A discussion between three clinicians who are talking in the hallway will provide food for thought. They are expressing frustration about their experiences with their supervisors.

> GLORIA: It's time for me to go find Frieberg (supervisor). She is never there when I'm supposed to meet with her. I wonder if she'll even show up today.
>
> TOM: Yeah. I get angry sometimes too. I feel like I have a lot of good ideas. As soon as I start to say something, Mr. Elton interrupts and then tells me what he thinks I should do. It makes me feel like an idiot.
>
> LINDA: Me too! I don't think the supervisors give us credit for what we know. It isn't like this is the first time we've done therapy. They mean well but . . .

Several issues relating to effective conferencing are raised here: respect for the supervisees' time, power messages, supervisor control of conference talk, and passive supervisee participation. The topics that follow will address these concerns and provide strategies to increase the quality of supervision.

Supervisee Expectations

The first factors to weigh in preparation for the conference are the viewpoints of those to be supervised. That is, what are the supervisees' expectations for the conference? An important consideration in regard to these anticipations is the level of the supervisee. The clinician in training is likely to have significantly different needs than the employed professional, although some basic concerns are likely to be similar. (The supervision of the employed professional is addressed in Chapter 7.) According to Pickering (1987a), clinicians expect supervisors to instruct, to share perceptions and past experiences with them, and to encourage their development and independence by providing a safe, secure, stimulating environment. Hatfield (Hatfield, Bartlett, Caven, and Ueberle, 1973) indicates that the supervisor must function as a teacher in assisting the supervisee to bridge the gap between theory, principle, and application. Student teachers report that supervisors are not perceived as helpful unless they provide valuative feedback (Brown and Block, 1975). Further, this evaluative information is thought to be most beneficial when the supervisee is first asked to self-evaluate. The student teachers also cite the use of support—viewing the supervisee as an individual with potential—as a critical behavior. Evans (1998) also sees support as a key supervisor behavior. Finally, a sample of graduate students' responses at the end of their clinical training identifies the following as desirable supervisor behaviors: being supportive, enhancing trainees' confidence, providing honest feedback, interacting in a collegial way, being helpful, responding interpersonally in a sensitive way, valuing supervisee's independence, and offering them praise (Dowling, 1999).

Dowling and Wittkopp (1982) describe a survey of supervisees, graduate and undergraduate students in speech-language pathology, at six universities. The resulting data identify five valued behaviors in regard to the student conference: (1) regularly scheduled individual conferences; (2) the availability of additional meetings, as needed; (3) active supervisee–supervisor problem-solving in the conference; (4) mutual decisions as to diagnostic and therapeutic techniques; (5) the supervisees' receipt of both positive and negative feedback about their clinical behavior. In particular, supervisees object to conferences in which there is no feedback. Larson (1981) has also polled supervisees in training, and reports that experienced clinicians, those with more than 150 earned clock hours, expect to assume an active role in the conference with opportunities to express their opinions and to suggest ideas. Further, such students envision a supervisor who is supportive but who also listens and values their contributions. Peaper and Mercaitis (1989) confirm this finding with trainees with clock hours in excess of one hundred. Inexperienced supervisees want to be vigorously involved in the exchange, but they differ in that they expect the supervisor to identify more weaknesses in their clinical behavior. Both groups have a strong desire for the supervisor to exhibit supportive communicative behaviors (Larson, 1981). In addition, Tihen (1983) reports exploring the domain of expectations at three levels of clinical experience: no experience, 25–150 completed clock hours, and more than 176. Supervisees with less than 150 clock hours expect the supervisor to assume an active role in the conference, with the clinician being more passive. The more experienced supervisees, who have more than 176 hours, anticipate the opposite: They expect the supervisor to talk less, while the supervisee assumes greater control. Goodyear and Bernard (1998) also note differences between supervisees based on their level of experience. Beginning trainees express a need for more support, structure, and encouragement, while those who are more advanced want to emphasize personal issues that affect their work and acquire higher level clinical skills.

Wagner and Hess (1997) explore how supervisees feel about the supervisor's use of power in the supervisory relationship, and found that supervisees prefer three types of power: expertise, reward, and referent. They want supervisors to share their expertise with them, to be reinforced in a positive manner, and to identify with the supervisor. In contrast, they *do not like* it when supervisors use coercive power. That is, they do not want to feel obligated to accept supervisors' views only because of their superior position or be forced to act in a specific way. Nelson (1997) observes that women benefit from supervisory relationships in which power is shared and there is mutual striving for the growth of both participants.

Important points emerge from the work cited above. Supervisees want to be actively involved in the conference, particularly as they gain in experience, and do not want to assume a passive stance in which they are simply told what to do. They do expect and appreciate feedback as well as expert guidance from the supervisor. They also want the opportunity to contribute their thoughts and to have those ideas incorporated, respected, and responded to in a thoughtful manner. In sum, they ask to be valued as individuals and as emerging professionals who have potential.

Typical Conferences

In a traditional view of the supervisory relationship, one assumes that the superior teaches and the supervisee learns. This is reminiscent of the "jug and mug" language approach in which the content to be learned is poured into the passive recipient (Muma, 1977). If it were possible to observe a conference selected randomly, one might have the opportunity to view this process in action. Research demonstrates that the majority of conferences are directive in nature. The supervisor tells, the supervisee listens and reports the events that have occurred in therapy. The supervisor then analyzes that information and suggests future strategies (Smith and Anderson, 1982; Roberts and Smith, 1982; Culatta and Seltzer, 1976; Dowling and Shank, 1981).

Pickering (1987a, 1989–90) states that supervisors expect students to be actively involved in the supervisory process and to share their perceptions of events occurring in both the clinical and supervisory interaction. But, the behaviors supervisors say they expect of supervisees and what they allow or encourage the supervisee to do in the conference can vary. If a supervisor verbalizes that the supervisee should be an active participant but, in the actual conference, assumes a direct, telling style, the supervisee will be nudged into a passive stance. The discrepancy between what one thinks one does and what actually occurs is likely to be greatest for those individuals who have not studied the supervisory process.

In contrast to what continues to occur in the conferences of untrained supervisors, theorists stress the importance of active supervisee participation in the conference (Anderson, 1988; Farmer and Farmer, 1989). In order to foster the development of self-supervisory skills and to optimize clinical/teaching performance, the supervisees need to be increasingly involved in data collection, analysis, and problem-solving in regard to the client and themselves (Dowling, 1998). Anderson (1988), Costa and Garmston (1994), Casey, Smith, and Ulrich (1988), Mercaitis and Peaper (1989), Dowling (1979, 1998), and Shapiro (1998) all say that movement toward professional independence is the goal.

In sum, contrary to supervisory philosophy, the behaviors that occur in actual meetings may be the opposite of what is believed to be happening. In the typical conference then, it is safe to predict a superior/subordinate relationship. The supervisor will do most of the talking. Supervisees will provide the raw information about the previous session (Culatta and Seltzer, 1976). The supervisor will reflect on the input and engage in problem-solving and strategy development. In most circumstances, data will not have been collected (Roberts and Smith, 1982; Smith and Anderson, 1982). In addition, a planned agenda for the conference will be rare, although the supervisor may, at times, have prepared, as feedback, a list of items to tell the supervisee (Anderson, 1988).

Effective Conference Precursors

The preceding material discusses the theoretical purpose of the conference, the supervisees' expectations, and includes a description of interactions that typically occur. The following discussion will address the factors to be considered in planning supervision that ensures the convergence of theory and practice, and will result in effective, useful conferences.

Preconference Planning: Supervisor

Conference Focus. Conferences need to be planned. Numerous authors, (Anderson, 1988; Farmer and Farmer, 1989; Shapiro, 1998; Evans 1998) say that supervisee involvement in the planning process is critical. A first issue participants may wish to consider is whether the meeting will be client/service-focused or supervisee-oriented. Client/service-centered conferences are directed almost exclusively to the growth of the patient. There is minimal discussion of supervisee behavior, and what does take place relates to what the supervisee might or might not be doing to enhance the client's performance. In contrast, a supervisee focus is the reverse. Client behavior is discussed only as it relates to clinician functioning. Conferences at the extremes of these types are likely to be relatively ineffective and a balance between the two is more appropriate. The degree to which each component is included will fluctuate, depending on the given circumstances and the immediate concerns of those involved. In addition, the needs and goals of the facility in which services are provided are likely to be factors. Service delivery organizations lean toward client-oriented exchanges, while clinical training facilities are generally more supervisee directed, although, in order to compete successfully in the marketplace, the latter group is increasingly becoming a dual-focused entity, jointly client and supervisee oriented (Mercaitis, 1990). Evans (1998) observes that supervisors have the responsibility of holding in balance both the needs of the supervisees and the patients they serve.

There is an important factor to keep in mind when selecting the orientation of the conference. The goal, whether in a training program or a work environment, is to produce a professional who performs optimally and functions independently. To achieve this, people must learn to engage in evidence-based practice (Logemann, 2000). This means observing, self-evaluating, and problem-solving. Encouraging the clinician to present a hypothesis, implement a strategy, measure the outcome, and make modifications accordingly is critical. As clinicians learn these skills, treatment on a short-term basis may be less efficient than if the supervisor simply tells the clinician how to proceed. In the long run, however, future clients will benefit as supervisees will have developed the tools and strategies necessary to deal effectively with novel clinical experiences. An effective conference, independent of a basic client or supervisee orientation, will have at least a portion of each meeting oriented specifically to the growth of the supervisee. Thus, the supervisor and supervisee will discuss the nature of the supervisory process and how it relates to the development of the supervisee.

Conference Philosophy.   In relation to planning the conference, supervisors may find it helpful to reflect on their own philosophies regarding the supervisory exchange. This may include considerations of what occurs in the conference as well as what is to be achieved. Juhnke (1996) suggests that a solution- versus problem-focused style of supervision enhances the process. In any event, the purpose of the supervisor–supervisee meeting is to improve the quality of services provided and to increase clinical and supervisory process outcomes. Supervisor philosophies will vary. If supervisors have a sense of their own personal philosophies, conference planning is simplified. In particular, knowledge of one's intent makes it possible to consider the exchange during and after the fact to determine if the events were consistent with the global plan.

Style Selection.   A critical decision to be made in designing the conference is choosing the style appropriate for the interaction. The Anderson (1988) model, in Figure 4.1, identifies the strategies that may be chosen. The direct or telling style is appropriate for the supervisee who is inexperienced or is feeling overwhelmed.

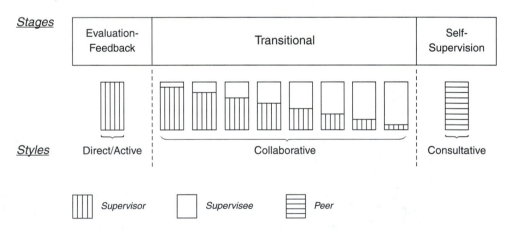

FIGURE 4.1   Composite of Stages of Supervision and the Appropriate Styles For Each Stage

Reprinted with permission from Anderson, J. *The Supervisory Process in Speech-Language Pathology and Audiology.* Austin, TX: Pro-Ed, 1988, 62.

This may include the beginning clinician who is having difficulty getting started, the individual struggling to survive clinically, or the employed professional with a type of client not previously encountered. The common denominator for the selection of this style is the perceived need for "telling" to assist the supervisee in obtaining control of the situation.

The collaborative style is suitable for a wide range of circumstances. Anderson (1988) states that this is the approach that will best facilitate supervisees' progress toward self-supervision, because clinicians gradually increase their volume of talk time, data collection, analysis, problem-solving, and strategy development in the conference. Accordingly, it is the style that is most appropriate in the majority of training circumstances and often the beginning point with employees. Note that, in this methodology, supervisor input decreases in response to an increase in the involvement of the supervisee. The supervisor listens and provides the volume and type of input cued by the supervisee. The essence of the collaborative style is that the supervisee and supervisor work as a team to foster the growth of all those involved.

Beginning clinicians, particularly those who have excelled academically and have been trained to participate in the supervisory process, often are able to move into the collaborative realm of supervision within a matter of weeks. The supervisor may stimulate this movement by collecting data initially, and then encouraging the supervisee to complete the analysis and related strategy development. In an analogous fashion, the supervisee can be nudged in this direction through open-ended questions that encourage him or her to reflect on events and to consider cause and effect.

More experienced trainees, as well as those completing the Clinical Fellowship Year, can be expected to participate in the collaborative mode of supervision. Employed professionals who have not had the opportunity or training for this type of supervision can also benefit from a collaborative approach. The appropriate point regarding expected degrees of supervisor/supervisee input within collaboration will need to be individually selected depending on the supervisee and supervisor's level of readiness. Anderson (1988) points out that, intermittently, it may be necessary to shift back to a directive style if circumstances warrant such a move. Similarly, there will be times when it is appropriate to switch to a consultative style.

Periodically, in the training environment, the supervisor will encounter the supervisee who is truly ready to function in the consultative stage. Obviously, this is a delightful opportunity when it presents itself. But, even in this circumstance, it may be necessary at times to shift back to collaboration or telling, as events warrant. A combination of collaboration and consultation is likely to be the most appropriate mode for the employed professional, although telling may be incorporated as needed.

The supervisor's task, then, in planning for the conference, is to assess oneself, the supervisee, and the tasks at hand to select the appropriate style for the conference interaction. Evans (1998) suggests that the choice of style is also affected by supervisee and supervisor interpersonal factors. The managerial grid

(Blake and McCanse, 1991) and the Mawdsley and Scudder (1989) strategy for use in speech-language pathology and audiology, discussed in Chapter 1, can also be used to assist in the selection of a style. Incorporating the supervisee's preferences is always a wise decision. The joint determination of an appropriate conference orientation is a critical aspect of effective conferencing.

An alternative conference option is to use cognitive coaching (Costa and Garmston, 1994). Its values are compatible with those of Anderson (1988). In particular, supervision is at the level of the supervisee's need. This approach guides supervisees as they gain increasingly accurate problem-solving skills. The supervisees are assisted in clearing defining concerns and then are directed to develop their own solutions. Key supervisor behaviors are pushing for precision and active listening. The supervisor using this style will also mirror the supervisees' verbal and nonverbal behaviors to increase communication effectiveness and to create trust.

Agenda Determination.   As mentioned earlier, most conferences just happen and are probably not preplanned. In reality, planning is critical to the implementation of an effective conference. The agenda may be formalized as a written plan or can exist more informally as a mental concept. For the individual who has not previously designed the conference on a conscious level, it may be helpful to outline the interaction in written form. Once it becomes part of a standard routine, it can then shift safely to a cognitive strategy.

Given the importance of agenda planning, it is surprising that research in this area remains limited. Peaper (1984) indicates that supervisee input to the agenda augments the clinician's sense of control in the interaction. Sbaschnig, Dowling, and Williams (1990) report a study that assesses the impact of shifting responsibility for agenda planning from the supervisor to the supervisee during the clinical term. The attributions made about successes and failure in therapy remain the same regardless of who plans the topics for the meeting. McLeod (1997) describes a self-appraisal strategy in which supervisees respond to a questionnaire about their entire practicum experience. Supervisees' responses serve as the agenda for a conference with their supervisors, and they report feeling empowered by this process.

The supervisor may wish to begin devising the agenda by selecting the topics to be addressed that day. Items can emerge from that week's observations and the related collected data, facility due dates, supervisee requests, or the supervisor's perceptions of areas needing discussion. Juhnke (1996) suggests a solution-focused orientation to agenda planning. The strategy is to have supervisees identify their strengths and then discuss ways to capitalize on those assets in treatment. Supervisees' needs should be paramount because the purpose of the conference is to assist them in enhancing their own performance and professional growth. Another factor to keep in mind in structuring the interaction is the number of issues that can realistically be handled, given the supervisee's readiness and the time available. A representative sample of conference topics for one supervisor/supervisee pair for one term appears in Table 4.1.

TABLE 4.1 Conference Topics That Emerged from One Supervisor after One Term with One Supervisee

Conference 1
Discussed perceptions of the assigned client and the planned assessment

Presented and talked about lesson plan expectations

Conference 2
Discussed clinician impressions of client

Addressed the supervisee's self-perceptions of strengths and weaknesses in test administration and client management

Identified additional aspects of client performance needing assessment

Began an initial discussion of the test findings and related interpretations

Considered areas in which the supervisee desired information and feedback

Conference 3
Discussed client test data
  a. Is the assessment complete? Baseline data?
  b. What does the supervisee need from the supervisor to assist her in the writing of the test analysis?

Considered client objectives

Engaged in dialogue regarding beginning treatment plans

Conference 4
Discussed client objectives, test analysis

Requested input as to information needed by the supervisee to complete the above

Operationalized client objectives, jointly

Considered lesson plan writing
  a. Proposed content
  b. Format of plan

Conference 5
Discussed treatment
  Considered supervisor and supervisee perceptions of what was and was not working in treatment
  Role-played one aspect of therapy of concern to the supervisee
  Analyzed treatment data
  Considered supervisee concerns
  Addressed lesson plan refinement in regard to task focus

Conference 6
Viewed and discussed videotape of supervisee providing treatment

Conference 7
Diagnosed supervisee
  Supervisee self-perceptions of strengths and liabilities shared
  Supervisor perceptions of supervisee as a professional conveyed

Selected, jointly, supervisee professional goals for the semester

Discussed data collection strategies to monitor the above objectives.

Conference 8
Conveyed midterm evaluation of supervisee

Discussed issues raised by supervisee

Analyzed data regarding supervisee performance

Conference 9
Discussed first draft of case summary

Addressed issues of concern to supervisee

Conference 10
Reviewed progress toward supervisee's professional objectives

Refined the related data collection procedures and selected targets for the following week

Discussed supervisor comments on lesson plans and evaluation forms as it related to the implementation of therapy

Conference 11
Viewed videotapes of second therapy taping

Discussed collected data

Talked about client end-of-term recommendations

Addressed issues raised by supervisee

Conference 12
Reviewed collected data and selected behaviors to be observed for the following week

Dealt with supervisee concerns

Assessed supervisee progress toward own professional goals

Discussed final case summary

Conference 13
Completed final supervisee evaluation

Several additional events or factors may affect the planning process. In some cases, the supervisee will bring an audiotape or videotape to the meeting, which provides a natural structure for the conference. Many times, collected data, either from the supervisee or supervisor, will be a primary focus. In other instances, the supervisee may offer a report draft or other relevant documentation for discussion. Each of the above will influence the format of the dialogue between the participants.

Additional factors relevant to agenda planning are scheduling and timeliness. Clinical trainees need regularly scheduled conferences at a time specifically set aside for them. Once conferences are scheduled, the timely arrival of both participants to the meeting is expected. Failure to do so is disrespectful and denies the importance of the other person's time. Scheduling on a "catch me if you can" basis and late arrival of participants will negatively affect the establishment of trust, the quality of the interpersonal relationship, and the effectiveness of the conference.

Supervisee Variables.   Once basic issues such as agenda items have been identified, the supervisor's thoughts may move to other conference considerations. For example, is the supervisee primarily a visual or auditory learner? To informally assess the learner's orientation, Farmer (1985–1986) suggests focusing attention on the verb types the person uses. A supervisee who says things such as "I see what you mean" or "It looks fine to me" is likely to be visually oriented. In contrast, the auditory learner is more apt to say "I hear you" or "It sounds good." Once this learning style is discovered, specific measures may be taken in the conference to adapt to the supervisee's needs.

If the clinician learns best through the visual mode, it is helpful to structure the conference around what may be seen. In this circumstance, a written agenda can help structure the supervisee's learning. Data can be graphed or shown in its original written form. It may also be appropriate to ask supervisees to list the strategies they agree to use during the following week. In contrast, the auditory learner needs information presented predominantly in the auditory mode. Written or collected data are preferably analyzed verbally and conclusions generated through discussion. It may also be helpful to have supervisees verbally restate impressions and commitments so that they have the opportunity to hear the information.

Cashwell, Looby, and Housley (1997) note that one's learning style can also by culturally influenced. This can include expectations for organizational structure, supervisor style, and preferred mode of learning. There are also gender preferences to be considered (Crespi, 1995; Sells, Lichtenberg, Goodyear, and Polkinghorne (1997). As can be seen, a variety of supervisee factors need to be considered so that appropriate accommodations can be made to enhance the quality of the conference.

In all instances, agenda planning will incorporate both a clinical and supervisory process focus. According to Anderson (1990), Strike-Roussos (1988) identifies three basic components: (1) reviewing the agenda for the current meeting, (2) planning for the clinical session, and (3) planning for the supervisory conference. Key points are that the agenda is open to modification and that it includes items from both the supervisor and supervisee. Planning for the clinical session involves both a clinician as well as a client development component. Thus, data will be analyzed and strategies for growth will be included for both the supervisee and client. Planning for the supervisory conference encompasses an analysis of data from the previous conference, goal development for the current and future interactions, a determination of the types of data to be collected during future observations, and the strategies for doing so. Therefore, in reviewing the effectiveness of the planning process, a key consideration will be whether each of the three components is incorporated: (1) Was the agenda reviewed and did both members contribute? (2) Did clinical planning focus on both the clinician and client? (3) Was the last conference analyzed and did planning for the supervisory process occur? An additional factor is to determine if accommodations for supervisee learning style, cultural differences, and gender were incorporated in the planning process.

Supervisee Diagnosis.   Similarly, diagnosis of the clinician's levels of ability, experience, and readiness assists in planning. Rockman (1977) states that the supervisor/supervisee relationship is parallel to that of the clinician/client. Patients are routinely tested prior to therapy. Correspondingly, it is fitting to diagnose the trainee or employed professional as part of the supervisory process. After two or three weeks of treatment, it is beneficial to engage in a formal assessment of the supervisee. The form in Table 4.2 is based on Rockman's ideas and will be useful in this analysis. In considering the form, the first segment is intended to identify the skills and experiences that the supervisee brings to the interaction. Subsequently, strengths and weaknesses that have emerged from the first weeks of treatment, from both the supervisee and supervisor's point of view, will be identified. Following the analysis, goals for supervisee growth can be developed that will give the supervisor a sense of the areas in which support or guidance will be most valuable in upcoming conferences. Therefore, the appraisal of the clinician becomes an important part of planning for the conference.

Site Selection.   In regard to planning, the site of the meeting, furniture arrangement, and the power relationships reflected in these choices are issues to consider. Typically conferences are held in the supervisor's office but, in given circumstances, particularly if the supervisee is feeling threatened, it may be helpful to meet on the supervisee's turf. This is particularly true in the professional work environment, where the supervisor may be making a conscious effort to reduce the superior–subordinate impression.

Furniture and Seating Arrangements.   Similarly, the placement of furniture sends power messages. Most supervisors choose to sit behind a desk with the supervisee seated in front, which dramatically identifies the superior and subordinate in the relationship. The desk is also a physical barrier that is likely to impede communication. A more desirable arrangement is to have both the supervisee and supervisor

TABLE 4.2   Supervisee Diagnosis Form

This form is to be completed jointly by the supervisor and supervisee.

_____   _____
    Supervisee   Supervisor

Information relating to the client:
    Age:
    Type of disorder (e.g., hearing impaired)
    Primary clinical problem (e.g., language)

Information relating to the supervisee:
    Number of previously earned clock hours _____
        A. Clock hours earned with preschool children _____
            Number of clients seen _____
        B. Clock hours earned with school-age children _____
            Number of clients seen _____
        C. Clock hours earned with adults _____
            Number of clients seen _____

Coursework completed relating to the current clinical problem:

Clinical experience relevant to the current clinical problem:

Supervisee's perception of own clinical strengths:

Supervisee's perception of areas needing growth:

Supervisor's perception of supervisee's clinical strengths:

Supervisor's perception of supervisee's areas needing growth:

This form is based on the ideas presented by Rockman (1977).

seated in an open area with no objects separating them. Side-by-side seating is defined as the most intimate and indicative of cooperation (Sommer, 1969). A compromise arrangement is turning the supervisor's desk to the wall so that the supervisee can sit beside the supervisor without a barrier between the two.

The seating of the supervisee in a chair comparable to that of the supervisor reflects equality in power. Physical comfort facilitates communication. In this regard, the supervisee should not be expected to stand or to sit in an uncomfortable chair if the goal is to foster discussion. In addition, the supervisor may choose to sit close to the supervisee, without violating personal space, as this too enhances the quality of the interaction. A distance of between two and one-half to four feet is typical in U.S. culture for the discussion of personal concerns.

Planning Summary. Conference planning crosses a variety of parameters. It is hoped that the focus of the conference and the style selected will reflect an understanding of both the supervisor and supervisee's levels of readiness in regard to the supervision continuum described by Anderson (1988). In all cases, the preparation of an agenda is critical to successful conferencing. This includes topic selection and decisions regarding the incorporation of data collection or videotapes in the exchange. Supervisee learning styles, cultural and gender issues, and a formal diagnosis of the supervisee also need to be taken into account. Similarly, site selection and the physical arrangements for the conference need to be planned.

It is falsely implied here that the supervisor is totally responsible for agenda preparation. This may be true only at the beginning of an interaction with a particular supervisee. The responsibility should begin to shift to the clinician as soon as possible. In fact, supervisees should be expected to contribute agenda items early in the relationship. Toward the end of the collaborative stage and in the consultative stage, trainees and employed professionals may appropriately design the conference plan independently. This shift is important to the growth of the supervisee. Unless supervisees become actively involved in topic selection, the probability that their needs are being met will be very small. Also, deciding what needs to be discussed is an important component of self-assessment. In essence, identifying what one does or does not do well and the related selection of topics for discussion is critical to the emergence of the professional self.

Preconference Planning: Supervisee

To maximize outcomes, supervisees also benefit from engaging in planning prior to the conference. Clinicians profit from reflecting on previous interactions to determine whether or not their needs have been met. If trainees or employees leave the conference feeling satisfied and confident that they have the tools for preparing for the following week(s), it is helpful to identify the supervisor and supervisee behaviors that led to this sensation. Similarly, if the individuals did not acquire necessary information, they need to think about what occurred and why. In essence, what did they do or not do that allowed this to happen?

Crago (1987) presents excellent guidelines (see the Appendix) to assist supervisees in preparing for the conference. She suggests that supervisees identify three therapy segments as possible topics for discussion: one activity that went well, one that was less successful, and one that was a surprise. Crago then guides trainees to reflect, for each segment, on their (1) skill as a clinician, (2) feelings and reactions, and (3) the effect the treatment had on the client. After completing this task, they then select one of the three parts to present in the conference and identify the purpose for doing so. They also determine what they want to achieve in and from the meeting. This includes the ways in which the supervisor can be most helpful. Supervisees also engage in and communicate this planning during the meeting to steer the conference in the direction necessary to meet their needs. Following the exchange, Crago also encourages supervisees to self-evaluate to determine if their concerns were addressed and to plan strategies for future encounters to increase overall effectiveness.

Supervisees may also use the previously discussed information presented by Rockman (1977) as a tool for preparing for the conference. Once the supervisees' diagnoses have been completed and related objectives developed, they will want to plan so that the content of conferences aids movement toward their own professional goals. For example, supervisees may request that data relevant to a personal objective be collected for analysis and discussion in the conference, or they may want to view a videotape segment with a specific purpose in mind. Or, supervisees may wish to discuss overall progress at a given point as a means of validating their own perceptions. This ongoing self-evaluation and diagnosis will provide a solid foundation for supervisee planning.

Supervisee planning is an essential element of effective conferencing. The focus is different than that of the supervisor but of equal, if not greater, importance. The primary concern is that the supervisory process affect the supervisee's growth optimally. It is both the supervisor's and supervisee's responsibility to see that it does so.

Conference Initiation

Initiating the conference by discussing the agenda is an effective way to begin. This gives the supervisee an opportunity to add or substitute topics. Then, as clinicians take more responsibility for this aspect of supervisory process planning, they are expected to contribute increasing amounts of the agenda or plan it in its entirety. In the latter case, the supervisor is asked if he or she has other items to add.

In conjunction with the structuring of the conference, the supervisor strives to actively build a working relationship with the supervisee. Farmer (1985–1986) indicates that the first five minutes of each conference sets the tone for the entire interaction. The continuing establishment of rapport begins with contact between the supervisor and clinician and continues throughout the relationship. Cogan (1973) and Costa and Garmston (1994) talk at length about the importance of establishing trust. At a minimum, supervisees need to sense that the content of discussions in the conference is confidential and that the information revealed will not be used to their detriment. Consistency in the supervisor's behavior also promotes trust as the supervisee is able to predict the other's response in various circumstances. McBride and Skau (1995) say that the foundations for trust in a relationship are "confidentiality, consistency, risk-taking, honesty, sincerity, and a climate of mutual exchange." In contrast, Nelson (1997) notes that criticism without nurturance undermines trust. It is important to remember that trust is earned. In addition, the support of risk-taking, independent of outcome, generates the feeling of trustworthiness. Pickering (1977) talks about the importance of encouraging taking chances, the willingness to try a new strategy that may or may not succeed, as a tool to foster development and to strengthen the supervisory relationship. Costa and Garmston (1989) state that it is important to foster risk-taking in supervisees as exceptional learners function at the edge of their competence. Therefore, risk-taking is critical to further growth.

Facilitative Conference Behaviors

Verbal/Nonverbal Pacing

Effective conferences begin in the planning stage. Once completed, several of the following strategies may also be incorporated in the conference to expedite the interaction: (1) verbal/nonverbal pacing, (2) facilitative interpersonal demeanor, (3) active listening, and (4) assistive nonverbal behaviors. Verbal/nonverbal pacing is an interesting concept. According to Costa and Garmston (1994), research on outstanding communicators indicates that these speakers engage in both verbal and nonverbal pacing with listeners. Verbally, they match the characteristics of a listener's utterances. This may include, for example, pitch, intensity, and phrasing patterns. Farmer (1985–1986) suggests that the mirroring may also be linguistically specific. For example, the supervisor might use the same verb types used by the supervisee. In the nonverbal realm, Costa and Garmston (1994) also suggest duplicating the listener's body movements and positions. During the exchange, as the listener shifts body position or gestures for emphasis, the effective communicator moves into a parallel stance and may even incorporate the supervisee's gestures into the conversation. Farmer (1985–1986; 1989) indicates that such nonverbal pairing encourages interaction, creates joint reference, and facilitates turn-taking and can include mirroring of the other participant's head and/or body orientation and movement, eye contact, facial expressions, and the position and motions of the trunk, arms, hands, legs and feet. Costa and Garmston (1989) suggest that communicators wait to make the shift until their next turn at talking, while Farmer says that the coinciding adjustments in movement or position can be made immediately or delayed for a brief time. In implementing such a strategy, the supervisor must take care to insure that the mirroring is subtle and does not cause discomfort to the supervisee. Costa and Garmston (1989) graphically describe the impact of an abrupt mismatch in the nonverbal domain. Communication is disrupted and listeners show uneasiness and a concern that they are doing something wrong.

Along these same lines, Brooks (1989) writes that rapport occurs when people perceive that others behave as they do. The more people resemble each other verbally and gesturally, the greater comfort they feel, which, in turn, stimulates a sense of immediate liking. He states that individuals enjoy being around people who exhibit attitudes and behaviors that parallel their own.

He goes on to say that people can be classified by their preferred modality for interacting with the world. He reports that 20 percent of the population is auditorily oriented, 20 percent is kinesthetically inclined and 60 percent prefer the visual mode. According to Brooks, people show dominance for one sense although they may use alternate modalities at certain times and in specific circumstances. For example, the person who processes auditorily tends to prefer information that provides auditory images, but he or she may have a visual leaning for scheduling the workday.

To establish rapport with individuals, Brooks suggests focusing on people's speech to determine their preferred modality, because a person's processing preference is likely to reflected in his or her utterances, and the words he or she uses will frequently show a bias for the auditory, visual, or tactile mode. Brooks provides numerous examples of how people's language choices likely reflect their preferred mode of interaction. People who interact visually with the world are likely to use words such as *see, look, bright, colorful, appear, perspective, foggy*, and their descriptions will reflect their reliance on visual metaphors: "Do you **see** how **clear** it is?" "Let's **focus** in on that point of **view**." "Can you **picture** what I mean?" In contrast, individuals who represent their world auditorily might say "**Tell** me how you like it." "That's **clear** as a **bell**." "Keep your **ear** to the ground." "I'd like to go to the beach today; how does that **sound** to you?" and use words that reflect their preference for sound and hearing in their descriptions, e.g., *listen, loud, melodious, discuss, harsh, resonance, be heard, off-key*. People in the third group, the kinesthetics, might say "I have a gut **feeling**." "I **sense** you are right." "Let's get a **handle** on things." Representative words in their vocabulary might be *exciting, firm, secure, clumsy, fits, touch, aware, feeling*.

As Brooks observes that, in interacting with others the first task is to identify the person's primary representational set. Once her or his style is identified, rapport and liking are readily attainable if the speaker mirrors and responds in kind to the other's word choices. Costa and Garmston (1989) and Farmer (1985–1986; 1989) encourage a similar strategy. In particular, they encourage the use of key words and gestures previously heard or observed. The greater the parallel between the speaker and listener's verbal and nonverbal behaviors, the more comfortable the participants are likely to be. The gains in attraction and rapport are likely to translate into increased communicative effectiveness.

Farmer (1983) reports a study of communication disorders in which trained and untrained observers were randomly assigned to watch four videotapes that showed varying degrees of verbal and nonverbal pacing during the first five minutes of a conference. Tape 1 showed the supervisor pacing the clinician's verbal behavior but not the nonverbal; in Tape 2, the nonverbal behavior was paced but not the verbal; in Tape 3, both the clinician's nonverbal and verbal behavior were paced; on Tape 4, the supervisor did not pace either the nonverbal or verbal behavior. The trained coders were able to identify the key pacing features of the four tapes more readily than those who had not been trained. In addition, the trained subjects found that the conferences in which both verbal and nonverbal pacing were used were more effective, followed by nonverbal pacing only, verbal pacing only, and no pacing. Farmer's study supports the value of the supervisor strategy of matching the supervisee's physical movements and verbal patterns and his findings are consistent with the views of Costa and Garmston (1994).

Perhaps an anecdote will best illustrate the importance of pacing in establishing and maintaining rapport. A supervisor once approached me about a problem with a supervisee who was often hostile, rude, and appeared not to hear feedback. The relationship was strained and the supervisor felt that it could not continue as it was. I provided the supervisor with information about Costa and Garmston's and Farmer's research. Subsequently, the supervisor began to mirror many of the supervisee's behaviors, both verbally and nonverbally. For example, the clinician would flip her hand through her hair and verbally interrupt the speaker, so the supervisor would also engage in these, as well as other, supervisee behaviors. In a short time, a radical change in the supervisee's actions occurred and the hostility disappeared. As the relationship improved, the supervisee confided that she "thought that earlier, the supervisor had been out to get her." In this case, the verbal and nonverbal pacing strategies clearly worked.

Positive Interpersonal Behaviors

A second strategy to enhance the conference is to use effective interpersonal behaviors. Two works in our field indicate that supervisory talk, in the samples studied, are interpersonally non-facilitative. The first, McCrea (1980), uses the McCrea Adapted Scales, based on the work of Carkuff (1969), to consider the interpersonal tone of the conference. She examines the occurrence of supervisee self-exploration in relation to the levels of respect, empathic understanding, genuineness, and concreteness provided by the supervisor. The volume of supervisor utterances in these categories is so low that supervisee self-exploration does not occur. Hence, McCrea indicates that the supervisors who are examined are not using facilitative interpersonal styles during meetings with supervisees.

Similarly, Pickering (1984) examines forty 10-minute samples collected from the conferences of two supervisors and ten clinicians over the length of a semester. The supervisors in this study also keep journals to record their observations and impressions of the conferences. The tapes are analyzed from the perspective of "sensitizing concepts" such as "sharing aspects of one's humanness," and the findings are integrated with the notations in the supervisors' journals. Pickering reports that the conferences tend to be cognitively rather than interpersonally focused. Neither feelings nor the relationship between the supervisor and supervisee are addressed, except rarely, and supervisors do not reveal their personal selves. Pickering's impression is that supervisors lack skill in the interpersonal domain.

In contrast to these two studies, Caracciolo, Rigrodsky, and Morrison (1978a) find that trained supervisors can provide a facilitative interpersonal climate. The eight supervisors in the study completed both a survey course and a practicum in supervision. Forty graduate students participated in the nine-week study with these eight supervisors. The Barrett-Lennard Relationship Inventory (1962) was used to identify the supervisees' perceptions of the supervisors' level of regard, the unconditionality of that regard, their empathic understanding, and congruence of verbal and nonverbal behavior. The instrument was administered at the beginning and end of the study along with two other research tools designed to assess changes in professional self-esteem and clinical growth, which shows that supervisors exhibited more positive than negative interpersonal behaviors during the study. As a result, growth occurred in supervisee self-esteem as well as in their clinical performance.

These studies indicate that engaging in facilitative interpersonal behavior requires effort and thought. The provision of a positive, growth-oriented interpersonal environment for the supervisee is important. Evans (1998) notes that, to do so, supervisors need to be aware of their own preferred style of interacting as well as those areas in which they need to grow. In addition, Wagner and Hess (1997) say that supervisees prefer that supervisors use three types of power in supervision: expertise, referent and reward. Laden and Legumen-Waterman (1999) suggest that the more a supervisor self-discloses, the stronger the emotional bond and agreement between the supervisor and supervisee about the goals and tasks of supervision will be. In addition, Ladany, Ellis, and Frielander (1999) find that the stronger the emotional bond between the supervisor and supervisee, the more the latter will be satisfied with the process. Thus, for the supervisor who does not have the opportunity for training in interpersonal effectiveness or a formal supervision course with a portion focusing on the interpersonal domain, it would be beneficial to read the literature in this area, particularly the work of Farmer and Farmer (1989), Pickering (1977, 1987a, b; 1989–1990), Caracciolo, Morrison, and Rigrodsky (1978b), Moses and Shapiro (1992), McCready, Roberts, Bengala, Harris, Kingsley and Krikorian (1996), and Evans (1998). Pickering (1989–1990), for example, highlights the importance of considering supervisor and supervisee personal needs and feelings in the supervisory process. In particular, she feels it is important to appreciate each person's individuality and to ponder and appreciate the meaning each participant attributes to events and behaviors.

Several interpersonal dimensions that are thought to improve conference interactions are frequently cited in the literature (Dussault, 1970; Caracciolo, Rigrodsky, and Morrison, 1978b; Pickering, 1977, 1989–1990; Farmer, 1989): unconditional positive regard, contact, empathy, congruence, authenticity, genuineness, and concreteness. Positive regard is a sincere liking and respect for an individual. In essence, it means accepting people as they are and valuing their humanity. To be unconditional, the regard or esteem must be constant, independent of the person's behavior. The second dimension, contact, means that the communicators are affecting each other on an interpersonal or psychological plane. In contrast, empathy is the ability to engage in perspective-taking, being able to see the other's point of view. Congruence is typically defined as a match of the supervisor's verbal and nonverbal behaviors, although it should be noted that nonverbal behaviors are less socialized and tend to be a truer index of one's intent. Often supervisors will state a willingness to talk but, at the same time, send the contradictory nonverbal message that they need to leave. In particular, if the verbal communication and facial expression conflict, the exchange is typically perceived as counterproductive (Long, 1978; Babad, 1992). Therefore, to be congruent both the verbal and nonverbal must convey the same meaning.

Authenticity is a concept discussed by Pickering (1977), who defines it as accepting one's feelings, perceptions, and experiences as one's own, even when they do not match one's desired self-image. To be authentic, one must also be willing to share aspects of self when it is appropriate in a relationship. Genuineness (McCrea, 1980) parallels authenticity. It is a natural, open expression of one's thoughts and feelings, unlimited by specific role definition. Finally, concreteness (McCrea, 1980) is defined as being specific when one communicates.

Caracciolo, Rigrodsky, and Morrison (1978b) postulate that if the conditions of unconditional positive regard, contact, empathic understanding, and congruence are conveyed by the supervisor and perceived by the supervisee, positive change can occur: The supervisee will be less defensive and preceive his or her professional behavior more objectively and realistically; the gap between the real and ideal personal and professional self will narrow; the clinician's own positive self-regard will increase, and the trainee will be less likely to model the supervisor and develop an individualized therapy style instead. In addition, Pickering (1977) states that the supervisor's reflection of authenticity enhances communication by facilitating the exchange of a true dialogue. Finally, McCrea (1980) hypothesizes that the use of respect, empathy, genuineness, and concreteness increases supervisee self-exploration, and Pickering (1989–1990) says that supervisees value support from their supervisors.

Conflict management is also a factor in the interpersonal domain. McCready and associates (1996) studied supervisors' projected responses to a clinician who had not completed an assigned task. The supervisors indicated the likelihood of their using fifteen different responses reflecting three conflict management strategies: avoidance, competition, and collaboration. The findings show that supervisors are likely to vary their response depending on the reason clinicians give for not completing the assignment. If the reason related to an event is outside the supervisee's control, the supervisor is more likely to respond in a collaborative manner. In general, supervisors tend to choose collaborative approaches to manage conflict, followed by avoidance and then competition. These researchers also note that supervisors are more likely to manage conflict effectively if they are aware of three things: (1) the options they have for dealing with conflict, (2) their own tendencies in conflict-management situations, (3) and the likely outcomes of various strategies in resolving the impasse. Farmer (1987), too, feels that being aware of and having options for managing conflict is a key to success.

The interpersonal domain is less concrete than many other areas in supervision and yet may be the factor that either enhances or undermines the conference. Supervisee performance and development are accentuated by positive, accepting, growth-oriented behaviors from the supervisor. One can begin by discussing the meanings of behaviors and the feelings generated by events. In addition, respecting the supervisee independently of the specific behaviors exhibited and communicating this esteem both verbally and nonverbally improves supervision.

Encouraging risk-taking is also constructive. Empathy is important and on a practical level, conveys the supervisor's ability to see the supervisee's perspective and even, at times, to say that he or she is sorry that particular circumstances exist. It also involves letting supervisees know that the supervisor cares about them as people and sincerely believes that they have the potential for professional growth. In sum, positive interpersonal verbal behaviors mean talking to supervisees openly, honestly, supportively, and specifically, even if what one has to say is not always positive.

Promotive Nonverbal Behaviors

Another aspect of effective supervision relates to the nonverbal component of communication. The importance of nonverbal behavior is well documented. Spangler (1995), summarizing nonverbal research, notes differences between men and women on almost every nonverbal variable, while Birdwhistle (1970) estimates that 65 percent of a message is conveyed nonverbally. Babad (1992) observes that when verbal and nonverbal behaviors do not match, the nonverbal is viewed as more valid, truthful, and revealing. There are two significant, although isolated, aspects of communication that the supervisor may choose to consider in the conference: kinesics, movements of the eye, head, hand, leg, and foot, and proxemics, the distance and angles between communicators (Wilbur and Wilbur, 1980).

Kinesics and proxemics influence how communication is perceived and interpeted. Head-nodding, along with minimal verbal reinforcers such as "uh huh," tend to increase verbal output from others, although it should be noted that women use head-nodding to nurture and encourage further talk, men perceive it as conveying agreement or confirming the content of the message (Langellier and Natalle, 1987). Women also smile more than men (Spangler, 1995), while eye contact is used to reduce psychological distance and to signal an open communication link, and, used during listening, reflects attention or consensus. It typically consists of brief glances of two- to three-seconds duration and should be focused on different parts of the face (Arygle, 1988). The avoidance of eye contact and a high frequency of looking away, in contrast, are interpreted as conveying uncertainty or disagreement with what is being said (Wilbur and Wilbur, 1980). Interestingly enough, feedback, negative or positive, is viewed more favorably when it is accompanied by frequent eye contact (Ellsworth and Carlsmith, 1968; Exline and Eldridge, 1967), but eye contact held longer than ten seconds is likely to trigger feelings of aggression, anxiety, and discomfort on the part of the listener (Nichols and Champness, 1971).

Active Listening

Another important set of supervisor conference behaviors is the use of active listening and open questions, strategies that characterize the skilled communicator and augment the quality of the supervisory exchange. Active listening is indicated by requesting additional information, clarifying, restating, or paraphrasing ideas the supervisee has expressed to insure the accuracy of one's interpretation (Farmer, 1989). Similarly, expanding on the comments of the clinician and incorporating verbal "greasers" such as "uh huh" encourage the trainee to elaborate. The supervisor's appropriate use of open-ended questions further stimulates active supervisee participation.

Active listening fosters effective communication in all environments (Costa and Garmston, 1994), and includes the use of silence, restating, and summarizing. It lets the supervisee know that her or his thoughts are important and that the listener truly wants to hear them. First, the appropriate use of silence is helpful. It means giving the speaker time to think and the opportunity to respond without interruption from the other participant. Unfortunately, it is a human tendency for the listener to begin to preplan her or his response instead of truly listening. Second, restating what the supervisee has said forces the listener to attend rather than drifting off into her or his own thoughts. In addition, it insures that the message sent was the one received. The supervisor may choose to rephrase the content of the clinician's utterance to make sure that it was understood. The supervisee may also be asked to reiterate to insure that a point was accurately heard. Third, summarizing the content of the meeting and highlighting tasks to be completed or strategies to be implemented increase the likelihood that they will be attained. Shapiro and Anderson (1989) indicate that this is particularly true if the commitments are written down.

Conference Content

Now that the extrinsic parameters of the conference have been defined, it is appropriate to shift to the content of the discussion. Independently of whether the exchange is clinician- or client-focused, direct or collaborative in style, the heart of the interaction, at its best, is data-based analysis, problem-solving, and decision making. The ideas discussed in Chapter 2, on data collection, will be helpful in assisting the supervisor and supervisee in gathering and analyzing data to be considered in the meeting. The goal is to identify critical incidents and to test hypotheses in regard to cause and effect (Cogan, 1973; Moses and Shapiro, 1996). This process provides the foundation for making logical decisions. Costa and Garmston (1994) indicate that, ultimately, the teaching of decision making is the critical consideration: The supervisor must guide the supervisee toward increasing independence. This is particularly true in the areas of data collection, analysis, problem-solving, and decision making because these are the prerequisite skills for a supervisee to function independently and competently in novel clinical situations. Such strategies empower clinicians as they increase and use their own personal power for professional growth (McBride and Skau, 1995).

In regard to talk in the conference, the volume of supervisor talk may fluctuate, depending on the stage of supervision being implemented. In general, though, the goal is to reduce supervisor talk while increasing that of the supervisee

(Anderson, 1988). Thus, the supervisee is encouraged to progressively engage in more of the data analysis, problem-solving, and future strategy development. Extensive supervisee talk devoted to the description of past therapy is thought to be of less value (Culatta and Seltzer, 1976). In terms of the use of questions, a balance of usage between both participants is optimal (Roberts and Smith, 1982). In addition, questions used by the supervisor are best if they are predominantly open-ended.

Three final considerations are important in the supervisor–supervisee exchange: feedback, supervisory process planning, and evaluation of the conference. In regard to feedback, one intent of the conference is to provide this type of information (a topic discussed at length in Chapter 3). In the ideal world, the supervisee will be taught the skills necessary for accurate self-assessment, thereby minimizing the need for direct supervisor input.

The second issue, planning for the supervisory process and active supervisee participation in the conference, is critical. It was alluded to earlier in this chapter in regard to developing conference agendas. It includes four activities: (1) suggesting agenda items for the next conference, (2) deciding what is to be observed the following week, (3) determining who is to gather and analyze the data, and (4) discussing the supervisory relationship. Brasseur and Jimenez (1996) suggest that supervisors should discuss their expectations for supervisee involvement in each of these activities to increase the probability of their occurrence. In regard to the supervisory relationship, the skilled supervisor will also want input from the supervisee in regard to supervisory strategies or approaches perceived as most and least beneficial to the clinician. In essence, the supervisor is asking "What can I do that will be of the most value to you?" An ideal growth environment for all participants—supervisee, client, and supervisor—is best achieved when the supervisory relationship is preplanned, actively discussed, and then evaluated.

A final facet of the conference, then, is to evaluate it. It is a reflection on the content and effectiveness of the exchange. The assessment is very similar to that done in regard to treatment. It is based on data collection, analysis, and problem-solving. The tools to gather information may be observation systems or informal data collection strategies. (As an example, the conference data collection instrument [Dowling, 2000] in Appendix B of Chapter 9 can be used for this purpose.)

All aspects of the conference are open to review. Who and how much are important in regard to participant's talk time, problem-solving, strategy development, and question type and usage. A consideration of the interpersonal tone of the interaction is also a significant part of this process. Typically, the objectives for the meeting are reviewed to see if they were met. Of even greater value is assessing whether the supervisee's needs were addressed.

Anderson (1988), Brasseur (1989), and Cogan (1973) all suggest that both the supervisee and supervisor should be involved in the evaluation of the conference. As the supervisor grows in her or his role, it is helpful to ask the supervisee for input. Of particular value is whether clinicians perceive that the meetings are addressing their needs. It is also beneficial to find out which specific aspects of the conference are of value as well as those that are not, and to determine if additional behaviors on the part of the supervisor would assist the supervisee. The greater the interchange about the supervisory process, the more effective the outcomes are likely to be.

Optimal Conference Summary

Numerous aspects of the conference have been discussed in this chapter. If one has the opportunity to observe an ideal conference for a supervisee at the collaborative stage of supervision (Anderson, 1988), the following will be evident. First, the supervisor and supervisee will arrive in a timely fashion. The meeting place will be arranged to facilitate communication and both participants will be seated comfortably with no barriers between them. The chairs will be arranged so that the supervisor and supervisee are close to each other without violating culturally determined personal space. The supervisor will be relaxed and maintain appropriate eye contact while engaging in periodic head-nodding to encourage supervisee participation. The supervisor will enhance supervisee self-exploration by making psychological contact and exhibiting unconditional positive regard, empathy, genuineness, and congruence of verbal and nonverbal messages. The supervisor will pace the supervisee's verbal and nonverbal behaviors. The interaction will be solution-focused and have a combined clinician/client orientation. Supervisee growth will be stressed. In that regard, evidence of ongoing diagnosis and planning for the supervisee will be observable. From listening, it will be obvious that both supervisor and supervisee preplanning for the conference has taken place. An agenda for the meeting will be evident. The supervisory style will be predominantly collaborative although shifts toward directness or consultation will occur as needed. The supervisor will exhibit active listening by restating key points, asking for clarification, and prompting supervisee elaboration. The supervisor will also encourage the supervisee to engage in risk-taking. Finally, the content of the conference will be predominantly data-based analysis, problem-solving, and decision making in regard to both the clinical and supervisory process.

An optimal conference for supervisees at other levels of development will be similar in most ways. The aspects that can be expected to vary relate to the supervisee's stage along the continuum of supervision (Anderson, 1988). For example, for the beginning supervisee, more telling is likely to occur while consultation will predominate for the more experienced individual. The remaining issues—room and seating arrangements, verbal and non-verbal pacing, planning for the conference as well as the growth of the participants, active listening, and the fostering of appropriate risk-taking—will be similar independently of the level of the supervisee.

Conference Insights

As we draw to the close of this chapter, a return visit to the clinicians we met at the outset would be useful. The three clinicians are near the end of their practicum experience and are talking among themselves.

LINDA: Hey Gloria and Tom. Do you have time for lunch?

GLORIA: Sure.

TOM: I'm starved.

LINDA: Remember earlier when we were talking about how frustrated we were with our supervisors?

Gloria and Tom nod.

LINDA: I have been really surprised by Ms. Griffer. She's new and really into supervision. I didn't really understand what I was supposed to do in conferences until I worked with her. Last week when she observed, she even transcribed my directions to Mary Lou. She gave the data to me and that's what we talked about in our conference. I feel like I'm a partner working with her. A lot of times, after she puts data in my box, I see how successful I've been. I like being able to figure out a problem. And when we meet, I always have something ready to discuss with her.

GLORIA: Ms. Frieberg's OK too. She gives me a lot of positive feedback. She's a good listener, too. It's still hard though, never knowing when I'm going to meet with her.

TOM: Mr. Elton tries. We just aren't a good match. Maybe I'll get Griffer next time.

Linda is very pleased with the supervision she has received. Her supervisor, Ms. Griffer, has incorporated many aspects of effective supervision into her relationship with Linda. Gloria appreciates Ms. Frieberg's use of active listening. Tom, on the other hand, has been disappointed. His supervisor's behaviors have not matched his expectations. Their exchange highlights the impact of supervisor behavior on supervisee contentment with the process. Strategies in this chapter emphasize opportunities to improve the quality and productivity of supervision as well as increase supervisee satisfaction.

Relationship of Effective Conferencing to the Specified Supervision Tasks

The conference is the context in which the thirteen tasks of supervision are achieved. A constructive working relationship is built from the interactions that occur when the supervisor and supervisee confer. Trust and respect are a natural outgrowth. A major thrust of initial conferences is to assist the supervisee in thinking through and refining the assessment process. Then, thoughts typically shift to the analysis of the collected data as a means of forming the basis for selecting appropriate client objectives. Once goals are set, discussions tend to shift to the implementation and refinement of management skills. A key component is the honing of the supervisees' observation and then their analysis skills. This typically includes talk about accurate charting of client performance and the related record-keeping. This same mechanism also leads to supervisee self-analysis and the evaluation of performance in the clinical process. Strategies for asking clinical questions and observing events typically evolve into basic clinical and supervisory research skills. Clearly, conferences are most effective when supervisees have an active role in planning the topics to be discussed and then function as an active member of the dyad when the meeting takes place. As time elapses, clinical reports are submitted, providing the supervisor the opportunity to guide the supervisee in the refinement of writing and editing skills through written feedback and consultation regarding that information. Also during conferences, ethical, legal, regulatory, and reimbursement issues relating to clinical work are likely to emerge. Throughout the supervisory relationship, the supervisor has numerous opportunities to model professional behavior and to assist the supervisee in exhibiting professionalism and ethical behavior. This is particularly true if goals are set for both the supervisor and supervisee. In sum, the conference is the focal point in contributing to and/or achieving each of the thirteen tasks of supervision.

Summary

This chapter focuses on the supervisory conference. It begins with a review of the literature offering differing perceptions of the purpose of one-to-one interactions between the supervisor and supervisee. Clinicians' expectations for this process are then presented as are those of the supervisor. A dialogue among clinicians is described and is followed by an extensive section on the precursors for effective conferencing. These include preconference planning by the supervisor in the following areas: (1) conference focus, (2) conference philosophy, (3) style selection, (4) agenda determination, (5) supervisee variables, (6) clinician diagnosis, (7) site selection, and (8) furniture and seating arrangements. The supervisee is also expected to plan for the exchange. Strategies for initiating the meeting are then presented. These ideas are followed by a discussion of behaviors that facilitate communication: (1) verbal/nonverbal pacing, (2) positive interpersonal, and (3) active listening. The actual content of typical conferences is discussed and is then followed by a description of an optimal supervisory conference. The last segment of the chapter relates aspects of the conference to the realization of the thirteen tasks of supervision.

REFERENCES

Anderson, J. *The supervisory process in speech-language pathology and audiology.* Austin, TX: Pro-Ed, 1988.

Anderson, J. Personal communication, 1990.

Barrett-Lennard, G. "Dimensions of therapist response as causal factors in therapeutic change." *Psychology Monograph,* 76 (1962).

Blake, R., and McCanse, A. *Leadership grid.* Houston: Gulf Publishing, 1991.

Brasseur, J. "The supervisory process: A continuum perspective." *Language, Speech and Hearing Services in Schools 20,* (1989): 274–295.

Brasseur, J., and Jimenez, B. "Novice supervisees' attitude changes after active participation in the supervisory process." In B. Wagner. *Proceedings of the 1996 Conference on Clinical Supervision: Partnerships in Supervision: Innovative and Effective Practice.* Grand Forks, ND: University of North Dakota, 1996: 80–89.

Brooks, M. *Instant rapport.* New York: Warner Books, 1989.

Brown, E., and Block, F. "Evaluating supervision." Paper presented at the Annual Convention of the American Speech-Language and Hearing Association. Washington, D.C., 1975.

Caracciolo, G., Rigrodsky, S., and Morrison, E. "Perceived interpersonal conditions and professional growth of master's level speech-language pathology students during the supervisory process." *American Speech Hearing Association, 20* (1978a): 467–477.

Caracciolo, G., Rigrodsky, S., and Morrison, E. "A Rogerian orientation to the speech-language pathology supervisory relationship." *American Speech Hearing Association, 20* (1978b): 286–290.

Carkuff, R. *Helping and human relations: A primer for lay and professional helpers-I.* New York: Holt, Rinehart and Winston, 1969.

Casey, P., Smith, K., and Ulrich, S. *Self-supervision: A career tool for audiologists and speech-language pathologists.* Rockville, MD: National Student Speech Language Hearing Association, 1988.

Cashwell, C., Looby, E., and Housley, W. "Appreciating cultural diversity through clinical supervision. *The Clinical Supervisor, 15* (1) (1997): 75–85.

Cogan, M. *Clinical supervision.* Boston: Houghton-Mifflin, 1973.

Costa, A., and Garmston, R. "The art of cognitive coaching: Supervision for intelligent teaching." Workshop presented at the conference, "Supervision: Innovations" of the Council of Supervisors in Speech Pathology and Audiology. Sonoma County, 1989.

Costa, A., and Garmston, R. *Cognitive coaching: A foundation for renaissance schools.* Norwood, MA: Christopher Gordon Publishers, 1994.

Crago, M. "Supervision and self-exploration." In M. Crago and M. Pickering, *Supervision in communication disorders: Perspectives on a process.* San Diego, CA: Singular Publishing Group, 1987: 137–168.

Crespi, T. "Gender sensitive supervision: Exploring feminist perspectives for male and female supervisors." *The Clinical Supervisor, 13* (2) (1995): 19–29.

Culatta, R., and Seltzer, H. "Content and sequence analysis of the supervisory session. *American Speech Hearing Association, 18* (1976): 8–12.

Dowling, S. "Developing student self-supervisory skills in clinical training." *Journal of National Student Speech and Hearing Association, 7* (1979): 37–41.

Dowling, S. "Facilitating Clinical Training: Issues for Supervisees and their Supervisors." *Contemporary Issues in Communication Science and Disorders, 25* (1998): 5–11.

Dowling, S. "Students' perceptions of supervision at the end of clinical training." Unpublished, 1999.

Dowling, S. Conference Analysis. Working Document. University of Houston, 2000.

Dowling, S., and Shank, K. "A comparison of the effects of two supervisory styles, conventional and teaching clinic, in the training of speech and language pathologists." *Journal of Communication Disorders, 14* (1981): 51–58.

Dowling, S., and Wittkopp, J. "Student's perceived supervisory needs." *Journal of Communication Disorders, 15* (1982): 319–328.

Dussault, G. *Theory of supervision in teacher education.* New York: Teachers College Press, Columbia University, 1970.

Evans, M. "Supervision: A developmental–relational approach. *Transactional Analysis Journal, 28* (4) (1998): 288–298.

Farmer, S. *Supervisory conferences in communicative disorders: Verbal and nonverbal interpersonal communication pacing.* Doctoral dissertation, University of Colorado, 1983. *Dissertation Abstracts International, 44,* 2715B. (University Microfilms No. 84-00, 891).

Farmer, S. "Relationship development in supervisory conferences: A tripartite view of the process." *The Clinical Supervisor, 3* (4) (1985–1986): 5–21.

Farmer, S. "Conflict management and clinical supervision. *The Clinical Supervisor, 5* (1987): 5–28.

Farmer, S. "Communication competence." In S. Farmer and J. Farmer, (Eds.), *Supervision in Communication Disorders.* Columbus, OH: Merrill, 1989: 94–153.

Farmer, S. and Farmer, J. *Supervision in Communication Disorders.* Columbus, OH: Merrill, 1989.

Goodyear, R., and Bernard, J. "Clinical supervision: Lessons from the literature." *Counselor Education and Supervision, 38* (1) (1998): 6–22.

Hatfield, M., Bartlett, C., Caven, C., and Ueberle, J. "Supervision: The supervisee speaks." Paper presented at the Annual Convention of the American Speech-Language and Hearing Association, 1973.

Juhnke, G. "Solution-focused supervision: Promoting supervisee skills and confidence through successful solutions." *Counselor Education and Supervision, 36* (1996): 48–57.

Ladany, N., Ellis, M., and Friedlander, M. "The supervisory working alliance, trainee self-efficacy, and satisfaction." *Journal of Counseling and Development, 77* (1999): 447–455.

Ladany, N., and Lehrman-Waterman, D. "The content and frequency of supervisor self-disclosures and their relationship to supervisor style and the supervisory working alliance." *Counselor Education and Supervision, 38* (1999): 143–160.

Larson, L. Perceived supervisory needs and expectations of experienced vs. inexperienced student clinicians. (Doctoral dissertation, Indiana University, 1981). *Dissertation Abstracts International, 42,* 4758B. (University Microfilms No. 82-11, 183).

Logemann, J. "What is evidence-based practice and why should we care?" *ASHA Leader, 5* (2000): 3.

Long, L. *Listening/responding: Human Relations Training for Teachers.* Monterey, CA: Brooks/Cole, 1978.

Mawdsley, B., and Scudder, R. "The integrative task-maturity model of supervision." *Language, Speech, and Hearing Services in Schools, 20* (3) (1989): 305–315.

McBride, M., and Skau, K. "Trust, empowerment, and reflection: Essentials of supervision." *Journal of Curriculum and Supervision, 10* (3) (1995): 262–277.

McCrea, E. *Supervisee ability to self-explore and four facilitative dimensions of supervisor behavior in individual conferences in speech-language pathology* (Doctoral dissertation, Indiana University, 1980). *Dissertation Abstracts International, 41,* 2134B. (University Microfilms No. 80-29, 239).

McCready, V., Roberts, J., Bengala, D., Harris, H., Kingsley, G., and Krikorian, C. "A comparison of conflict tactics in the supervisory process." *Journal of Speech and Hearing Research, 39* (1996): 191–199.

McLeod, S. "Student self-appraisal: Facilitating mutual planning in clinical education." *The Clinical Supervisor, 15* (1) (1997): 87–101.

Mercaitis, P., and Peaper, R. "Strategies for helping supervisees to participate actively in the supervisory process." In D. Shapiro, (Ed.), *Supervision: Innovations A National Conference on Supervision.* Cullowhee, NC: Western Carolina University, 1989: 20–28.

Mercaitis, P. Personal communication, 1990.

Moses, N., and Shapiro, D. "Assessing and facilitating clinical problem solving in the supervisory process. In S. Dowling, (Ed.), *Proceedings of the 1992 National Conference on Supervision.* Houston: University of Houston, 1992: 70–77.

Moses, N., and Shapiro, D. "A developmental conceptualization of clinical problem solving." *Journal of Communication Disorders, 29* (1996): 199–221.

Muma, J. "Language intervention strategies." *Language Speech and Hearing Services in the Schools, 8* (1977): 107–125.

Nelson, M. "An interactional model for empowering women in supervision. *Counselor Education and Supervision, 37* (2) (1997): 125–138.

Peaper, R. "An analysis of student perceptions of the supervisory conference and student developed agendas for that conference." *The Clinical Supervisor, 2* (1984): 55–64.

Peaper, R., and Mercaitis, P. "Satisfactory and unsatisfactory supervisory experiences: Contributing factors." In D. Shapiro, (Ed.), *Supervision: Innovations A National Conference on Supervision.* Cullowhee, NC: Western Carolina University, 1989: 126–140.

Pickering, M. "An examination of concepts operative in the supervisory process and relationship." *American Speech Hearing Association, 19* (1977): 607–610.

Pickering, M. "Interpersonal communication in speech-language pathology supervisory conferences: A qualitative study." *Journal of Speech and Hearing Disorders, 49* (1984): 189–195.

Pickering, M. "Expectation and intent in the supervisory process." *The Clinical Supervisor, 5* (4) (1987a): 43–57.

Pickering, M. "Interpersonal communication and the supervisory process: A search for Ariadne's thread." In M. Crago and M. Pickering, *Supervision in Human Communication Disorders: Perspectives on a Process.* San Diego, CA: Singular Publishing Group, 1987b: 203–226.

Pickering, M. "The supervisory process: An experience of interpersonal relationships and personal growth." *National Student Speech Language Hearing Association Journal, 17* (1989–1990): 17–28.

Rassi, J. *Supervision in Audiology.* Baltimore: University Park Press, 1978.

Roberts, J., and Smith, K. "Supervisor–supervisee role differences and consistency of behavior in supervisory conferences." *Journal of Speech and Hearing Research, 25* (1982): 428–434.

Rockman, B. "Supervisor as clinician: A point of view." Paper presented at the Annual Convention of the American Speech and Hearing Association, Chicago, 1977.

Sbaschnig, K., Dowling, S., and Williams, C. "Causal attributions for clinical successes and failures in speech-language pathology treatment sessions." Paper presented at the Annual Convention of the American Speech-Language and Hearing Association. Seattle, WA, 1990.

Sells, J., Lichtenberg, J., Goodyear, R., and Polkinghorne, D. "Relationship of supervisor and trainee gender to in-session verbal behavior and ratings of trainee skills." *Journal of Counseling Psychology, 44* (4) (1997): 406–412.

Shapiro, D. "Professional preparation and lifelong learning: The making of a clinician." In D. Shapiro, (Ed.), *Stuttering Intervention: A Collaborative Journey to Fluency Freedom.* Austin, TX, Pro-Ed, 1998: 474–571

Shapiro, D., and Anderson, J. "One measure of supervisory effectiveness in speech-language pathology and audiology." *Journal of Speech and Hearing Disorders, 54* (4) (1989): 549–557.

Smith, K., and Anderson, J. "Relationship of perceived effectiveness to content in supervisory conferences in speech-language pathology." *Journal of Speech and Hearing Research, 25* (1982): 243–251.

Sommer, R. *Personal space.* New Jersey: Prentice-Hall, 1969.

Strike-Roussos, C. *Supervisors' implementation of trained information regarding broad questioning and discussion of supervision during their supervisory conferences in speech-language pathology.* Doctoral Dissertation, Indiana University, Bloomington, IN, 1988. *Dissertation Abstracts International 49,* 09B. (University Microfilms No. DEW 8824185, 3710).

Tihen, L. *Expectations of student speech/language clinicians during their clinical practicum.* (Doctoral dissertation, Indiana University, 1983). *Dissertation Abstracts International, 44,* 3048B. (University Microfilms No. 84-01, 620).

Wagner, B., and Hess, C. "Supervisees' Perceptions of Supervisors' Social Power in Speech-Language Pathology." *American Journal of Speech-Language Pathology, 6* (3) (1997): 90–94.

APPENDIX 4-A
Guidelines for Supervisees
on Preparing for Supervision

A. Pre-Supervision

1. Choose one case. Videotape or audiotape a clinical or supervisory session.
2. Watching and listening to the tape, choose three segments, each about 5 minutes long:
   If you observed the session
   a. One segment in which the session was effective
   b. One segment in which the session was ineffective
   c. One segment that surprised you
   If you conducted the session
   a. One segment in which you were satisfied with your performance
   b. One segment in which you were dissatisfied with your performance
   c. One segment that surprised you

3. For each segment, write down your impressions concerning:
   If you observed the session
   a. What you learned from this segment
   b. Your feelings/reactions during this segment, that is, the impact of the patient/client on you
   c. The effect or impact of the therapist's intervention on the patient/client
   If you conducted the session
   a. Your skill as a clinician in this segment
   b. Your feelings/reactions during this segment, that is, the impact of the patient/client to you
   c. The effect or impact of your intervention on the patient/client

4. Choose one of the three segments to present during supervision. Write down why you have chosen this segment.

B. In-Supervision

1. Present the case, the clinical or supervisory segment, and why you chose it.
2. Identify the "problem" you want to deal with.
3. Define your objectives vis-à-vis this segment and this supervision session (e.g., want to determine a clear plan of what to do next time).
4. Identify your expectations of your supervisor (e.g., want confirming feedback that you handled the situation well).
5. Choose the method by which you feel you can best be helped in this supervision session (e.g., tape review, discussion, role-play).
6. Using the method chosen, go over the interview segment with the supervisor and self-evaluate a, b, and c.
7. Check your self-evaluation with your supervisor's feedback on a, b, and c.

Crago, M. "Supervision and self-exploration." In M. Crago and M. Pickering, (Eds.), *Supervision in Human Communication Disorders: Perspectives on a Process.* San Deigo, CA: College Hill, 1987: 162–163. Reprinted with permission of the authors.

8. Work out incongruent evaluations.
9. Explore with your supervisor alternatives for strategies whereby you can change certain behaviors or ways of interacting with patient/client.
10. Try out alternative chosen in role-play situation.
11. Self-evaluate "new behavior" and check out with supervisor's feedback.
12. Evaluate the supervision session (e.g., What did you learn? What plan of action resulted from it? Did this session respond to your needs?)

C. Post-Supervision

1. Write down what you learned from the supervision session.
2. Determine what you will do about the feedback you received.
3. Identify what you should be working on this week to improve or maintain your performance.
4. If the supervision session did not respond to your needs, identify the reasons for this (e.g., you did not present your objectives for this session clearly enough, therefore, time was spent on material that was unimportant to you).
5. Identify how you can prepare for the next session so that you get the feedback you need.
6. Set up goals for next supervision session.

PART THREE

Supervising People

CHAPTER

5 Supervising Clinical Training

Clinical Supervision Tasks Relevant to Supervising in Clinical Training

Task 1: Establishing and maintaining an effective working relationship with the supervisee;

Task 2: Assisting the supervisee in developing clinical goals and objectives;

Task 3: Assisting the supervisee in developing and refining assessment skills;

Task 4: Assisting the supervisee in developing and refining clinical management skills;

Task 5: Demonstrating for and participating with the supervisee in the clinical process;

Task 6: Assisting the supervisee in observing and analyzing assessment and treatment sessions;

Task 7: Assisting the supervisee in the development and maintenance of clinical and supervisory records;

Task 8: Interacting with the supervisee in planning, executing, and analyzing supervisory conferences;

Task 9: Assisting the supervisee in evaluation of clinical performance;

Task 10: Assisting the supervisee in developing skills of verbal reporting, writing, and editing;

Task 11: Sharing information regarding ethical, legal, regulatory, and reimbursement aspects of professional practice;

Task 12: Modeling and facilitating professional conduct; and

Task 13: Demonstrating research skills in the clinical or supervisory process.

Clinical experience is at the heart of preparing individuals to work as speech-language pathologists and audiologists. Generally, practicum experiences are divided between a university training facility and externship sites. The needs of supervisees will vary depending on their level of experience, competence, and site of service. The nature and practice of supervision will change in response to the above variables. Following background information and a discussion of general issues relating to the supervision of trainees, the progression of the supervisee from the initial practicum to the externship experience will be used as the organizational structure for this chapter. This will include the acculturation of the supervisee to various settings and variations in supervision appropriate for supervisees at differing levels of competence. The chapter will end with a discussion of the relationship of the thirteen tasks of supervision to the supervision of clinicians at varying stages of skill development.

Supervisor Beginning Thoughts

A discussion among three supervisors highlights some of the issues relating to the supervision of trainees at different levels of experience and skill.

> **JOHN:**   I just picked up my supervisee/client assignments. I really have a mix of clinicians this time. I have been debating about the best way to get them all off on the right foot.
>
> **SALLY:**   Me too, although all of mine are new clinicians. They are so scared at the beginning. I am hoping that at least part of them will become active conference participants by the end of the term. I am concerned about one in particular because she has just scraped through on her coursework.
>
> **STEPHANIE:**   I have two who are just wrapping up their clock hours. I want them to function as independently as possible. I am going to need to think about how to do that.
>
> **SALLY:**   Supervision is always a challenge. I wish I had more information about differences among clinicians and ways to make my supervision more effective for them.
>
> **JOHN:**   Me too.

The concerns expressed by these supervisors are frequently voiced. The material that follows will be helpful to them.

Literature

Theory

Numerous theorists suggest that supervision should be an active, changing process responding to the level of the supervisee. Cogan (1973), a proponent of clinical supervision in education, proposes the idea of molding the process to fit the needs of the person being supervised. In business, Hersey and Blanchard (1988) discuss the life-cycle model, which suggests the use of four different styles of supervision, depending on the individual's level of readiness. A determination of the supervisees' level of development is based on task-relevant skills/education, their level of personal maturity, and their need for achievement. Mawdsley and Scudder (1989) subsequently adapt the Hersey and Blanchard model for speech-language pathology and integrate it with the Cogan (1973) model of supervision. Anderson (1988), in speech-language pathology, proposes a continuum of supervision with supervisor styles ranging from direct to consultative, paralleling the supervisee's evolution through three stages: evaluation/feedback, transition, and self-supervision. Farmer (1989) proposes a multiple-strand style matrix for use with supervisees performing at varying levels of competence. Dowling (1992), and each of the above scholars, suggest that the content of supervision should vary depending on factors such as supervisor/supervisee skill levels, the participants' interpersonal styles, and the nature and complexity of given clients' management.

Practice

In contrast to the goal of varying supervision in response to supervisee need, research in speech-language pathology demonstrates that the supervisory styles of untrained supervisors tend to be static across time, clinician, and the clinician's level of development. Roberts and Smith (1982) find that supervisors dominate conferences by controlling topic initiation and talk time with no evidence of variability in response to individual supervisees. Similarly, Smith (1979) reports that supervisors maintain control by asking numerous questions. Ingrisano, Guinty, Chambers, McDonald, Clem, and Cory (1979) show that supervisory conference behaviors are stagnant from one training site to another and across varying levels of supervisee clinical experience. Further, Culatta and Seltzer (1976, 1977) determine that supervisor talk tends to be direct and unchanging across time or clinician, even when the supervisor has expressed a desire for change, and Cimorell-Strong and Ensley (1982) note that, even with feedback from supervisees about their behavior, supervisors do not alter their conference talk. Joshi and McAllister (1998) suggest that untrained supervisors do not modify the supervision they provide because they are unclear about the behaviors that characterize a given style such as direct or indirect. Thus, even if supervisors desire change they may not know which behaviors will enhance their conferencing skills. In sum, the research documents a discrepancy between desired and actual supervision practice.

In the field of education, Zahorik (1988) examines university student teacher supervisors, their methods, and supervisory styles, and finds them to be constant and unchanging, independently of the individual being supervised. He goes on to acknowledge the importance of varying supervisory approaches depending on the goal of supervision and the supervisee's stage of learning, and indicates that the ideal is to alter the manner of supervision in relation to the given circumstance. Thus, if individual supervisors exhibit a fixed style and are unable to make modifications as needed, he suggests matching the supervisors, based on their methods and goals, to supervisees who can best benefit from that approach. As a result, supervision will not be a random type of assignment. Rather, supervisors and student teachers will be matched to create optimal pairs.

There is also a body of research demonstrating that training in supervision enhances the quality of supervision. Sbaschnig and Williams (1983) demonstrate that supervisors can become more consistent in the evaluation of supervisees by establishing guidelines for them and making active efforts to modify their behavior. Hagler (1986) shows that supervisors can decrease their talk time in the conference if given a directive to talk less through a "bug-in the ear" during the actual conference. Dowling (1986) finds that trained supervisors do supervise differently in response to individual supervisees, and Barrow and Domingo (1997) note that trained supervisors are able to change their conference behavior. According to their research, supervisors who receive ten hours of training relating to supervision research, supervisory models, conferencing, and the ASHA competencies for supervisors modify their conference behavior. The trained supervisors and their supervisees rate subsequent conferences as having more supervisor behaviors classified as indirect, fewer that are direct in nature, and an increase in the supervisees' expressions of their supervisory process needs. Trained supervisors also rate themselves as being more supportive and better able to help supervisees set realistic goals. Brasseur (1989) determines that supervisory training allows participants to add behaviors not previously in their repertoires and Dowling (1991, 1994) demonstrates that supervisors in training who set goals and then strive to meet them are able to modify their conference talk behavior. Thus, with training, supervisors can use a supervisory style more compatible with theory. Educating the supervisee may also be a factor as work by Dowling (1988) indicates that training affects supervisee attitudes toward supervision.

Summary

Theory indicates that supervision is at its best when supervisors alter their behaviors in response to the needs of supervisees; in practice, however, supervision is often static and unchanging. With supervisory training or specific guidance, supervisors are able to change their behavior. This ability to modify behavior is critical to the implementation of the ideas to be considered in this chapter as the purpose is to discuss the supervision of supervisees at different levels of development. Therefore, to meaningfully address this topic, two assumptions must be made. The first is that supervisors recognize differences among supervisees. The second is that supervisors have the potential to modify their own behavior in response to different individuals and circumstances.

Continuum of Supervision

Anderson's (1988) continuum of supervision is an excellent framework for considering variations needed to supervise people with differing levels of experience and ability. She identifies three stages of supervision: evaluation/feedback, transition, and self-supervision. During the evaluation/feedback phase, she suggests a direct or active supervisory style, which means that a significant amount of telling occurs. In essence, the supervisee is given specific directives on how to proceed.

She then encourages the supervisor to introduce a collaborative approach as quickly and in as much depth as possible. The intent is to assist the supervisee in moving into the transitional stage of supervision. In this stage, both participants are actively responsible for the clinical and supervisory interaction. This includes planning, observing, analyzing, problem-solving, and decision making. The key characteristic is the joint assumption of responsibility for both the clinical and supervisory process with decreasing direct supervisor involvement. The final stage of supervision is self-supervision. The supervisor's role, at this point, then shifts to one of consultation. Anderson's (1988) model appears in Figure 5.1.

A unique aspect of this model rests in its fluid nature. Supervisors will actively teach, stimulate, and guide the development of supervisees to foster their movement through the continuum of supervision. Anderson further stresses that shifts in supervisory style—*direct/active, collaborative, consultative*—should be responsive to variations in the needs and abilities of the supervisee. For example, if a supervisee in the evaluation-feedback stage exhibits the ability to analyze a specific type of behavior, the supervisor should adopt a collaborative style in regard to that particular domain. Similarly, if the clinician who is in the transitional or self-supervision stage requires specific, direct input, the supervisor will move into a direct/active style to address a given area or situation of concern.

The points along the Anderson continuum appropriate for use in supervising clinicians at various levels of experience and skill will be identified as each group is discussed in this chapter. Indeed, this model provides the framework for the discussion of supervisees at varying stages of development. It is important to note that supervisees functioning at the three levels of performance—marginal, average, and outstanding—also cut across other methods of categorization of them,

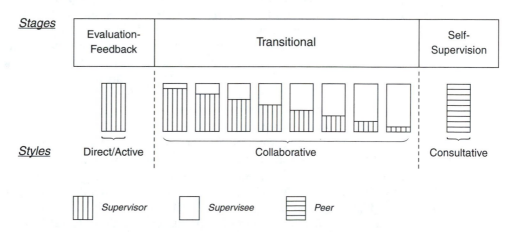

FIGURE 5.1 Composite of Stages of Supervision and the Appropriate Styles For Each Stage.

Reprinted with permission from Anderson, J. *The Supervisory Process in Speech-Language Pathology and Audiology.* Austin, TX: Pro-Ed, 1988, 62.

such as beginning, advanced, or undergraduate and graduate clinician. In addition, supervisees can shift among the levels. The average performer may evolve to be one who is exceptional. Likewise, the marginal clinician may improve. In other cases, supervisees may, initially, be so overwhelmed that they are unable to function. With sufficient structure, they may gain control of the situation and evolve into strong clinicians. Thus, people must be viewed and interacted with on the level at which they are performing at a given time, and great care must be taken to accurately diagnose their level of development and to select the appropriate supervisory approach (Anderson, 1988; Rockman, 1977).

Recall also the classic work in education that identifies teacher expectation as a key to performance (Rosenthal and Jacobson, 1968). When teachers are told that specific children, who have been randomly selected, will "bloom" that year, the designated children significantly outperform their classmates. The only difference is the attitude held by the teachers toward them. Thus, independently of initial performance, supervisees benefit from supervisors who sense, anticipate, and communicate to them that they will be competent and will improve. Similarly, literature in goal-setting has demonstrated that expectations that are slightly out of reach but are perceived as achievable enhance overall performance (Taylor, Fisher, and Ilgen, 1984; DeShon and Alexander, 1996).

Characteristics of Supervisees

According to the work of Moses and Shapiro (1996), variations in problem-solving skills differentiate clinicians at varying levels of clinical development. Beginning clinicians see the clinical process predominantly from their own perspective and assume that they are entirely in control of client learning, consider limited number of variables in their approach to an issue, and tend to generate only one solution to the problem. In contrast, an experienced clinician is more likely to see the clinical process from the client's perspective as well as his or her own, understands that multiple factors relate to a problem, and can generate multiple options for dealing with a projected event during treatment. Thus, cognitive style levels are one factor that differentiates groups of supervisees, and Tryon's (1996) work documents that growth in thinking, autonomy, and self-awareness do occur as supervisees move through the training process.

Another factor is the supervisee's level of clinical skill. In regard to marginal, average, and outstanding trainees, Hagler, Madill, Kampfe, and Mitchell (1990) found that 64 percent of student scores on the W-PACC evaluation tool (Shriberg, Filley, Hayes, Kwiatkowski, Shatz, Simmons, and Smith, 1975) can be predicted by four traits: (1) ability to use coping strategies and seek support; (2) grade-point average; (3) age; (4) marital status at the time of the clinical practicum.

To clarify the characteristics of supervisees at different skill levels, Dowling (1985), using a tool validated by Dowling and Bliss (1984), asked forty-three supervisors to complete two clinician evaluation scales, one for a hypothetical outstanding clinician and another for one who is failing. According to the respondents, outstanding clinicians are competent in all areas evaluated. The middle category, average, are seen as exhibiting satisfactory performance throughout or having a weakness in isolated areas, such as diagnosis, time usage, or writing, but having acceptable or better performance in the remaining aspects. Failing clinicians, in contrast, are viewed as weak across the board. Chamberlain and Gallagher (1974) discuss strategies for identifying and dealing with the marginal clinician. They report that poor academic performance and/or weak interpersonal skills increase the probability that the supervisee will have trouble clinically, but they stress that it is difficult to predict the quality of a student's performance prior to direct involvement. A consistent characteristic of the marginal clinician is difficulty in applying academic material to actual clinical situations. The responding supervisors' comments (Dowling, 1985) about this latter group included: "cannot work independently," "unable to formulate goals and procedures," "basic gaps in conceptual understanding," and "difficulty following through with suggestions."

Impressions of Supervisees

One would like to think that supervisees who come through a similar training sequence will perform comparably in a clinical environment. In practice, this does not always prove to be true. In this regard, Schermerhorn, Gardner, and Martin (1990) state that three primary factors contribute to the quality of individual performance: ability, effort, and available support. The performance of clinicians, then, may diverge markedly for varying reasons. For example, they may differ in innate ability and/or level of commitment. They may complete the same coursework but have diverged in effort and time applied to learning. They may attach differing degrees of importance to the value of learned information, or vary in their ability to translate classroom content into clinical application. External circumstances, such as the presence/absence of personal support systems or financial problems, may further fragment the focus of their efforts. A lack of perceived support from supervisors can also be a factor.

In general, the assumption is made that those who are strong academically will perform better clinically. Conversely, those who demonstrate marginal performance in the classroom often have significant difficulties in clinical practice. In practice, there are exceptions to these generalizations. In isolated instances, weak students are superb in practicum, and an individual who excels academically may be unable to translate that knowledge into acceptable clinical performance.

Supervisors, in discussing clinicians of varying ability levels, often express concern about the amount of time devoted to the respective groups, *marginal, average* and *outstanding*. They feel a disproportionate amount of effort is directed to supervisees having significant difficulties, often at the expense of the outstanding performer. This dilemma, from a supervisory and ethical perspective, is not easy to resolve.

Potential for Bias

It is safe to assume that supervisees will bring differing levels of cognitive development, ability, and skill to their practicum experience, but supervisors may also bring biases to the same interaction that can affect ultimate outcomes. Variability in supervisor evaluation of treatment is documented in the literature. For example, Blodgett, Schmitt, and Scudder (1987) report significant differences in the valuative rating of the identical videotape of therapy among supervisors from three different programs, and hypothesize that the degree of familiarity with the clinician may have affected ratings. Further, recognizing the variability inherent in supervisor evaluations, Sbaschnig and Williams (1983) have developed a training protocol to reduce this variation, and report that three terms of work are necessary to reduce these discrepancies to an agreed-on level.

Andersen (1981) has unequivocally demonstrated the potential for supervisor bias. Anderson studied the ratings of fifty-six supervisors who were given varying written information about a supervisee. For example, the clinician was said to have a grade-point average of 2.5 or 3.5, had earned 23 or 210 clock hours, and had an acceptable or outstanding record of past clinical and conference behavior. After being given the written information, the supervisors were shown a videotape of therapy that they were asked to evaluate. The ratings of the supervisors were found to increase with the clinician's grade-point average and previous evaluations of outstanding clinical and conference behavior. Higher grades also enhanced the supervisors' perceptions of the person's clinical performance although the number of clock hours did not affect the scorings. Less favorable data has the reverse effect in that the supervisee was viewed more negatively.

Given the susceptibility to bias, it behooves supervisors and classroom teachers to minimize the information exchanged about current or future supervisees. This includes academic performance, interpersonal style, impressions of and experiences with the individual. Withholding opinions at times creates ethical dilemmas and may result in weak supervisees being placed in a clinical assignment significantly beyond their abilities. On the other hand, sharing of past experiences sets the stage for predisposing supervisor attitudes toward that person. In situations in which it is critical to share information for the well-being of a supervisee, supervisors will need to make a conscious effort to minimize biases that may color their interactions with the supervisee.

With the background information now in place, thoughts will turn specifically to the supervision of supervisees at different levels of experience and skill. Although this discussion is oriented to the supervisee in training, some of the same methods can be used with working professionals performing at similar levels of skill.

Supervision of the Beginning Clinician

Supervisee Acculturation

As they begin their first practicum experience, supervisees need to feel they are an integral part of the clinical program in which they are participating. They are often new to a facility and feel adrift. An orientation to discuss general clinical operation is helpful. This may include procedures for getting assignments, selecting a treatment room, signing out materials and files, scheduling appointments with supervisors, contacting clientele, and learning to use evaluation instruments. In addition, a tour of the facility and the provision of a personal mailbox, and work and lounge areas will assist new clinicians in becoming acclimated.

A broad discussion of the clinic philosophy early in the relationship is also helpful to students. This may include a statement of organizational values such as: "Our goal is to guide you as you develop into the finest clinician possible." "Our mission is to provide the highest quality of service to patients." It will be important to show supervisees how they fit into this organizational mission. Understanding how they contribute will help them establish their own professional identity. In addition, to increase the satisfaction of individuals within a facility, trainees need to feel valued and respected, and to perceive that they are integral members of the clinical service team.

To aid in the acculturation process, it is helpful to identify basic competencies that supervisees need to exhibit to successfully begin the clinic process. The following is a list of examples: how to learn a test protocol; how to order a clinic file appropriately; how to administer an oral–peripheral examination and compare it to normal structure and function; how to write a clinic objective with a progression of steps in task difficulty that will achieve the goal; how to write a lesson plan; how to use at least four behavior management strategies; how to administer and interpret a defined group of assessment tools; how to define an appropriate assessment protocol for a client; how and when to use the mainstream language in both its spoken and written form; how to use reinforcement strategies appropriate for children and adults; and how to comport oneself appropriately with clients and caregivers. Taylor and Horney (1997) add to this list the ability to self-evaluate how their own behavior affects client performance.

As part of the orientation process, trainees may be told that prior to the onset of clinic they need to pass a proficiency examination in each of the above areas. If they do not demonstrate proficiency, their clinic practicum will be delayed until they possess the appropriate skills. This strategy will alert the trainees to fundamental skills and require them to take responsibility for acquiring those they do not have prior to clinic enrollment. Having these basic skills will enhance their clinic performance, safeguard services to clients and minimize staff frustration.

There are two additional acculturation strategies that may be useful. To facilitate a supervisee's entrance into clinical practice, Perkins and Mercaitis (1995) use a clinical practicum guide (see Chapter 3, Appendix A) with the expected competencies broken down into progressive weekly increments. The first four weeks of the guide focus on planning and the remainder on treatment strategies and the provision of closure at the end of sessions. These guides are then used to structure the supervisee's treatment planning, to organize supervisor feedback from observations, and to provide the basis for discussion in the conference. Perkins and Mercaitis report that supervisees who used the guides perceived greater clinical growth than those who did not.

The other strategy is the use of a clinical competency portfolio, developed at the University of Alberta (Pickering, Rassi, Hagler, and McFarlane, 1992), that

provides a source of integration for both a clinician's academic and clinical training. It is a valuable tool for the acculturation of new clinicians because it contains
an ongoing record of the trainee's professional development in addition to his or
her academic training in an area and relevant experiences. It is introduced during orientations and used to focus discussion on relevant experiences and competencies and the areas in which continuing growth is needed. This profile then
follows the trainee throughout his or her training experiences, including externships, and is continually updated to present a "cumulative portrait of a student's
knowledge and skills" (p. 58.) Both tools aid new clinicians as they begin their
journey into clinical training. Rassi and McElroy (1992) have described a similar
strategy for use in training audiologists.

Goals

New clinicians begin with a clean slate and several goals they are expected to
achieve. During their first term, they are expected to learn to function clinically,
that is, how to assess their clients accurately and provide the appropriate treatment. In addition, they have to become accurate observers of their own behavior
and that of their clients (Dowling, 1998), and learn how to analyze the impact
of their own behavior on the clinical process (Taylor and Horney, 1997). Self-
evaluation becomes particularly important when a strategy is not working
because it provides the basis for active problem-solving. Another objective for new
clinicians is that they begin the process of professional development and make a
commitment to lifelong learning in order to build and maintain their clinical
competence (Kamhi, 1995; Goldberg, 1995). Finally, they must become increasingly active participants in the supervisory process and partners in their own
professional development.

Strategies

Several strategies are appropriate for the beginning clinician. On a global level,
a discussion of the supervisory process, supervisee diagnosis, data collection,
and goal-setting will be of value. On a more specific level, joint planning,
demonstration of therapy techniques, audio- and videotape, verbatim recordings, and a dialogue regarding tools to be used for supervisee evaluation are
helpful.

Prior to and as part of the first practicum, discussion of the supervisory
process is useful and the Anderson continuum of supervision may be used as a tool
to discuss the nature of supervision. Talking with them about this plan for growth
empowers supervisees. Initially, beginning clinicians will be in the feedback stage
of the model, and they need to understand that it is in their best interest to move
along the continuum of supervision toward collaboration. This means they will be
expected, as they are able, to take increasing responsibility for problem-solving
and active participation in the conference. After this discussion, it will be helpful
to diagnose both the supervisee's and the supervisor's levels of development to

ascertain where, on the continuum, supervision will begin. After the supervisee has settled in and is demonstrating the beginnings of proficiency, data collection will be introduced as a tool for problem-solving and as a mechanism to begin the supervisee's movement toward collaborative discussions in the conference. In addition, supervisee goals will be set to foster growth along the continuum toward professional independence.

In their first practicum experience, clinicians are likely to need greater structure and support than they will later in their careers (Harris, Ludington, Ringwalt, Ballard, Hooper, Buoyer, and Price, 1991–1992). Joint planning, even some joint lesson plan writing, and demonstration of therapy techniques may be useful. Audio- and videotapes of their own performance during sessions treatment, used in appropriate amounts, will help beginning clinicians to perceive their treatment behaviors as others might.

They are also likely to need concrete, frequent feedback in the early phases of their first practicum. This feedback can take the form of checklists, verbatim recordings of events in treatment sessions, and, later, collected data. Joint discussions of the perceived importance and meaning of the items on evaluation forms will assist supervisees in targeting those behaviors that will improve their performance; they also benefit from evaluating their own performance first and then comparing it to the supervisor's evaluation of the same treatment session. The latter practice increases the accuracy of the supervisee's self-evaluation. Donnelly and Glaser (1992) have shown that providing a structure for and training in self-evaluation enhance the supervisee's ability to do so.

Conference

In considering the Anderson continuum of supervision, beginning clinicians will generally begin in the evaluation/feedback stage in which the supervisor does a lot of telling. For many clinicians, a movement into the transitional state with reasonable amounts of collaboration will occur before the end of that first term. Supervisors will need to be sensitive to the signs that signal readiness in the supervisee. When appropriate, the supervisor will introduce data collection and encourage the supervisee to analyze events occurring in treatment and propose strategies. Thus, the nature of the conference is likely to change during this first clinical experience from supervisor dominance to one reflecting more equality. Supervisee factors, such as competence and personal development, will determine the nature of conferences and the rate of movement toward collaboration for clinicians in the first practicum.

Outcomes

By the end of the first practicum, most supervisees will have a clinical foundation on which to build, but some will still be struggling. Differences among clinicians, related to their general skill level, will have emerged. The question is then, How does one supervise clinicians who have differing levels of skill?

Supervision of the Marginal Clinician

Identification

Dowling (1985) reports that marginal clinicians cannot work independently, are unable to formulate goals and procedures, have basic gaps in conceptual understanding, and cannot follow through with suggestions. The following descriptions of hypothetical supervisees show how the traits frequently exhibited by marginal clinicians can be identified by supervisors.

> Sue had difficulty assessing her client. In particular, she had trouble recognizing significant behaviors and did not identify areas that needed additional testing. Numerous errors in both administration and scoring were evident. Once she had obtained accurate information, she was unable to translate the data into meaningful objectives for her clients. After goals had been established, her therapy implementation consistently lacked focus.

> Mary Lou typically arrived at the audiology suite just as patients arrived in the waiting room. At times, she had not read the case history information beforehand. She was able to assess pure tone hearing acuity adequately but often forgot to follow up by testing spondee words. On more than one occasion, she failed to examine the tympanic membrane before attempting to insert the probes used to obtain a tympanogram. Mary Lou, if asked, would indicate that her performance was better than average.

> Tom collected incomplete test data but did not realize that he had done so. Some of the objectives he selected were not only inappropriate but were based on hunches rather than data. Subsequently, his treatment proceeded in an illogical manner, and his reinforcement patterns were erratic. His implementation of language therapy, in particular, did not parallel legitimate theory or consist of accepted procedures. Ironically, Tom did not ask questions, ask for suggestions, or apparently perceive that he had a problem.

> Chris was minimally aware that her therapy was poor but did not know what to do about it. Frequently, she did not grasp the need for change, although she did make modifications if she were told to do so. She often persisted in inappropriate behavior, and seemed unable to see the total therapy picture. Thus, when she made an improvement in one area, she thought all aspects of her therapy were better, even though the area changed may have been minimally important in the overall picture. Her writing skills were in the average range.

> Sally was enthusiastic and felt that her treatment skills were at least average or better, but she did acknowledge that some sessions were better than others. For those that were weak, she consistently identified an external cause for the weakness, such as the client didn't feel well or she had been tired. When the supervisor provided collected data in the conference or provided it to her at the end of an observation, she would look at it but show little or no comprehension of the meaning of the data or its application for her day-to-day strategy development. Even with guidance from the supervisor, Sally exhibited little evidence that she could analyze her therapy techniques. Her problem-solving skills were minimal in regard to not only what had occurred but, also in relation to potential alternatives and future strategies.

Sam was floundering in all aspects of treatment. Planning, implementation, and behavior management were marginal at best. His writing was an area in which he openly indicated he was having difficulty. His reporting of data was incomplete and did not follow in a logical manner. Spelling and grammatical errors were scattered throughout his work. Even when these were repeatedly marked by the supervisor, the same mistakes intermittently reappeared when the reports were resubmitted. In addition, a grammatical or spelling error corrected early in the report continued to surface in other places.

In practice, the marginal supervisee rapidly surfaces as being representative of this category. Difficulties typically emerge during initial testing or become clearly evident within the first few weeks of therapy. With time, the pervasiveness of the problem becomes increasingly obvious. Tom, Chris, and Sally are prime examples of an issue that often emerges with marginal clinicians: They are unable to accurately self-evaluate and often misperceive their level of competence (Kruger and Dunning, 1999).

Goals

Goals for supervisees at this level of development vary significantly. The primary thrust is to assist them in functioning at least at a minimally acceptable level. A further reasonable aspiration is that they will evolve into qualified professionals. For those who do not grow and whose performance remains in the incompetent range, career counseling with the intent of helping them to choose an alternate profession becomes an important focus.

Strategies

A first step in considering a strategy is to determine the appropriate supervisory approach. The supervisee functioning in the marginal range fits best in the Anderson evaluation–feedback stage of supervision in which a direct/active supervisor style is appropriate. This directive style of supervision means that the supervisor is likely to ask questions, give both positive, negative feedback, engage in problem-solving, actively generate strategies and give the supervisee concrete guidance in both the assessment and treatment realms (Smith and Anderson, 1982).

With the supervisee at this level of development, data collection may prove to be more of a hindrance than a help. Supervisors may choose to collect data for documentation purposes or use it themselves to give the supervisee concrete feedback. The supervisee is likely to feel overwhelmed, however, even bordering on the inability to function. Requests by the supervisor for the supervisee to collect data are likely to be viewed as an increased burden with minimal return for the effort. Because such clinicians are functioning on a need-to-know basis, they may be unable to see the relevance of the collected data to the upcoming therapy session. The supervisor's presentation of this type of information with the expectation that the supervisee will problem-solve may be equally meaningless.

There are exceptions, of course. The rare struggling supervisee may be able to take objective feedback and translate it into improved performance. It is almost as if it serves as the missing key they are seeking to unravel the therapy puzzle. For this reason, it may be useful to present data initially and, depending on the supervisee's reaction to and use of this information, make a decision about the appropriateness of this as an ongoing strategy.

For the supervisee functioning at the marginal level, specific supervisor strategies are likely to be beneficial. These may include joint planning, role-playing, demonstration therapy, structured observations, videotape/audiotape, and selected verbatim illustrations. In addition, data collection and analysis should be incorporated as soon as it can be used meaningfully. The first of these methods, joint planning, may vary in content. Initially, it may be the actual writing of a lesson plan or objectives. It may even be a step-by-step map for carrying out a specific therapy activity. Following the formulation of the plan, the supervisee may find it helpful to role-play the procedure with the supervisor while assuming either the position of the client or clinician. This approach allows the supervisee to practice a skill in a safe environment in which feedback is readily available. Often joint planning will of necessity focus on one aspect of treatment. As areas of difficulty are resolved, planning can then shift to other concerns.

Demonstration therapy, or assistance by a clinician with the use of specific skills, is also extremely helpful. Provision of therapy by another person allows the supervisee to observe a successful interaction and provides concrete guidance for future implementation. A person in the role of model who is particularly skilled in an area, such as behavior management, may demonstrate or guide the supervisee within the context of the therapy session. This shows struggling clinicians how to work with their own clients. Demonstration therapy, whether by the supervisor or a clinical assistant, is most acceptable to the supervisee when it is preplanned and/or requested by the clinician. Research shows that supervisees strenuously object to unannounced interruptions (Dowling and Wittkopp, 1982).

Structured observations may be extremely helpful to at-risk supervisees. They may be encouraged to watch other clinicians who exhibit a strength in an area in which they are having difficulty, for example. Observing others work successfully often provides them with ideas and strategies for resolving the problem in their own therapy. While watching, supervisees can also benefit from recording or charting the behaviors that they are being asked to observe. The informal data collection methods described in Chapter 2 or the Mawdsley's Kansas Inventory of Self-Supervision (1987) might be used to achieve this end. Incorporating a limited amount of data will assist these people in identifying cause and effect. It will also help them begin to see the value of accurate observation and the relevance of collected data for strengthening their clinical performance. Feedback regarding the accuracy of their observations and data collection will aid them in becoming more proficient.

Videotape and audiotape are also excellent tools for the marginal supervisee. With these tools as an aid, they may begin to step out of themselves and start to view their therapy as others might. It also allows them the opportunity to identify their own strengths and areas needing growth. In conferences, the actual behaviors can be observed so that examples of skills or weaknesses are available for discussion. This may also lead to concrete discussions of how to amplify or change behavior. Further, during the observation of the tape, the supervisor may demonstrate the collection and interpretation of data critical to the supervisee's success. The application of this information on a concrete level can then be discussed.

A selected verbatim approach (Acheson and Gall, 1992) might also be used with audio- or videotape. For example, the supervisor or supervisee might transcribe the supervisee's directions or models during an activity as a means for feedback. Anderson (1988) suggests that transcribing the session might also be used to bring home the quality of the total interaction. The purpose to be served and the projected benefits need, as with any procedure, to be weighed against the time required for either the supervisor or supervisee to carry out this strategy.

Documentation by the supervisor of the supervisee's performance is significant for all supervisees but is critical for those with marginal performance. Great care must be taken to collect concrete evidence of work quality. This may take several forms: (1) a written, ongoing log, (2) valuative rating forms or other types of feedback instruments, (3) collected data, (4) copies of notes on lesson plans or communications to the supervisee, (5) drafts of written materials, and (6) records of interactions. The ongoing log can be informal notations about the quality of lesson plans and/or reports as well as significant events. With regard to information concerning observations, the supervisor needs to be very careful that supervisees have not only been adequately observed but that they have received feedback about their performance. Thus, the supervisor may choose to keep a journal of the dates and times of observations as well as the types of feedback provided. In addition, having supervisees initial and return observation instruments becomes an important aspect of the students' records. Similarly, midterm and final evaluations are best initialed or signed by supervisees and then included in their permanent files.

Conference

As indicated earlier, the supervisory style most appropriate for the marginal clinician in the evaluation–feedback stage is direct/active (Anderson, 1988). The need for directness that influences the feedback given to the supervisee following observations affects the conference as well. During meetings, the supervisee will need specific feedback based on data collected by the supervisor regarding performance, and concrete assistance in planning and strategy development. Additional strategies cited above, such as role-playing, can also be incorporated as appropriate.

In regard to conferencing, Kruger and Dunning (1999) note that the potential for conflicting supervisor–supervisee views about the quality of the latter's performance. Persons who lack competence often are unaware of their skill level. Kruger and Dunning hypothesize that the same skills underlying effective performance also are the basis for accurate self-evaluation. Thus, not only are poor performers ineffective but they also lack the ability to accurately self-evaluate. Efforts will need to be made during the conference to resolve the differences between perceived performance and reality.

It is important with all supervisees, but particularly for those who are having significant problems, to let them know they are valued as persons independently of their clinical ability. Emotional support of the supervisee may become an increasingly critical aspect of the exchange as the realization of an inability to perform surfaces. Resistance to supervision is likely to build in direct proportion to performance anxiety (Liddle, 1986). Unfortunately, most persons, in a circumstance in which they are failing, have great difficulty taking responsibility for their own behavior. The anger and frustration that emerges often is directed toward the supervisor. This is likely to be particularly true as supervisees begin to hunt for alternative "causes." Generally, the longer the failing experience continues, the greater the associated emotion.

As the term progresses, conferences with failing clinicians may, at times, become volatile. If this occurs, it is important to document outbursts and to have supervisees initial the transcript of the exchange indicating that it is an accurate description of the events that occurred. They may also attach their own rebuttal. In some cases, openly tape-recording meetings as a record for both the supervisor and supervisee may help keep the situation from erupting. In extreme cases, a neutral third party may need to be invited to meetings to serve as a buffer. Hopefully, the supervisee will be voluntarily removed from the experience before this level of emotion is generated.

Outcomes

In general, there are three potential outcomes for the person who functions in the marginal range. The best is that with intensive supervision they are able to sufficiently strengthen their work to an acceptable or higher level. The second result is one in which the supervisee is removed from the clinical experience to develop specific skills before reattempting clinical work. This might consist of additional coursework and/or structured learning experiences designed to fill in informational gaps and/or be oriented to the development of specific clinical skills such as behavior management. The least palatable, but often necessary alternative for the truly marginal/failing clinician is the provision of support in seeking an alternate vocation. Referrals for formal career counseling are highly appropriate to assist them in finding their niche in life.

Legal Implications

The marginal supervisee has more potential for legal implications than any other group of trainees. The possibility of a legal action, although unusual, is very real. Documentation becomes increasingly critical. Facilities may wish to include the exact procedures to be implemented when a supervisee is identified as "at risk" in the clinic manual. This may include observations of the clinician's therapy by other supervisors, regular videotaping of treatment, an outline of the documentation to be accumulated, and timelines for improvement or removal from the practicum experience. Minimally, supervisors need to take great care to ensure that specified due process procedures are carefully observed and that the supervisee has not been treated arbitrarily. In addition, records of clinicians who have had significant difficulties should be retained for a reasonable period. In particular, they should be kept long enough to deal with a delayed decision to litigate.

Finally, more than one supervisor should be involved in the supervision of supervisees who are having significant problems. Thus, if the person who does clinical assignments is aware of supervisees at risk, every effort should be made to split those persons' assignments so that they simultaneously have more than one supervisor. If this does not occur, the assigned supervisor may wish to have another person observe this clinician's cases in the event that the question of bias emerges.

Supervision of the Average Clinician

Identification

In general, average clinicians will exhibit satisfactory performance throughout their clinical experience or have significant difficulties in isolated areas such as report writing, diagnosis, time usage, or, possibly, behavior management. Their remaining skills are likely to be at least acceptable or better (Dowling, 1985). It is important to note that the idea of what is average performance is somewhat misleading as it includes people exhibiting skills just above the marginal level up to the borderline for outstanding. To focus the discussion for this group of individuals, the person truly in the middle of the range will be considered, but it is done with the understanding that alternate strategies, those more suited to the marginal or outstanding clinician, will be incorporated, as appropriate, in response to the performance of a given supervisee. Descriptions of typically average clinicians will indicate how supervisors can identify this group.

> Marisa exuded enthusiasm. Her initial testing was thorough, although she made scoring errors on two different measures. Her objectives were generally on-target, and her behavior management skills were strong. Lesson plan content was acceptable but was frequently lacking in task variety. Periodic errors were made in planning task difficulty for her client. Report writing was very difficult for her in terms of both content and style.

> Bob began the term with a flourish. His initial planning was excellent and treatment was structurally appropriate. His sessions seemed to move well and to be organized. Approximately three weeks into therapy, however, his client refused to perform some tasks and often did not appear to understand what was expected. Bob had great difficulty isolating the problem. When given collected data regarding the sequence of events within activities and a transcription of his directions, he saw the relevance of the information but was unclear about a strategy for resolution. He was concerned that he could not crystalize alternatives, but consistently

demonstrated willingness to do whatever was necessary to improve his clinical work.

Jim's work was average throughout his practicum. Lesson plans were adequate and consisted of varied procedures, although they often appeared hastily written. Previous and upcoming sessions were not integrated. He tended to treat aspects of the client without considering the complete therapy picture. His behavior management was appropriate but somewhat variable. He was responsive to feedback but did not actively seek out information to enhance his work. His work was acceptable but appeared to be significantly below his potential. When this was pointed out, he indicated that he probably could do better but was satisfied with his current level of performance.

Betsy was excited about her enrollment in her audiology practicum. She did a good job of reviewing a client's case history information and in selecting an appropriate test battery, but her implementation was somewhat variable. She had a tendency to present stimuli at equal, predictable intervals, which may have distorted some of her findings. Her interpretations were often not a logical extension of the assessment results. With feedback, she adapted appropriately. She was able to establish an effective relationship with most patients although young children were more difficult for her.

Lucille was initially overwhelmed by her predominantly nonverbal client's manipulative behavior. She consistently displayed positive regard for her client but expressed extreme frustration to her supervisor. Therapy was well-organized but periodically lacked therapeutic benefit. Lucille gradually improved pieces of her therapy until an increasing number of sessions were quite good. Unfortunately, her performance was erratic from day to day. In addition, accurate, meaningful data collection eluded the clinician until well beyond midterm. Throughout the experience, Lucille maintained a constructive attitude and worked diligently to resolve areas of weakness.

The classification of a supervisee as an average clinician is likely to emerge over time and may not be immediately evident. Often, a supervisee who starts out strong in the structured environment of assessment may settle into more ordinary performance when confronted with the less concrete aspects of therapy. Similarly, supervisees who struggle initially may strengthen their performance as they settle into the more routine aspects of the clinical process. An underlying characteristic of this group of supervisees is that they have the basic potential to perform at a minimal or better level of clinical competence.

Goals

Objectives for the average clinician focus on maximizing their professional development, enhancing patient treatment, and increasing their involvement in the supervisory process. For people who enter with somewhat shaky skills, the intent will be to assist them in becoming consistently competent, that is, functioning at an average or higher level. In contrast, the goal for individuals who enter with truly average achievement will be to enhance that performance to a level bordering on highly skilled. A final goal for this group is for them to assume as active a role in the supervisory process as they can.

Two additional points are relevant to goal-setting for the average supervisee. First, the intent, as in all supervision, is to move them along the continuum of supervision toward self-supervision. Independently of where they are at a given point in time, the desire is for them to develop further. Therefore, if they are in the direct/feedback stage, the intent is to guide them into the transitional phase. Similarly, if they are demonstrating abilities reflective of the transitional level, the objective is to increase their collaborative involvement and, if appropriate, lead them into self-supervision. Second, supervisees have the right and responsibility to themselves to be actively involved in decisions regarding their objectives and personal growth. In sum, objectives for supervisees are not formulated in a vacuum by the supervisor. In particular, supervisees with at least average skills have the capability to be actively involved in decisions affecting their development.

Strategies

In considering the Anderson continuum of supervision, the average supervisee may be in the evaluation–feedback stage at some times but in the transitional level at others. In addition, a given clinician may begin at the evaluation–feedback level but gradually shift to the transitional phase. Others may be ready for a collaborative interaction from the outset with periodic needs for directness. As a result, the supervisor's style may include telling but will also incorporate varying degrees of collaboration as appropriate. The clinician at this level of development will test the supervisor's ability to accurately read the supervisee and situation to arrive at the most effective supervisory style.

Some of the supervisory strategies suggested for the marginal supervisee continue to be appropriate, in a modified form, for the average clinician. These may include joint planning, demonstration therapy, directed observations, selected verbatim, audio- or videotape, and data collection and analysis. Joint planning is likely to take the form of discussions of objectives and potential procedures rather than the concrete writing of a lesson plan. The average clinician generally can comfortably translate these ideas to a written plan. Once the objectives and initial plans have been developed jointly, the supervisee is often able to move forward with increasing independence, although ongoing specific feedback in response to the clinician's planning is likely to be needed.

Demonstration therapy and directed observations continue to serve a valuable function. Ideally, the provision of demonstrations will be preplanned and will typically be directed to specific aspects of treatment that elude the clinician's grasp or will relate to alternatives discussed in the conference. Rarely will whole sessions need to be modeled. Similarly, the observation of peers proficient in a specific facet of treatment will assist the supervisee in developing certain skills and will facilitate the generation of new ideas and alternate treatment strategies. This is particularly true if supervisees collect and analyze data while they are watching.

Selected verbatim (Acheson and Gall, 1992) is also potentially helpful to the average clinician. Directions, reinforcements, off-task verbalizations or other aspects of treatment might be transcribed to provide specific feedback to the supervisee. The focus of this approach may be strengths and/or weaknesses and may be documented by either the supervisor or supervisee. Transcriptions increase the participants' awareness of specific aspects of therapy and provide the foundation for change. In some instances, particularly individuals whose performance fluctuates markedly, the recording of a large segment of a particularly poor session may heighten their awareness of the extremes of their professional performance (Anderson, 1988).

Audiotape, and particularly videotape, are potent tools for the average supervisee. When they view their tapes, they generally can identify aspects of therapy that were successful and those that were less so, even though they may not be able to delineate the cause of a strength or weakness or be able to suggest a solution. Awareness, however, is significant, as it is the first step toward growth. Others, with the aid of the tapes, will be able to identify critical incidents and be able to modify their behavior independently. In sum, the use of audio- and videotape frequently allows average supervisees to step out of themselves and view their behaviors as others would.

Collected data, in varying amounts, is often valuable to average clinicians, but their readiness for and ability to use this information may vary. Initially, the focus may be, of necessity, very concrete. The supervisor may even want to take responsibility for collecting this information and then providing it to the supervisee. The supervisor may also need to demonstrate problem-solving on the basis of the data. As supervisees mature, they will be expected to take increasing responsibility for data collection, analysis, and the problem-solving process.

As mentioned earlier, some average supervisees will be able to use collected data to markedly enhance their performance while others can only grasp its value on a superficial level or in regard to specific behaviors. Thus, the use and appropriateness of this strategy may vary markedly across individuals. In the same vein, the supervisees' involvement in planning for and actually collecting data will vary, depending on their level of interest and ability. Their active participation in deciding what is to be observed, strategies for gathering information, and interpretation of the results should, in all cases, be encouraged and rewarded. In addition, as related to data collection, continuous process improvement and critical thinking skills (addressed more fully in the section on the outstanding clinician) may also be useful in fostering the growth of the average clinician.

Once average supervisees have treatment procedures under control, the setting of objectives for their professional growth becomes a consideration. An assessment of readiness to focus on client performance as well as personal professional development is best completed in conjunction with the supervisee. A decision is needed regarding not only the appropriateness of the objectives but, if they are to be used, the magnitude to be targeted. Some individuals will feel that a client focus is all they can handle at the time; others will select in-depth goals. For example, some supervisees may set an objective to read four articles relevant to the treatment of their clients. Others might actively work to improve the quality of their directions, while even others may strive to increase awareness of their clinical strengths. Supervisees who choose to work toward specific, personal goals will also want to be involved in the planning for and the collection of data to determine if they have achieved those goals. The critical outcome is that average supervisees leave the supervisory experience with a sense of the value and importance of personal, professional objectives in their long-term development.

Documentation of performance remains important in working with average supervisees. Objective record-keeping by supervisors reduces the potential for any bias that might creep into evaluation. The types of data collected are identical to those for marginal supervisees: (1) observation checklists/forms and midterm and final evaluations, all initialed by the clinician; (2) a log regarding the timeliness and quality of lesson plans and written reports; (3) drafts of the supervisee's reports; (4) a list of the dates on which the supervisor observed the clinician and the type of feedback provided; (5) informal notes about the supervisee's clinical effectiveness and interactions in the supervisory process. The types and format of the above information is often largely determined by individual supervisors, facilities, and specific events that have shaped the policies that have emerged.

Conference

In considering the Anderson continuum of supervision, the appropriate conference style may vary significantly, depending on the given average supervisee, the length of time the supervisory relationship has existed, and the particular issues under consideration. At times, direct telling will be highly appropriate. At other times, the beginnings of collaboration will be evident. In some instances, true collaboration, marked by minimal supervisor input, may even occur. Marked variations in method may also be evidenced within and across conferences with a particular supervisee. As indicated earlier, the supervisor will need to take great care in assessing the situation to select a facilitative supervisory style.

In actual conferences, the supervisor will want to foster supervisee independence and active involvement in the supervisory conference. Joint consultation regarding the agenda for the current, as well as future meetings, facilitates supervisees' development. As clinicians grow in skill and confidence, they may wish to take increasing responsibility for planning the agenda of the meeting. In addition, the analysis of collected data, problem-solving, and the resulting strategy development will constitute as much of the conference as appropriate to a given supervisee. Initially, as well as when needed, the supervisor may be the primary person engaged in these endeavors, but the intent is to involve the supervisee as rapidly and as in-depth as possible. Finally, as in all conferences, confidence in the individual's ability to grow and a positive interpersonal climate, such as that described by Caracciolo, Rigrodsky, and Morrison (1978) and Pickering (1989–1990), maximize the outcomes of the interactions. This is particularly true for the supervisee who appears to be resisting the supervisory process (Liddle, 1986).

The average clinician should also begin to become actively involved in the supervisory process. Expectations in this realm will need to be tempered, based on the ability and the interest of the individual being supervised. As part of this process, feedback may be solicited regarding supervisor behaviors/strategies that have been perceived as most beneficial and those actions that have not been helpful. The clinician may also choose to be involved in or actually complete the plans for the content, timing, and assignment of responsibilities for data collection. Similarly, decisions regarding the division of tasks in data analysis and interpretation may also be influenced or determined by the supervisee.

Outcomes

Average supervisees demonstrate the potential for a diverse range of outcomes. In rare cases, as case-load assignments increase in diversity and in complexity, clinicians at this level may begin to function marginally. Generally, the majority will achieve minimal or better levels of clinical competency. A joy in supervision are those who evolve into consistently capable or outstanding professionals who increasingly engage in self-supervision.

Legal Implications

Litigation resulting from the supervision of the average clinician is less of a concern than is the resolution of disputes regarding evaluations and the related assignment of a grade. Careful, objective documentation, as described previously, generally is sufficient when contention emerges. If supervisees demonstrate the ability and willingness to engage in ongoing data analysis and problem-solving, they typically have a clearer picture of their own levels of performance. As a result, their formal grades are not a surprise to them. Supervisee frustration can be minimized by documentation and supervisee involvement in data collection and self-analysis.

Supervision of the Outstanding Clinician

Identification

This group of clinicians is readily identifiable because they excel across the board. Supervisors report that these supervisees are competent in all the areas on which they are evaluated (Dowling, 1985). These clinicians exhibit strength in assessment and in the implementation of treatment. The following descriptions illustrate the characteristics that identify outstanding performers.

> Sandy approached her clinical assignment with marked enthusiasm, although she confided she was nervous. Prior to test selection, she came to the conference with appropriate questions that reflected extensive consideration of her client's disorder, and her assessment battery was well-reasoned. Before she turned in the results of the testing to her supervisor, she carefully checked the scoring and reviewed the

logic underlying her interpretations. The objectives that followed were appropriate, and her therapy was consistently sound.

Don often requested the most difficult clients because he felt that the challenge increased his growth. His test selection was innovative and insightful, while his manner with his clients was delightful to observe. Mel's sessions were always goal-oriented, well-implemented, and creative. When a difficulty arose, he quickly gathered data to identify the source of the problem. Generally, he was able to resolve problems with a minimum of input from the supervisor. When asked, he could identify both his areas of strength and those he wanted to improve.

Rose initially was unsure of herself. In response to her anxiety, she engaged in extensive planning. As a result, her treatment was well-organized and implemented. Early in the term she was concerned that she seemed unable to think "on her feet" or to resolve problems on the spot. She was aware, almost from the outset, when a procedure was less than optimal. To deal with this problem, she began planning alternate strategies to use if the first did not work. By the end of the term, she was able to spontaneously lower or increase task difficulty when her client's performance deteriorated.

Jerry was an exceptional audiological diagnostician. He planned the evaluation battery well and implemented the procedures skillfully. He continually monitored the patient's and his own performance and made adjustments as needed. He consistently interpreted findings accurately. His ability to convey the results to his patients in a thorough and sensitive manner was excellent.

Typically the outstanding supervisee is readily identifiable and rapidly emerges as having the characteristics of this group of persons. At times, a strong average performer will evolve into the exceptional. This is particularly true for the inexperienced supervisee. But, even then, glimmerings of excellence often peek through at an early stage of their work.

Goals

The objectives for outstanding clinicians are focused on maximizing their potential, including their ability to provide treatment that optimizes their clients' growth. They also center on fostering the supervisee's own professional development and problem-solving skills. Finally, they are intended to ensure the supervisee's fullest participation in and contribution to the supervisory process.

Strategies

On the Anderson continuum of supervision, the outstanding supervisee is likely to enter the process at the transitional stage, already exhibiting readiness for collaboration. The degree of supervisor input is likely to decline over the term as the supervisee's contributions increase. A direct/active style may be appropriate at times, but the need is likely to be infrequent. Some supervisees in training, particularly those near completion of their degree, may demonstrate increasing abilities to engage in self-supervision. Thus, with the outstanding supervisee, the supervisor is most likely to engage in collaboration, but can also incorporate telling and consultation, as appropriate.

Some strategies described for the average clinician may be appropriate for the outstanding supervisee, although the intent is likely to be different. For example, if joint planning of treatment is done, rather than being concretely focused, it will be designed to generate speculation about alternate, creative treatments. An inclusion of an estimate of the likely outcomes is also beneficial (Cogan, 1973). In a similar fashion, demonstration therapy, video- and audiotape and selected verbatim (Acheson and Gall, 1992) can be used. If demonstration therapy is used, however, it should be offered as a food for thought, not as how-to instruction.

Outstanding clinicians may choose to use audio- or videotape extensively as a vehicle for their own growth. Typically, in observing a tape, they will readily identify areas of strength as well as those that can be modified. With a limited amount of assistance, they are often able to consider the content of their sessions objectively. This is particularly true if they engage in data collection as they consider the tape. In addition, they become increasingly aware of critical incidents and cause/effect in the treatment process. They may also choose to select specific recorded events as a springboard for discussion in the conference. This strategy, in particular, may serve as a potent tool, assisting the supervisee to move toward self-supervision.

Selected verbatim may be extremely helpful to clinicians who excel. For example, if they want to maximize their directions to a client, a listing of those specific verbalizations may be used to gauge progress toward that goal. Depending on previous planning, outstanding supervisees and/or their supervisors may be responsible for gathering the verbatim data. This information would then be used by the clinicians for self-analysis or for joint consideration. Hence, selected verbatim may serve as an extremely valuable tool for enhancing professional development.

Data collection will become a critical tool for the outstanding supervisee. After a period of initial training in data gathering and analysis, and having the opportunity to see the application of that information to their clinical work, they will be able to use the process in an increasingly independent manner. Most of these people will rapidly see the link between data and the determination of cause and effect in therapy. As they grow in skill, they are likely to invent a variety of methods for gathering information specifically tailored to their own needs. Once they are successful in accumulating and analyzing clinical information, they further benefit from being encouraged to use the same strategies, with a focus on their own professional development. In practice, data collection and the related analysis, problem-solving, and strategy development are likely to serve as the primary mechanisms for assisting the supervisee through the transitional supervisory stage to that of self-supervision.

The establishment of ongoing professional objectives are critical for the optimal development of outstanding supervisees. As with all clinicians, these supervisees have the right to decide if they would like to work toward selected professional goals. Almost always, a desire for maximum growth is characteristic of the exceptional performer.

Again, a good starting point is for both supervisors and supervisees to make a list of the supervisee's professional strengths and weaknesses. After discussion of the items, supervisees may select as many or as few of these items as they wish as targets for professional development. A discussion of relevant data collection methods to document his or her growth will also be helpful. The general division of responsibility for data collection may also be discussed as part of the goal-setting process, including anticipated changes in roles/tasks as the supervisee develops. Once established, outstanding supervisees will be able to use this method to foster their ongoing professional growth.

In addition to the concrete strategies cited above, such as videotape and script taping, some specific philosophical stances benefit the outstanding supervisee. These include fostering risk-taking, maximizing growth, implementing continuous process improvement, encouraging critical thinking, and increasing autonomy. Pickering (1977) discusses the importance of encouraging supervisees to take risks. Failing and learning from one's errors underlies creative growth. Rewarding individuals for their creative failures is a means to foster innovation (Peters and Waterman, 1982). Thus, acknowledging the potential for either success or failure and then rewarding both is necessary to stimulate risk-taking and encourage optimal supervisee development.

Growth is further maximized by encouraging supervisees to stretch their skills a little further than they initially think they can. This may mean guiding them to set professional objectives slightly beyond their reach. The intent is that the goals are potentially achievable but that their attainment will require concerted effort. These high, but reasonable expectations, optimize development.

Continuous process improvement is a potent tool for professional growth (Bruce and Dowling, 1994; Dowling and Bruce, 1996). The underlying idea is that clinical work is ongoing and that throughout the process, the goal is to maximize outcomes. The plan–do–study–act cycle (Leebov and Ersoz, 1991) provides a framework for this method. First, clinicians state the result they desire, and then consider the inputs to the process. This will include client variables such as background information and presenting behavior and clinician factors such as knowledge, skill, and experience. After considering this data, clinicians can engage in planning how to achieve the desired outcomes. The plan is implemented and data gathered to assess the result. Supervisees then study the data and make changes to improve the outcomes for the next time. Continuous process improvement provides a structure for problem-solving and maximizing clinical effectiveness. It also allows supervisees to measure the efficacy of their diagnosis and treatment on a continuous basis.

The refinement of critical thinking skills will further enhance the growth of the outstanding clinician. Moses and Shapiro (1996) and Shapiro (1998) indicate three skills that are characteristic of the advanced clinician: viewing the treatment process from both the client and clinician perspective; understanding that multiple factors contribute to a clinical problem; and considering multiple potential solutions. These parallel the ideas that Nelson (1990) and Dowling and Bruce (1997) suggest. According to Nelson (1990), there are four distinct but sequential developmental levels of thought: (1) answers are either right or wrong; (2) there may be more than one answer and the one selected is a matter of opinion; (3) a logical decision is made on the basis of reasoned arguments; and (4) a logical decision is made with the understanding that the decision can be appropriate in one circumstance but not in another. The outstanding clinician will, in most cases, engage in logical problem-solving. The use of data in the conference as the basis for problem-solving and strategy development regarding clinical issues will strengthen this skill. In addition, having supervisees generate multiple alternatives for dealing with a given problem, and deciding in which circumstances one or more might work better than another, will foster thought process development. Fong, Borders, Ethington, and Pitts (1997) indicate that the gains in cognitive development are paralleled by increases in clinical effectiveness. As a result, growth can be predicted in the quality of the supervisees' treatment and in their active participation in the conference. Indeed, through developing their ability to think critically, they will learn mental strategies that will speed their movement into self-supervision.

The final philosophical orientation for outstanding clinicians is fostering their autonomy. For example, once lesson plans are consistently proficient, clinicians can be given the opportunity to engage in planning without formally submitting a written document to the supervisor. Similarly, supervisors can decrease the volume of their data collection and guide supervisees to take most of the responsibility for this task, as well as for the subsequent analysis, problem-solving, and strategy development. Supervisees can also assume primary responsibility for planning the conference agenda, or choose to decrease the frequency of actual meetings with the supervisor as they move toward self-supervision.

Anderson (1988) discusses the joint responsibility of the supervisor and supervisee for the outcomes of both the clinical and supervisory process. Both members of the dyad should grow as a result of the relationship. Of the three groups of supervisees, failing, average, and outstanding, the latter has the greatest potential for maximally influencing both processes. Clearly, if growth is to occur, supervisees will need to be actively encouraged and rewarded for contributing to the supervisory process.

Active supervisee involvement in the supervisory process may take several forms: planning for data collection, contributing to the conference agenda, goal-setting for the supervisory relationship, and giving supervisors feedback about behaviors that maximally or minimally assist supervisees. In the best circumstance, their participation will also include providing their perceptions of their supervisors' professional strengths and weaknesses. These will be incorporated with the views of the supervisors as a foundation for developing professional objectives for supervisor growth.

Documentation of supervisee performance for the outstanding individual will be similar to that gathered for clinicians performing at other levels of ability.

Observation checklists, written notes, collected data, and drafts of written work will be collected for the supervisee's file. In addition, dates of observations and a record of the type of feedback provided, and a running log regarding performance in both the clinical and supervisory process will be kept.

Conference

In regard to the continuum of supervision, the most useful conference style appropriate for the outstanding supervisee is collaboration, with consultation incorporated whenever appropriate. At times, direct telling may occur, but it is likely to be infrequent. Over the span of the relationship, the volume of the supervisor's contributions during collaboration will gradually decrease with a parallel increase in supervisee input.

The nature of the conference is largely determined by the supervisee's readiness for assuming control. Increasingly, the clinician will be expected to contribute agenda items, to analyze data, and solve problems. An important part of all meetings will be the joint and gradual supervisee assumption of responsibility for the determination of the clinical and professional goals to be targeted during a specific observation, and the types of data to be collected, including the selection and division of tasks involved in the gathering and analysis of the information. Thus, the focus of exchanges may vary among aspects of the clinical and supervisory process depending on the needs of the participants at a given time.

Outcomes

This group, in particular, has the greatest potential for maximum benefit from and involvement in both the clinical and supervisory process. Even though this is true, three potential outcomes exist for the outstanding supervisee. In the best case, they become even better. In another, they maintain their level of skill but do not progress beyond that point. In the worst scenario, they regress to average performance. In practice, the majority of exceptional clinicians are likely to perform in the first two categories. Encouraging them to make a commitment to ongoing, lifelong growth assists these high performers in achieving and maintaining clinical excellence (Kamhi, 1995).

Legal Implications

Rarely is this topic an issue with the outstanding supervisee. As with all supervisees, normal documentation must continue to occur. This may include having the supervisee initial and return observation and/or valuative instruments, storing drafts of report-writing, and making notations regarding lesson-plan writing and clinical performance. If contention does arise with this group of supervisees, it is likely to be limited to grade assignment.

Supervisor—Later Thoughts

Late in the term, the three supervisors, John, Sally, and Stephanie, are once more talking in the staff lounge.

SALLY: This term has flown. Remember, in the fall, how concerned I was about the new clinicians assigned to me and hoping that at least some of them would become active participants in supervision by the end of the term? Well, I have been very pleased. All but one is now doing some conference agenda planning and all are collecting data. Talking with them about the Anderson Continuum and how it is used to guide their growth really helped them see their role in this process. Even the one I was really worried about has done okay.

JOHN: I agree. The continuum helped me too. I had such a mix of clinicians. This is the first term in which I consciously diagnosed each clinician to better understand their needs. In combination with the supervision continuum, it has been very effective. I feel like I was able to adjust my supervision to fit the clinician. It gave me a way to structure that made it so much easier.

STEPHANIE: Yeah. My supervisees had more experience coming into this term, and it has been fun to work with them. They have really gotten into data collection and problem-solving. Once they understood the idea of continuous process improvement, they began working as a team to figure out ways to optimize their treatment methods. They did a lot of videotaping and asked me to do some selective verbatim recordings when I observed. They have each grown a lot this term. I have really enjoyed supervising them.

JOHN: It has been a good term. I feel like I have had a variety of new tools to guide them. I have done everything from joint planning and demonstration therapy to guiding them to think logically within a context. I agree. It has been very productive.

The supervisors are excited about their experiences. The addition of new ideas and strategies has given them tools to deal with a variety of clinicians. They see growth in the clinicians and they, themselves, feel a sense of satisfaction with the process.

Supervision of the Externship Experience

Externship settings play a vital role in preparing professionals. Yet, it is becoming increasingly complicated for a supervisor and a facility to decide to become a partner in clinical training. The basic requirement from the American Speech-Language-Hearing Association is that 50 percent of diagnosis and 25 percent of treatment implemented by students must be directly observed in order for students to accrue clinical clock hours and to allow for the provision of services within the scope of the Association's code of ethics. In addition, managed-care funding issues, as well as types of observation and documentation required to charge for services provided by students in some settings, places increasing demands on the supervisor. Thus, the decision to accept an extern requires careful thought.

The externship experience is a unique experience for clinicians in training. The supervisee will have dual supervisors: They are responsible to a direct supervisor, but are also likely to report to a university supervisor who visits on a periodic basis. For many, it will be the first time they have treated numerous clients simultaneously. In the training clinic, they will have devoted hours preparing for an individual session. In the externship setting, they will no longer have this luxury. The work setting will also have a broader range of expectations with less tolerance for variations in performance. Client service is paramount; clinician growth becomes a secondary concern. Adaptability becomes a critical performance characteristic, as does the ability to work as an effective member of an interdisciplinary team.

In considering interns, it is important to note that all are not created equally. They are, in general, not a homogeneous group. This variability comes from several sources. First, they will have had varying amounts of diagnostic and clinical experience. In their university training experiences, they may have implemented treatment primarily in an individual format, whereas others will have worked with groups. They may have treated adults, but more likely they treated children. In addition, they will vary as individuals in their general level of clinical skill. Finally, some will have completed more externships than others before arriving at a facility. This variability in extern ability and experience can cause consternation on the part of the supervisor who expects that externs will arrive with a higher, more consistent level of competency/proficiency than they may in reality possess.

Supervisee Acculturation

When externs arrive at a facility, several tactics can be implemented to aid their transition into the setting. First, introduce them to others with whom they will interact and identify key individuals who will contribute to their success. For example, there may be an administrative person who handles supplies and organizational or procedural issues with whom the trainee needs to establish a working relationship. Second, a tour of the facility will be helpful so that the trainee knows where he or she is to go when told. In some facilities, services will be provided out of one location. In others, the point of service will vary, depending on the task at hand. Third, it is helpful to provide trainees with a work station or, minimally, a secure place to store their personal belongings. Fourth, they will need to be oriented to the types of services offered and the clientele typically served in that work setting. From the outset, the productivity of the relationship is enhanced by helping them feel that they are important members of the service team and not just visitors.

Expectations

An important part of orienting them to the externship site will be a discussion of expectations for their performance. Externs are often confused about the criteria that will be used to evaluate them: Are they being compared to the polished professional or to previous students? Are they expected to demonstrate competency with patients from the outset or is there an expected growth curve? Thus, it will be important to identify the level of competence to which they are being compared. In addition, it is best if the supervisor shares specific expectations for their performance. For example, if externs are expected to spontaneously complete a bedside evaluation with just the items they routinely carry, they need to be told that. Similarly, talking about the kind of skills externs need to demonstrate to function well in a given setting will assist them in getting off on the right foot.

Once the externs are in place, it is helpful to gradually transition them to patient/client care. It is helpful if they observe the professional with a client before they assume responsibility. It gives them a feel for that individual and the therapy the client is receiving as well as preferred practices in that setting. In addition, Teitelbaum (1998) notes that supervisees are more open to critical feedback if their strengths are acknowledged first.

Feedback

Once they begin to see clients, they benefit from feedback on their performance. Many supervisees report not getting enough feedback. Others feel they receive too much. At one extreme are individuals who, literally, get no feedback from their supervisors or receive a limited amount, and, in general, feel they are on their own. On the other end of the spectrum are those who are given copious notes after each observation. Students do need feedback, but the optimal type and quantity may vary, depending on the needs of the supervisee and the supervisor's view of what can realistically be provided in that setting. A joint discussion of perspectives about the desired frequency and type of feedback will enhance the relationship.

Conference

Similarly, supervisees need opportunities to meet with their supervisors. Informal, on-the-spot discussions are fine, but a formal meeting is needed periodically as well. This will include more structured feedback about performance, but also opportunities to problem-solve and generate strategies for the clientele they are treating. In particular, having the externs engage in as much problem-solving as possible will foster their growth and increase their satisfaction with the externship experience. For example, they can be asked to think about why a strategy did or did not work, and then encouraged to suggest strategies for future intervention. Collected data enhances this process. In addition, discussions of their professional goals and their progress toward attaining them are an important component of the conference. McLeod (1997) further suggests that conferences should also include a discussion of the overall placement experience and the site's role in assisting the supervisees in achieving their goals.

Diagnosing the supervisee will be an important tool for determining the most appropriate conference style for interacting with him or her. At the beginning of the externship, the supervisee may need a direct/active or a telling style from the supervisor because he or she is new to the setting, and probably unfamiliar with the population seen at the externship site. As soon as the supervisee is ready, a shift into increasing collaboration will benefit his or her development. Even after a move into collaboration has occurred, a new client type or a unique situation may necessitate that the supervisor be more direct on occasions. Other trainees, particularly those in their last externship experience, may be ready for collaboration throughout the relationship.

In general, trainees value supervisors who show respect for them as emerging professionals; they value a sense of support from their supervisor as well and like being given as much responsibility and independence as possible.

Outcomes

The desired outcomes of the externship experience are twofold. First, trainees should make a contribution to the worksetting in which they are placed. This may include the provision of quality service and an increase in the volume of people treated. Second, trainees should grow in clinical skill and breadth of experience. If they accomplish these goals, they will have taken another step toward professional competence and independence and the externship site will have benefited from their involvement in clinical training.

Feedback about Supervision Experiences

Students who were completing a course in clinical supervision at the end of their master's program at one university were asked to reflect on their supervisory experiences throughout their training experience, to identify the aspects they particularly enjoyed or disliked. They were are also encouraged to identify the predominate styles of supervision they have experienced. Although the sample is limited, it is helpful to view the training process through the eyes of the supervisee (Dowling, 1999).

Considering both in-house and externship experiences, most respondents indicated that the expectations for their performance often were not stated. In general, the requirements tended to become clearer as the experience evolved, and the conference styles were most often direct in nature, independently of the setting in which they took place.

Positive Perceptions

There are numerous aspects of the process that clinicians particularly like. They appreciate having the supervisor demonstrate with given client types before being asked to assume responsibility for their treatment. They also value being given support and time to adjust to the work in a new setting. A sense of support from the supervisor is reported as contributing to their feelings of confidence. They like the supervisor who not only gives them support but is then able to step back and allow them to take increasing responsibility and, even, make mistakes on their own. This latitude provides the opportunity for clinician growth and gives them a sense of independence. In addition, they like having someone to bounce ideas off, and value shared collaboration. Being treated as a partner in the process is important to them because they enjoy being given opportunities to problem-solve and to use collected data.

They like supervisors who are good listeners, have clear-cut expectations, and give them helpful suggestions and honest feedback, as well as supervisors who respect them and take their feelings into account. They appreciate situations in which feedback is ongoing and in which they are viewed positively. They appreciate the supervisor who assists them in setting goals for their own growth and discusses their progress throughout the term.

Negative Perceptions

The supervisees described several circumstances that they felt were negative. They did not like receiving mixed messages from different supervisors, for example. Insufficient conferences were also cited. Some had only one, and many said that their supervisors were unavailable for conferences. For others, conferences took place on the fly. Another source of complaint was infrequent observation of their clinical work, and particularly frustrating was an observation of minimal duration followed by a lengthy critique. Limited opportunities to problem-solve were also of concern.

There were numerous concerns about the feedback process. Not being given feedback is a major issue for some, while, for others, receiving predominantly negative evaluation was distressing. Supervisees expressed annoyance when they were graded down for not implementing a procedure requested by a supervisor when it was implemented but the supervisor had not seen it. Being critiqued critically without being asked the rationale for a particular strategy was also upsetting. Similarly, being told they could not implement a particular strategy without being given a reason was just as frustrating as being told what to do without their own input.

Several behaviors attributable to supervisors were said to be dissatisfying. The use of sarcasm was cited as were supervisors who are very critical and communicate in a domineering and/or disappointed tone. Supervisors' refusals to discuss the supervisee's valuative ratings were described as particularly frustrating, as were supervisors who gave "nasty" written feedback without discussing it with the supervisee.

From the supervisees' perspective, the clinical training process can be both a source of joy and dissatisfaction. Training in supervision for both the supervisor and supervisee should provide the participants with the tools to enhance their relationship and increase levels of satisfaction. Sadly, financial constraints and the demands of service delivery make it difficult to consistently optimize the supervisory process, even when it is the explicit desire of the participants. Teitelbaum 's (1998) citation of a supervisee's hopes for an enjoyable and productive supervisory experience, is an appropriate conclusion for this section on supervisees' views of the process: "What I look for in a supervisor is someone who is warm and accepting, generous and wise, and who can teach me the things I need to learn in an atmosphere that capitalizes on my strengths."

Relationship of the Thirteen Tasks of Supervision to Supervising in Clinical Training

In regard to the thirteen tasks of supervision, most are relevant to supervisees at various levels of experience and ability. Tasks one to six, for example, and the clinical aspects of seven, nine, ten, eleven, twelve are in this category because they are crucial in the establishment of an effective working relationship and for the clinician's development of various skills: meeting goals and objectives, assessing and managing clients, observing and analyzing the quality of therapy sessions, finding ways to self-evaluate, and becoming appropriately involved in the supervisory conference. Similarly, all clinicians must learn to write and edit reports and understand the ethical, legal, and regulatory aspects of clinical practice regardless of the level of their experience or ability. In addition, supervisors will demonstrate and/or participate with the supervisee in the clinical process. In sum, the thirteen tasks form the basis of effective clinical training independently of the experience or skill level of the supervisee.

However, it is vital to note that many of the tasks can vary in regard to the depth of implementation or achievement, depending on the experience or competence level of the supervisee. For example, the beginning and marginal clinician may benefit from concrete directives based on the supervisor's analysis of a treatment session. In contrast, the average clinician and those functioning at a higher level, the outstanding trainee, and the extern, are more likely to engage in their own data collection and analysis of clinical issues with less supervisor input. Similarly, the marginal clinician may only minimally contribute to the planning of observations and the related data collection, while clinicians with greater experience and skill can take primary responsibility for these tasks. The same is true of planning for the supervisory conference, involvement in clinical and supervisory process research, and the realization of competent clinical management and assessment skills. In summary, the thirteen tasks of supervision apply to all supervisees, but the form of implementation is likely to vary depending on the supervisee's experience level and status as a marginal, average, or outstanding professional.

Summary

This chapter began with a listing of the clinical supervision tasks relevant to training supervisees at varying levels of experience and ability. A review of literature relating to the supervisory topics in this chapter followed. Then, the utility of Anderson's continuum of supervision was cited as a foundation for supervising clinicians exhibiting different levels of experience and ability. The primary focus of this chapter has been the supervision of supervisees at two experience levels, beginning and extern, and three performance levels: marginal, average, and outstanding. Other topics, however, were explored in regard to both the new clinician and the extern. For the marginal, average, and outstanding clinician, the identification, of each supervisee's level of performance, the establishment of goals for differing levels of ability, the formulation of strategies for optimal treatment, the content of conferences as well as therapy outcomes and the legal implications of supervision were considered. Perceptions of the supervisory process from individuals at the end of clinical training round out this chapter, and it ends with thoughts about the thirteen tasks of supervision and clinical training.

REFERENCES

Acheson, K., and Gall, M. (3rd ed.). *Techniques in the Clinical Supervision of Teachers: Preservice and Inservice Applications.* New York: Longman, 1992.

Andersen, C. *The effect of supervisor bias on the evaluation of student clinicians in speech-language pathology and audiology.* (Doctoral dissertation, Indiana University, 1981). *Dissertation Abstracts International, 41,* 4479B. (University Microfilms No., 81-12, 499).

Anderson, J. *The Supervisory Process in Speech-Language Pathology and Audiology.* Austin, TX: Pro-Ed, 1988.

Barrow, M., and Domingo, R. "The effectiveness of training clinical supervisors in conducting the supervisory conference." *The Clinical Supervisor, 16* (1) (1997): 55–77.

Blodgett, E., Schmitt, J., and Scudder, R. "Clinical session evaluation: The effect of familiarity with the supervisee." *The Clinical Supervisor, 5* (1987): 33–43.

Brasseur, J. "The supervisory process: A continuum perspective." *Language, Speech and Hearing Services in Schools, 20* (1989): 274–295.

Bruce, M., and Dowling, S. "Continuous Process Improvement and Critical Thinking: Optimizing Clinical Training." Miniseminar presented at the Annual Convention of the American Speech, Language, Hearing Association, New Orleans, LA, Nov., 1994.

Caracciolo, G., Rigrodsky, S., and Morrison, E. "Perceived interpersonal conditions and professional growth of master's level speech-language pathology students during the supervisory process." *American Speech Hearing Association, 20* (1978): 467–477.

Cogan, M. *Clinical Supervision.* Boston: Houghton-Mifflin, 1973.

Chamberlain, M., and Gallagher, T. "Supervising the marginal student in clinical practicum." Paper presented at the Annual Convention of the American Speech-Language and Hearing Association, Detroit, Michigan, 1974.

Cimorell-Strong, J., and Ensley, K. "Effects of student clinician feedback on the supervisory conference." *American Speech Hearing Association, 24* (1982): 23–29.

Culatta, R., and Seltzer, H. "Content and sequence analyses of the supervisory session." *American Speech Hearing Association, 18* (1976): 8–12.

Culatta, R., and Seltzer, H. "Content and sequence analyses of the supervisory session: A report of clinical use." *American Speech Hearing Association, 19* (1977): 523–526.

DeShon, R., and Alexander, R. "Goal setting effects on implicit and explicit learning of complex tasks." *Organizational Behavior and Human Decision Processes, 65* (1) (1996): 18–36.

Donnelly, C., and Glaser, A. "Training in self-supervision skills." *The Clinical Supervisor, 10* (2) (1992): 85–96.

Dowling, S. "Clinical performance characteristics of failing, average and outstanding clinicians." *The Clinical Supervisor, 3* (3) (1985): 49–54.

Dowling, S. "Supervisory training: Impetus for clinical supervision." *The Clinical Supervisor, 4* (1986): 27–35.

Dowling, S. "Impact of preclinical supervisory training." Paper presented at the Annual Convention of the American Speech-Language and Hearing Association, Boston, MA, 1988.

Dowling, S. "Supervisory training, objective setting and grade contingent performance." Paper presented at the Annual Convention of the American Speech-Language and Hearing Association, Atlanta, GA, Nov. 1991.

Dowling, S. *Implementing the Supervisory Process: Theory and Practice.* Englewood Cliffs, NJ: Prentice-Hall, 1992.

Dowling, S. "Supervisory Training: Comparison of Grade Contingent/Non-contingent Objective Setting." In M. Bruce, (Ed.), *Proceedings: International and Interdisciplinary Conference on Clinical Supervision: Toward the 21st Century.* Burlington, VT: University of Vermont, (1994): 180–183.

Dowling, S. (1998). Facilitating Clinical Training: Issues for Supervisees and their Supervisors. *Contemporary Issues in Communication Science and Disorders, 25,* 5–11.

Dowling, S. "Students perceptions of supervision at the end of clinical training." Unpublished, 1999.

Dowling, S., and Bliss, L. "Cognitive complexity, rhetorical sensitivity: Contributing factors in clinical skill?" *Journal of Communication Disorders, 17* (1984): 9–17.

Dowling, S., and Bruce, M. "Improving Clinical Training through Continuous Quality Improvement and Critical Thinking." In B. Wagner, (Ed.), *Proceedings: Partnerships in Supervision: Innovative and Effective Practices.* Grand Forks, ND: University of North Dakota, (1996): 66–72.

Dowling, S., and Bruce, M. "Clinical Training: Enhancing Clinical Thought and Independence." Seminar presented at the Annual Convention of the American Speech, Language and Hearing Association, Boston, MA, Nov., 1997.

Dowling, S., and Wittkopp, J. "Students' perceived supervisory needs." *Journal of Communication Disorders, 15* (1982): 319–328.

Farmer, S. *"The trigonal model of communication disorders supervision: Concepts."* In S. Farmer and J. Farmer, (Eds.), Supervision in Communication Disorders, Columbus, OH: Merrill, 1989.

Fong, M., Borders, L., Ethington, C., and Pitts, J. "Becoming a counselor: A longitudinal study of student cognitive development." *Counselor Education and Supervision, 37* (2), (1997): 100–114.

Goldberg, B. "The transformation age: The sky's the limit." *American Speech Hearing Association 37* (1995): 44–50.

Hagler, P. *Effects of Verbal Directives, Data, and Contingent Social Praise on Amount of Supervisor Talk during Speech-Language Pathology Supervision Conferencing.* Doctoral Dissertation, Indiana University, Bloomington, IN, 1986.

Hagler, P., Madill, H., Kampfe, C., and Mitchell, M. "Students' coping strategies and prediction of practicum performance." Paper presented at the Annual Convention of the American Speech-Language and Hearing Association, Seattle, WA, Nov., 1990.

Harris, H., Ludington, J., Ringwalt, S., Ballard, D., Hooper, C., Buoyer, F., and Price, K. "Involving the student in the supervisory process." *National Student Speech Language Hearing Association Journal, 19* (1991–1992): 109–118.

Hersey, P., and Blanchard, K. *Management of Organizational Behavior: Utilizing Human Resources.* (5th ed.). Englewood Cliffs, NJ: Prentice-Hall, 1988.

Ingrisano, D., Guinty, C., Chambers, R., McDonald, J., Clem, R., and Cory, M. "The relationship between supervisory conference performance and supervisee experience." Paper presented at the Annual Convention of the American Speech-Language and Hearing Association, Atlanta, GA, 1979.

Joshi, S., and McAllister, L. "An investigation of supervisory style in speech pathology clinical education." *The Clinical Supervisor, 17* (2) (1998): 141–153.

Kamhi, A. "Research to Practice: Defining, developing and maintaining clinical expertise." *Language, Speech and Hearing Services in Schools, 26* (4) (1995): 353–356.

Kruger, J., and Dunning, D. "Unskilled and unaware of it: How difficulties in recognizing one's own incompetence lead to inflated self-assessments." *Journal of Personality and Psychology, 77* (6) (1999): 1121–1134.

Leebov, W., and Ersoz, C. *The Health Care Manager's Guide to Continuous Quality Improvement.* Chicago: American Hospital Publishing, 1991.

Liddle, B. "Resistance in supervision: A response to perceived threat." *Counselor Education and Supervision, 26* (2) (1986): 117–127.

Mawdsley, B. "Kansas inventory of self-supervision." In S. Farmer, (Ed.), *Clinical Supervision: A Coming of Age.* Proceedings of a national conference on supervision. Las Cruces, NM: New Mexico State University, 1987, 171–175.

Mawdsley, B., and Scudder, R. "The integrative task-maturity model of supervision." *Language, Speech, and Hearing Services in Schools, 20* (3) (1989): 305–315.

McLeod, S. "Student self-appraisal: Facilitating mutual planning in clinical education." *The Clinical Supervisor, 15* (1) (1997): 87–101.

Moses, N., and Shapiro, D. "A developmental conceptualization of clinical problem solving." *Journal of Communication Disorders, 29* (1996): 199–221.

Nelson, C. "Fostering critical thinking and mature valuing across the curriculum." Short course presented at the Annual Convention of the American Speech Hearing Association, Seattle, WA, 1990.

Perkins, J., and Mercaitis, P. "A guide for supervisors and students in clinical practicum." *The Clinical Supervisor, 13* (2) (1995): 67–78.

Peters, T., and Waterman, R. *In Search of Excellence: Lessons from America's Best-Run Companies.* New York: Harper & Row, 1982.

Pickering, M. "An examination of concepts operative in the supervisory process and relationship. *American Speech Language Hearing Association, 19,* (1977): 607–610.

Pickering, M. "The supervisory process: An experience of interpersonal relationships and personal growth." *National Student Speech Language Hearing Association Journal, 17* (1989–1990): 17–28.

Pickering, M., Rassi, J., Hagler, P., and McFarlane, L. "Integrating classroom, laboratory and clinical experiences." *ASHA, 34* (1992): 57–59.

Rassi, J., and McElroy, M. *The Education of Audiologists and Speech-Language Pathologists.* Timonium, MD: York Press, 1992.

Roberts, J., and Smith, K. "Supervisor–supervisee role differences and consistency of behavior in supervisory conferences." *Journal of Speech and Hearing Research, 25* (1982): 428–434.

Rockman, B. "Supervisor as clinician: A point of view." Paper presented at the Annual Convention of the American Speech-Language and Hearing Association, Chicago, IL, 1977.

Rosenthal, R., and Jacobson, L. *Pygmalion in the Classroom.* New York: Holt, Rinehart and Winston, 1968.

Sbaschnig, K., and Williams, C. "A reliability audit for supervisors." Paper presented at the Annual Convention of the American Speech-Language and Hearing Association. Cincinnati, OH, 1983.

Schermerhorn, J., Gardner, W., and Martin, T. "Management dialogues: Turning on the marginal performer." *Organizational Dynamics, 18* (4) (1990): 47–59.

Shapiro, D. "Professional preparation and lifelong learning: The making of a clinician." In Shapiro, D., (Ed.), *Stuttering Intervention: A Collaborative Journey to Fluency Freedom.* Austin, TX: Pro-Ed, (1998): 476–511.

Shriberg, L., Filley, F., Hayes, D., Kwiatkowski, J., Shatz, J., Simmons, K., and Smith, M. "The Wisconsin Procedure for the Appraisal of Clinical Competence (W-PACC): Model and data." *American Speech Hearing Association, 17* (1975): 158–165.

Smith, K. "Supervisory conference questions: Who asks them and what are they?" Paper presented at the Annual Convention of the American Speech-Language and Hearing Association, Atlanta, GA, 1979.

Smith, K., and Anderson, J. "Relationship of perceived effectiveness to content in supervisory conferences in speech-language pathology." *Journal of Speech and Hearing Research, 25* (1982): 243–251.

Taylor, M., Fisher, C., and Ilgen, D. "Individuals' reactions to performance feedback in organizations: A control theory perspective." In K. M. Rowland and G. R. Ferris, (Eds.), *Research in Personnel and Human Resources Management,* Vol. 2. Greenwich, CT: JAI Press, (1984): 81–124.

Taylor, C., and Horney, M. "A phenomenographic investigation of students' approaches to self-evaluation of their clinical practice." *The Clinical Supervisor, 16* (2) (1997): 105–123.

Teitelbaum, S. "The impact of supervisory style." *Psychoanalysis and Psychotherapy, 15* (1) (1998): 115–129.

Tryon, G. "Supervisee development during the practicum year." *Counselor Education and Supervision, 35* (1996): 287–294.

Zahorik, J. "The observing–conferencing role of university supervisors." *Journal of Teacher Education, 39* (2) (1988): 9–16.

6 Supervising Speech-Language Pathology Assistants

Clinical Supervision Tasks Relevant To Supervising Speech-Language Pathology Assistants

Task 1: Establishing and maintaining an effective working relationship;

Task 4: Assisting the supervisee in developing and refining clinical management skills;

Task 5: Demonstrating for and participating with the supervisee in the clinical process;

Task 6: Assisting the supervisee in observing and analyzing assessment and treatment sessions (note that analyzing and assessment are not within the purview of the assistant);

Task 7: Assisting the supervisee in development and maintenance of clinical and supervisory records;

Task 9: Assisting the supervisee in evaluation of clinical performance;

Task 10: Assisting the supervisee in developing skills of verbal reporting, writing, and editing;

Task 11: Sharing information regarding ethical, legal, regulatory, and reimbursement aspects of the profession;

Task 12: Modeling and facilitating professional conduct;

Task 13: Demonstrating research skills in the clinical or supervisory process.

This chapter is devoted to the supervision of speech-language pathology assistants. The employment of paraprofessionals is a relatively new component of clinical practice in this field, and significant confusions exist among practitioners and assistants about supervisory requirements and the boundaries of ethical practice for assistants. The American Speech-Language Hearing Association provides guidelines for the training and supervision of these paraprofessionals. These guidelines provide a framework for understanding the functions they perform.

The Speech-Language Pathology Assistant's Scope of Practice

Speech-language pathology assistants are a type of support personnel recognized by the American Speech-Language Hearing Association. A national mechanism administered by the American Speech-Language Hearing Association for registering assistants is expected to be in place by 2002. The requirements to be specified are likely to include completion of an appropriate training program, supervised assistant placements, and a competency assessment (ASHA, 1996b; Council on Professional Standards and Council on Academic Accreditation, 1999).

Individual states and countries that endorse the use of paraprofessionals have differing approaches to delimiting the scope of practice for assistants and the standards for their licensing. The Board of Examiners in North Carolina has taken a leadership role in the delineation of the role of the speech-language pathology assistant and, together with the North Carolina Association of Supervisors in Speech Pathology and Audiology (NCASSPA), is working to train speech-language pathologists to supervise the assistants (McCready, 1999). On a national level, the American Speech-Language and Hearing Association has published "Guidelines for the Training, Credentialing, Use, and Supervision of Speech-Language Pathology Assistants" (ASHA, 1996a), which include a sample curriculum and suggested competencies for assistants. (See Appendix A for the curriculum and competencies formulated by ASHA and the competencies developed in Canada by Hagler and McFarlane [1997].) These documents specify the tasks that may be assigned to assistants if they are adequately trained and supervised.

The tasks they may implement follow:

1. Conduct speech-language screenings (without interpretation) following specified screening protocols developed by the supervising speech-language pathologist;

2. Provide direct treatment assistance to patients/clients identified by the supervising speech-language pathologist;

3. Follow documented treatment plans or protocols developed by the supervising speech-language pathologist;

4. Document patient/client progress toward meeting established objectives as stated in the treatment plan and report this information to the supervising speech-language pathologist;

5. Assist the speech-language pathologist during assessment of patients/clients, such as those who are difficult to test;

6. Assist with informal documentation (e.g., tallying notes for the speech-language pathologist to use), prepare materials, and assist with other clerical duties as directed by the speech-language pathologist;

7. Schedule activities, prepare charts, records, graphs, or otherwise display data;

8. Perform checks and maintenance of equipment;

9. Participate with the speech-language pathologist in research projects, in-service training, and public relations programs (ASHA, 1996a, p 25).

ASHA's guidelines also stipulate the aspects of the profession that the assistant cannot engage in and those that are solely in the domain of the professional speech-language pathologist. In general, "The speech-language pathology assistant should not perform any task without the express knowledge and approval of the supervising speech-language pathologist." In particular, speech-language pathology assistants cannot engage in the following activities:

1. Perform standardized or nonstandardized diagnostic tests, formal or informal evaluations, or interpret test results;

2. Participate in parent conferences, case conferences, or any interdisciplinary team without the presence of the supervising speech-language pathologist or other ASHA-certified speech-language pathologist designated by the supervising speech-language pathologist;

3. Provide patient/client or family counseling;

4. Write, develop, or modify a patient/client's individualized treatment plan in any way;

5. Assist with patients/clients without following the individualized treatment plan prepared by the speech-language pathologist or without access to supervision;

6. Sign any formal documents (e.g., treatment plans, reimbursement forms, or reports; the assistant should sign or initial informal treatment notes for review and co-signature by the supervising professional);

7. Select patients/clients for services;

8. Discharge a patient/client from services;

9. Disclose clinical or confidential information either orally or in writing to anyone not designated by the supervising speech-language pathologist;

10. Make referrals for additional services;

11. Communicate with the patient/client, family, or others regarding any aspect of the patient/client status or service without the specific consent of the supervising speech-language pathologist;

12. Represent himself or herself as a speech-language pathologist (ASHA, p. 26).

Further, these guidelines define those aspects of the clinical process that are completely in the domain of the speech-language pathologist:

1. Complete initial supervision training prior to accepting an assistant for supervision and upgrade supervision training on a regular basis;

2. Participate significantly in hiring the assistant;

3. Document preservice training and credentials of the assistant;

4. Inform patients/clients and families about the level (professional versus support personnel), frequency, and duration of services as well as supervision;

5. Represent the speech-language pathology team in all collaborative, interprofessional, inter-agency meetings, correspondence, and reports. This would not preclude the assistant from attending meetings along with the speech-language pathologist as a team member or drafting correspondence and reports for editing, approval, and signature by the speech-language pathologist;

6. Make all clinical decisions, including determining patient/client selection for inclusion/exclusion in the case load, and dismissing patients/clients from treatment;

7. Communicate with patients/clients, parents, and family members about diagnosis, prognosis, and treatment plan;

8. Conduct diagnostic evaluations, assessments, or appraisals, and interpret obtained data in reports;

9. Review each treatment plan with the assistant at least weekly;

10. Delegate specific tasks to the assistant while retaining legal and ethical responsibility for all patient/client services provided or omitted (ASHA, 1996a, p. 26).

As these guidelines indicate, the purpose of assistants is not to take the place of certified professionals but to provide the more routine aspects of treatment and to extend services as needed. Assistants are technicians not decision-makers, and the supervising speech-language pathologist has all the ethical and legal responsibility for the assistant's performance and patient care, including liability in the event that the assistant makes an error, engages in unethical behavior, or something unforeseen occurs.

Guidelines for Assistant Supervision

In some instances, people supervising assistants may not have had any or only minimal training in supervision. Administrators often mistakenly assume that the master's degree in speech pathology is a sufficient qualification. In other instances, without being aware that they are being unethical, some new employees are encouraged to begin supervising while they are still completing the clinical fellowship year (French, 1997; Anonymous, 1999).

Ten hours of continuing education, at minimum, is required to assume a supervisory role with assistants. Individuals without supervisory training have no information about supervision other than their personal experiences. What they discover about supervising is the result of struggling through the process rather than approaching it from an informed perspective (French, 1995), and the supervision they provide is likely to mirror that of any supervisor who has evolved into the role without supervisory training. It is likely to be direct and inflexible, which leads to minimal supervisee development (Anderson, 1988; Farmer and Farmer, 1989; Dowling, 1992). Radaszewski-Byrne (1997) suggests that master's level preservice training in supervision will make supervisors aware of their ethical and legal responsibilities in this relationship and will enhance the quality of assistant service delivery.

According to the ASHA guidelines, supervisors of speech-language pathology assistants must hold the certificate of clinical competence, have two years of experience after certification, and at least a one-credit course (minimum of fifteen contact hours) or ten hours of continuing education in supervision prior to the supervision of assistants. Supervisors are further encouraged to continue updating their supervisory skills beyond the basic stipulations. The ASHA position statement (1985) delineating the competencies of effective supervision—the thirteen tasks—serves as a guide for supervisor professional development.

The guidelines (ASHA, 1996a) stipulate the level of supervision to be provided to assistants in general, and on the basis of employment length. During an assistant's first ninety days of work:

1. 30 percent documented direct and indirect supervision;
2. No less than 20 percent must be direct, documented supervision accounting for a minimum of 20 percent of patient/client contact time;
3. Each patient must have some direct contact with the certified speech-language pathologist, at least once every two weeks;
4. Data on each client/patient treated by the assistant must be reviewed by the supervisor weekly;
5. Additional indirect supervision is required to be no less than 10 percent of actual patient/client contact time.

After an assistant's first ninety days of work:

1. The volume of supervision may be adjusted, dependent on assistant competency and client needs;
2. A minimum of 20 percent supervision must be maintained, of which at least 10 percent is direct (ASHA, 1996a, pp. 27–28).

In addition, at no time can a given individual supervise more than three assistants. Within the appropriate scope of practice for an assistant, the nature and complexity of tasks performed will necessitate varying degrees and types of supervision as well. Thus, the person who does scheduling, material preparation, and the most routine aspects of treatment may only need the minimum supervision specified. As treatment increases in complexity or when the assistant is given added responsibility, the intensity of supervision will need to expand accordingly. (Appendix 6-B provides a guide developed by McFarlane and Hagler (1997) to assist supervisors in determining the amount and type of supervision needed for given tasks.)

A meeting between an administrator and a supervisor illustrates typical misconceptions about the kind of tasks speech-language assistants are qualified to undertake and the roles they can legally perform:

Administrator to supervisor:

> I am glad we could meet today. You know we haven't been able to hire enough staff. There just isn't enough money. You keep telling me that there are populations we aren't serving and others we aren't serving well because there isn't enough of you or your staff to go around. I've been talking to administrators in other facilities and they have added speech-language pathology assistants to take up the slack. There is enough leeway in the budget to hire one or two and then we could expand services. Down the road we may be able to lay off one of your least productive staff members and replace that person with assistants who could each have their own caseloads. Just think how many more people we could serve and it would be a lot cheaper too. You won't have to spend so much of your time writing individual education plans and going to family meetings to approve them. It should make your job a lot easier and wouldn't take up much of your time.

This administrator is misinformed as he has voiced many of the misconceptions individuals have about the use of assistants and the extent to which hiring them will alleviate common service delivery problems. In practice, (1) assistants cannot have independent caseloads, (2) cannot legally perform the duties of professional staff, or (3) write individual education plans and present them for approval; likewise, (4) a supervisor cannot mentor an unlimited number of assistants, and (5) supervision demands increase with the addition of assistants.

The decision to include an assistant on a professional work team is one not to be made lightly. The scope of duties an assistant can perform is constrained and the amount of supervision required is significant. Assistants can and do make valuable contributions to a work setting, but their work must remain within the scope of ethical practice. According to Logemann (1999), assistants can do repetitive tasks but are not qualified to determine what comes next or what to do about it if a patient performs in a certain way. Assistants can also be very helpful in organizational areas, material development, and in implementing the routine aspects of treatment. They may, indeed, increase the intensity of treatment by allowing clients to be seen more often, giving them additional opportunities to practice the behaviors they are being taught, and assisting them in generalizing learned skills to new settings. An added benefit of assistants is that they are likely to be a part of the community in which services are provided, and, as such, serve as an important link culturally and linguistically to the families being served (Council of Exceptional Children, 1997; Longhurst, 1997).

As a result, in deciding to add an assistant to one's staff, the first step is to decide what the facility expects the assistant to do, and then to determine how much and what types of supervision he or she will need to complete assigned tasks. Hagler and McFarlane (1998) say that it is critical to convey to administrators that different tasks require different levels of supervision. Thus, if administrators want assistants to engage in complex aspects of treatment, they need to understand that a larger proportion of the supervisor's time will be needed to guide the assistants as they assume and perform these responsibilities. The supervisor's workload needs to be actively negotiated with administrators as assistants are added to the staff.

Supervisors and assistants work in a very close personal relationship. Due to the assistant's scope of practice, joint case management, and supervision requirements, it is critical that the supervisor and assistant like and respect each other. To increase the probability of having an effective working relationship, it is important to have the supervisor actively involved in the hiring and retention, and, if it becomes necessary, the firing of assistants with whom they work. French (1993), however, notes that supervisors frequently have little or no control in these events. Assistants are often hired in central administration or by a building principal rather than the speech-language pathologist. Such a situation is made worse when the supervisor cannot control assistant assignments (French, 1997). To make the relationship productive, the professional staff needs to actively educate administrators about supervision requirements and the importance of involving the supervisor in the hiring, review and placement process.

Nature of Assistants

Speech-language pathology assistants are likely to be a diverse group of people. The guidelines for training assistants remain in flux; the amounts and types of pre-employment training for these individuals is and is likely to remain variable. In addition, applicants for an assistant position also diverge in levels of ability and professionalism, their personal need to grow as a person, and in the effort they are willing to expend.

In response to this diversity, supervision will need to vary accordingly. The Anderson continuum of supervision model will be an effective tool for structuring supervision in response to assistants' needs. Of the three stages of the model, evaluation–feedback, transition, and self-supervision, only the first two are appropriate for assistants because they cannot ethically engage in self-supervision. In addition, supervisors must be directly involved in case management and observation of treatment by assistants throughout their work life. Thus, movement into a predominantly collaborative style, one in which the supervisee is problem-solving, developing strategies, and planning case management, is not appropriate. The evaluation–feedback stage, which involves a direct/active supervisory style, is likely to predominate in the relationship. Movement into the transitional stage with collaboration between the assistant and supervisor is desirable but will vary in degree, depending on the abilities of the assistant and the skill of the supervisor.

As the supervisory relationship with the assistant begins, it is important to discuss each person's expectations of the other. From the perspectives of the assistant and the supervisor, it is important to be explicit about the types of tasks the assistant will be expected to perform and general expectations for performance, to confirm the confidential nature of the relationship between them, and to be clear about the supervisor's philosophy of supervision. Finally, according to Hagler and McFarlane (1998), both individuals must understand that the supervisor is expected to provide the support the assistant needs to complete requested tasks. In particular, newly hired paraprofessionals need to be asked what they will need to know to perform successfully. Discrepancies in perceptions and a resolution of differences are important for establishing an effective supervisory relationship and for opening up the lines of communication.

Discussion of several other topics will enhance the relationship: (1) a strategy for communicating assignments and changes to tasks, (2) the frequency and nature of evaluation, and (3) guidelines for professional appearance, particularly if there is an unwritten code. In addition, whenever a new task is assigned, it will be important for the supervisor to provide a clear definition of the new responsibility so that the assistant knows what is expected.

Organizational Acculturation

In addition to talking globally about the supervisory process, it will be valuable to welcome new employees to the job setting and give them information that will assist them in getting settled, for example, introducing them to others in the facility and identifying who performs tasks that relate to the assistant's job or will make it easier for them to complete assignments. At the same, showing them where things are located is helpful. In particular, the restrooms, lunch area, and mailboxes should be pointed out. If possible, assistants should be given their own work space. At a minimum, they need a place to secure their personal belongings. An erasable board or a notebook for recording their schedule will assist them in knowing when and where they are expected, and planned supervision can also be noted in this organizational tool. If carried out or provided, such orientation activities will assist the assistant in adjusting to the job.

Goals and Strategies for Attainment

The goals for speech-language pathology assistants are diverse in nature. In regard to clinical practice, they should be able to perform their assigned tasks competently, assume increasing responsibility within their scope of practice, facilitate the provision of clinical services to clients/patients, and present themselves in a professional manner. They also need to identify themselves as assistants and be assertive in refusing to perform tasks beyond their scope of practice or letting people other than their supervisor assign them responsibilities. Finally, they need to like their job and feel that they are a contributing member of the team.

Competent Performance

The supervision of assistants shares components of the process typical to other supervisees. A factor that will vary will be the proportionally larger component devoted to the direct teaching and provision of support sufficient to enable the assistant to complete assigned tasks. Radaszewski-Byrne (1997) suggest, as guidelines and standards for assistant training develop, that the need for direct on-the-job training may decrease in some areas as assistants will start to arrive with more of the skills needed for basic job performance. Even then, the supervisor is likely to use a directive style, asking questions, giving both positive and negative feedback, demonstrating problem-solving, actively generating strategies, and giving the supervisee concrete guidance (Smith and Anderson, 1982).

For example, if the assistant is going to carry out speech and language screening, the procedures for screening, the screening instruments, and the recording of data will need to be reviewed. In addition, the assistant may need input regarding behavior management and strategies for guiding the behaviors of the population being screened. The organizational aspect of setting up a screening may also need to be considered. Once the assistant demonstrates competency, it is then appropriate to initiate the screening process with the supervisor monitoring the implementation and interpreting the findings.

Thus, for each new task the assistant is to undertake, the supervisor, with input from the supervisee, will determine the assistant's training and supervision needs. As the assistant grows in skill, confidence, and experience with a given task, less direct supervision will be required. Then, as the complexity of the assistant's assignments increases, further training and additional supervision will be needed. The charts developed by Hagler and McFarlane (1997) will be helpful tools in the determination and documentation of suitable levels of supervision in regard to task complexity (see Appendix B, Decision Matrix for Amount and Type of Monitoring and Assistant and Professional Planner).

Responsibility and Client Service

The overall goal is to increase the number and range of tasks that the assistant can competently perform while maintaining the integrity of the clinical process. Initially, assistants may perform support functions, routine aspects of treatment, and organizational tasks. As the assistant demonstrates the ability, and with appropriate levels of supervision, the complexity of tasks designated may increase. As this process evolves, the combined efforts of the supervisor and assistant will result in optimal treatment for patients/clients by allowing for increased intensity and/or frequency of service. In addition, having an assistant involved will facilitate the treatment process by allowing the supervisor to focus on case management, diagnosis, the more complex aspects of treatment, and those tasks only a certified speech-language pathologist can perform.

Professional Behavior

A key responsibility of the supervisor is guiding the assistant's development of an appropriate demeanor. One of the thirteen tasks of supervision is the supervisor's modeling of professional behavior, which includes confidentiality, appearance, ethics, and appropriate interaction with clientele and others in the working setting. Most assistants will come to the job with some information in these areas, and situations that arise in practice will provide opportunities to refine the assistant's professional posture.

Role Identification

It is critical to introduce and continually refer to the assistant as an *assistant.* Recipients of service and other professionals are often unclear about the status of a given service provider, and think that an assistant is a certified speech-language pathologist. Thus, when service is initiated, it is important to indicate to clientele that you have an assistant and clarify who will be providing their service and your role as the supervisor in that interaction. Clients/patients need to understand how and when they will see the certified speech-language pathologist and the proportion of their treatment that will be provided by an assistant. McFarlane and Hagler's 1995 Client Review Table (see Appendix B) will aid in planning and monitoring this process. Further, assistants need to reiterate that they are an assistant when anyone refers to them as a speech-language pathologist. A name badge with the title of assistant will help minimize this confusion.

Job Satisfaction

Speech-language pathology assistants will always be assistants unless they go back to school for additional education. The absence of a career path makes motivation for this level of personnel difficult. On the other hand, the limited training needed to become an assistant allows people a quick entry into a professional job. In school systems, individuals often enjoy being an assistant because it gives them prestige and a feeling of accomplishment. They feel valued as a contributing team member. Assistants who are parents also have an opportunity to work a schedule that parallels that of their children (Logue, 1993). Potential negative aspects of the job are

stress due to the complexity of assignments and the behavior management of difficult cases, inadequate training to perform assigned tasks, lack of respect by clientele, and low wages (Logue, 1993). Passaro, Pickett, Latham, and HongBo (1994)
note some of these issues but add three other sources of dissatisfaction: few opportunities for advancement, little administrative support, and inadequate benefits.
These negative aspects of the position contribute to a high assistant turnover rate.

To create job satisfaction and to minimize turnover, assistants must feel that
they are partners in the clinical process. They need to be valued and treated as
team members within the limits of their position. A big step toward this end is for
the supervisor to clarify the assistant's role to administrators and others in the
work setting. Then the assistants will not be asked to perform tasks outside their
range of expertise. Ideally, the assistant will only have one supervisor to whom to
report. If the assistant is working for more than one supervisor, the process needs
to be actively coordinated or one of the supervisors should assume a primary role.
This situation can create difficult circumstances and increased stress, especially if
the assistant is often being moved from one place or task to another, is being given
conflicting responsibilities, or is assigned more tasks than can be reasonably managed. A defined chain of command for supervision of the assistant is a requirement
for job satisfaction.

The permissible scope of practice for assistants has been defined. Within
those parameters, it will be helpful to show individuals a plan for their potential
development. It may begin with them doing organizational tasks and routine
aspects of treatment. Show them, as they demonstrate readiness, how they will
assume more responsibility and gradually increase the complexity of the tasks
they perform. As they evolve, the plan can be reviewed and their growth noted.
This ongoing process will allow them to see their progress and derive pleasure
from their achievements. To facilitate this process, the supervisor will provide the
support the assistant needs to take on new and complex tasks.

Interpersonal issues also contribute to job satisfaction. Being treated with
respect by everyone in the work setting is a key factor in fostering assistant contentment. In particular, a supervisory attitude of positive regard for the assistant
forms the basis for a productive working relationship. Saying "thank you" and
acknowledging his or her successes and contributions will make the assistant feel
valued. Likewise, being honest and constructive when there is a problem is vital.
It will be important to treat the assistant with respect when dealing with families,
caregivers and others in the work setting. Each of these strategies will contribute
to the assistant's sense of well-being.

Supervisory Tools

Several specific supervisory tools are likely to be beneficial to the assistant. These
may include joint planning, roleplay, demonstration therapy, data collection,
objective setting, structured observations, videotape/audiotape, and selected verbatim. Each makes a unique contribution to the assistant's development.

Joint Planning and Role-Playing

In regard to joint planning, the supervisor and assistant may organize the latter's work week or plan for upcoming events. More specifically, as a part of reviewing lesson plans, a step-by-step strategy for carrying out a specific therapy activity may be jointly outlined. The amount of joint planning will be adjusted depending on the assistant's needs and the complexity of the task. Following planning, the supervisee may find it helpful to role-play a procedure with the supervisor while assuming either the stance of client or clinician. The supervisor and assistant can then shift roles so that a direct model of therapy implementation can be provided. Role-playing allows the supervisee to practice a skill in a safe environment in which feedback is readily available.

Demonstration Therapy

Demonstration therapy may be used by the supervisor as a tool to train the assistant, and it is particularly helpful if the supervisor demonstrates some of the more difficult aspects of treatment with the clients for whom the assistant is sharing responsibility. The supervisor and the assistant may also jointly implement an activity or session so that the supervisor provides demonstration and guidance within the context of a specific therapy session. This is particularly helpful as it guides assistants in implementing aspects of treatment with their own clientele; it is often eye-opening to watch someone else successfully implementing a strategy that has been a source of personal frustration. Joint implementation of therapy may also relieve the pressure of having the assistant deal with all aspects of the session simultaneously, giving the individual time to absorb key information. Planned rather than spontaneous joint implementation or demonstration therapy is most acceptable to the supervisee. Most supervisees strongly object to unannounced interruptions (Dowling and Wittkopp, 1982).

Data Collection

Data collection and analysis should be incorporated as soon as it can be used meaningfully. Supervisors may choose to collect data for documentation purposes or use it to give the assistant concrete feedback. They can also collect data and show the supervisee how it relates to the solution of immediate concerns. Assistants will be collecting client data but may also gather data about their own performance. Decisions, based on data, to alter the direction of treatment remain in the domain of the supervisor.

Objective Setting

Objectives are excellent as a way to stimulate professional growth. Initial goals can be oriented to learning the job. For example, the assistant could review a specific number of client files per week to become acquainted with individuals constituting the caseload. Once the person has settled in, goals can be directed toward optimizing performance. Goals are particularly beneficial in combination with data collection. Then, once a goal has been identified, a strategy for collecting data to assess the assistant's achievement of that goal can also be planned. In general, goal development increases work satisfaction and commitment to an organization (Nelson, 1997). Attainment of goals is also likely to increase confidence in one's ability to perform well (Dowling, 1993).

Other goals that might be set for an assistant could relate to interactions with clients. To enhance therapy implementation, for example, the assistant could learn how to present stimuli in a preplanned manner, adjusting the use of visual and auditory stimuli as needed, or how to vary aspects of therapy to maintain the client's interest and willing participation. Or, the assistant could be shown how to implement an appropriate level of task difficulty during treatment activities for various clients. Other goals for assistants might include showing an understanding of behavior management strategies, completing tasks as assigned, preparing and organizing treatment materials prior to each treatment session, and organizing and filing client records. These are all tasks that speech-language assistants should be able to perform. Numerous other goals will be appropriate given the nature of the assistant's role in various settings.

Structured Observations

The supervisor may arrange for the assistant to observe other clinicians who are skillful in implementing specific aspects of treatment. The observation of another person allows supervisees to watch a successful interaction and to think about ways to incorporate these behaviors into their own work. It also increases the range of options they have for therapy implementation. While watching, supervisees will benefit from recording or charting the behaviors that they are being guided to observe. The informal data collection methods described in chapter three might be used to this end. Collecting data will assist the observer in identifying cause and effect. It will also help the assistant begin to see the value and relevance of data for strengthening clinical performance.

Videotape and Audiotape

Videotape and audiotape are also excellent tools for training assistants because they allow them to step out of themselves and start to view their therapy as others might. It also gives them the opportunity to identify their own strengths and areas for growth. When videotapes or audiotapes are incorporated into the conference, actual behavior can be observed so that examples of skills and weaknesses can be discussed. This can also lead to concrete discussions of how to amplify or change behavior. Further, during the observation of the tape, the supervisor can also demonstrate the collection and interpretation of data critical to the supervisee's success. In terms of picking a tape segment, either the assistant or supervisor may do so. Crago's (1987) idea of choosing segments that went well, created concern, or surprised the supervisee or supervisor may be used as a means of selection.

Selective Verbatim

Selected verbatim (Acheson and Gall, 1992) can also be used with audio- or video-tape. This is a written verbatim record of specific aspects of treatment. For example, the supervisor or supervisee might transcribe the supervisee's directions or models during an activity. The transcription often is enlightening. Individuals may think their directions are concise and clear when in fact they are long and confusing. The assistant may even want to rewrite the directions as a tool to improve them for future use. Selective verbatim is also effective during direct observation. The supervisor may become aware of a particular behavior and record it for discussion with the supervisee. Similarly, if supervisees express concern about an aspect of their work, verbatim recordings can be very helpful in defining the issue and providing a basis for change. Whether these recordings are spontaneous or preplanned, they will prove to be valuable supervisory tools.

Performance Documentation and Appraisal

Documentation of an assistant's performance is important to his or her development and ability to maintain performance integrity, and it can take several forms: (1) a written, ongoing log, (2) valuative rating forms or other types of feedback instruments, (3) collected data, (4) copies of notes on lesson plans or communications to the supervisee, (5) drafts of written materials, and (6) records of interactions. The ongoing log may be informal notations about the quality of lesson plan implementation and/or behavior management as well as significant events that may have occurred. In regard to information concerning observations, the supervisor needs to take care that supervisees are adequately observed, that they receive feedback about their performance, and have an opportunity to provide input from their perspective. Passaro and colleagues (1994) note that assistants' self-ratings of performance are often higher than a supervisor's rating of the same events. In order to take such discrepancy into account, the supervisor may choose to keep a journal of the dates and times of observations as well as the types of feedback provided and the supervisees' response. This will also be helpful in documenting the types and quantity of supervision suggested by the American Speech-Language Association guidelines and individual state or country requirements. The journal can be helpful for planning supervision as well. At a glance, a supervisor will know the time periods and patients yet to be monitored. It is always a good idea to have assistants initial and return observation instruments as a means to document performance. Other valuative information should also be initialed or signed by the supervisees and then placed in their personnel file. It is important to note that acknowledging receipt of a form does not signal agreement with the valuative content. It only demonstrates that it has been seen by those involved.

Feedback through checklists, written comments, and informal interactions are an expected part of the evaluation process. Due to the newness of the role of assistant, checklist tools are not widely available. In addition, the nature of the assistant's role will vary with time, across settings, and in relation to the types of tasks the assistant assumes. Due to this variability, it may be necessary to craft and adapt a valuative instrument as needed.

A more formal performance appraisal will need to occur on a regular basis. In the first year, relatively frequent appraisals may be appropriate, perhaps monthly. As the assistant gains skill, formal evaluations can be done on a quarterly or six-month schedule, and should include valuative feedback in each area of an assistant's responsibility, for example, specific support functions, treatment, and screening implementation, interactions with clientele, their families and other staff members, and professionalism. Evaluation can also address more personal issues such as initiative, timeliness, reliability, appearance, and use of grammatically correct spoken and written language.

Conference

Conferencing with the assistant may be a lot of short exchanges during joint interactions as well as more typical conferences. However such discussions occur, it is important to meet with the assistant on a regular basis to discuss client/patient performance and the ongoing development of the supervisee. The conference style is most likely to be direct/active with a significant amount of telling in the beginning of the relationship. Assuming the assistant grows in skill as tasks become repetitive, increasing amounts of collaboration may be appropriate. Expanding the quantity and quality of supervisee input in conferences will enhance the assistant's sense of competence and well-being. Discussions about the supervisee's perceived supervisory needs are an important component of the conference. Additional strategies discussed in Chapter 4 are also appropriate for implementation with assistants, for example, aspects of cognitive coaching (Costa and Garmston, 1994), verbal and nonverbal mirroring, active listening, and conscious control of power messages by adapting room arrangements.

Relationship of the Specified Supervision Tasks to Supervising Speech-Language Pathology Assistants

Ten tasks of supervision are identified as relevant to supervising assistants. Establishing and maintaining an effective working relationship is the foundation for effective supervision. This includes welcoming assistants to the position, valuing, respecting, and communicating honestly with them. Once they are situated, they should be assisted in developing and refining their clinical management skills, either by means of supervisor demonstration and/or cooperative participation in the clinical process. The supervisee should be guided to observe and analyze treatment. Data collection will aid such observations but it is also a useful tool for self-evaluation of clinical performance. Treatment, outcomes, and the documentation of the types and volume of supervision are required. Thus, assisting the supervisee in the development and maintenance of clinical and supervisory records will be important. Similarly, verbal reporting, writing, and editing are critical components of the assistant's role, so appropriate assistance in developing and refining these skills will be helpful. To function successfully, the assistant will also need to be informed about ethical, legal, regulatory, and reimbursement aspects of the profession. The supervisor can do this by providing information, mentoring, and modeling professional conduct. Finally, as assistants grow in skill, exposure and involvement in research relating to the clinical or supervisory process will increase their levels of involvement, and assist the supervisor in assessing outcomes to document treatment efficacy, a critical aspect of evidence-based clinical practice.

Summary

This chapter has covered an array of topics relating to the supervision of speech-language pathology assistants. Due to the continuing confusion about the role, training, and supervision of the assistant, the ASHA guidelines for each of the above serve as the starting point, followed by ideas to help the assistant become an effective participant in the work setting. Goals for the assistant were suggested along with supervisory strategies to aid attainment, and several supervisory tools were presented to assist the supervisor in guiding the assistant toward increasing competence. Performance evaluation and the supervisory conference were also addressed. The relationship of the thirteen tasks of supervision to effectively supervising the assistant conclude this section. The material in the appendices will be particularly helpful to the reader. It is hoped that the content of this chapter will be used to guide and enhance the contributions of speech-language pathology assistants in the workplace.

REFERENCES

Acheson, K., and Gall, M. (3rd ed.) *Techniques in the Clinical Supervision of Teachers: Preservice and Inservice Applications.* New York: Longman, 1992.

American Speech and Hearing Association. Committee on Supervision in Speech-Language Pathology and Audiology. "Clinical supervision in speech-language pathology and audiology: A position statement." *American Speech Hearing Association, 27* (1985): 57–60.

American Speech-Language Hearing Association. "Guidelines for the training, credentialing, use and supervision of speech-language pathology assistants." *ASHA, 38* (16) (1996a): 21–34.

American Speech-Language Hearing Association. Proposed Strategic Plan for Credentialing Speech-Language Pathology Assistants. Rockville Pike, MD, 1996b.

Anderson, J. *The Supervisory Process in Speech-Language Pathology and Audiology.* Austin, TX: Pro-Ed, 1988.

Anonymous. Personal Communication, 1999.

Costa, A., and Garmston, R. *Cognitive Coaching: A Foundation for Renaissance Schools.* Norwood, MA: Christopher Gordon Publishers, 1994.

Council of Exceptional Children. "Report of the consortium of education organizations on the preparation and use of speech-language paraprofessionals in early intervention and education settings." *Journal of Children's Communication Development, 18* (1) (1997): 31–56.

Council on Professional Standards and Council on Academic Accreditation. "SLP assistant forum: Proposed standards for credentialing SLP assistants." Seminar at the national convention of the American Speech-Language and Hearing Association. San Francisco, CA, Nov., 1999.

Crago, M. "Supervision and self-exploration." In M. Crago and M. Pickering, (Eds.), *Supervision in Communication Disorders: Perspectives on a Process.* San Diego: Singular Publishing Group, 1987.

Dowling, S. *Implementing the Supervisory Process: Theory and Practice,* Englewood Cliffs, NJ: Prentice-Hall, 1992.

Dowling, S. "Supervisory training, objective setting and grade contingent performance." *Language Speech Hearing Services Schools, 24* (1993): 92–99.

Dowling, S., and Wittkopp, J. "Students' perceived supervisory needs." *Journal of Communication Disorders, 15* (1982): 319–328.

Farmer, S., and Farmer, J. *Supervision in Communication Disorders,* Columbus, OH: Merrill Publishing, 1989.

French, N. "Are community college training programs for paraeducators feasible?" *Community College Journal of Research and Practice, 17* (1993): 131–140.

French, N. "Teachers and paraeducators: How they work together." Unpublished manuscript. University of Colorado at Denver, 1995.

French, N. "A case study of a speech-language pathologist's supervision of assistants in a school setting: Tracy's story." *Journal of Children's Communication Development, 18* (1) (1997): 103–110.

Hagler, P., and McFarlane, L. "Collaborative service delivery by assistants and professionals (Revised)." Alberta Rehabilitation Coordinating Council. Edmonton, Alberta, Canada, 1997.

Hagler, P., and McFarlane, L. "A field tested model for supervision of support personnel." Short Course presented at the Annual Convention of the American Speech-Language and Hearing Association, Nov., 1998.

Logemann, J. "The State of Our Profession." University of Houston, Houston, TX, Jan. 22, 1999.

Logue, O. "Job satisfaction and retention variables of special education paraeducators." Paper presented at the 12th Annual Conference on the Training and Employment of Paraprofessionals in Education and Rehabilitation, Seattle, WA, 1993.

Longhurst, T. "Career pathways for related service paratherapists working in early intervention and other education settings." *Journal of Children's Communication Disorders, 18* (1) (1997): 23–30.

McCready, C. V. Personal Communication, 1999.

Nelson, B. "Motivating people." *Executive Excellence, 14* (9) (1997): 16–418.

Passaro, P., Pickett, A., Latham, G., and HongBo, W. "The training and support needs of paraprofessionals in rural special education." *Rural Special Education Quarterly, 13* (4) (1994): 3–9.

Paul-Brown, D. Director, Speech-Language Pathology Practice: Clinical Issues. American Speech-Language and Hearing Association. Personal communication, 1999.

Radaszewski-Byrne, M. "Issues in the development of guidelines for the preparation and use of speech-language paraprofessionals and their supervisors working in education settings." *Journal of Children's Communication Disorders, 18* (1) (1997): 5–22.

Smith, K., and Anderson, J. "Relationship of perceived effectiveness to content in supervisory conferences in speech-language pathology." *Journal of Speech and Hearing Research, 25* (1982): 243–251.

APPENDIX 6-A

1. Sample Curriculum for the Speech-Language Pathology Assistant
2. Speech-Language Pathology Assistant Suggested Competencies
3. Approved Tasks for Communication Assistants

Sample Curriculum for the Speech-Language Pathology Assistant (ASHA, 1996)

Any of the three training options for the speech-language pathology assistant (i.e., an associate's degree, certificate program, equivalent course of study) could include the following core coursework and practicum experience. The coursework may vary depending on the setting within which the assistant will be working. For example, the curriculum may include a course in neurogenic disorders for those assistants whose anticipated employment setting is a hospital or clinic. Multicultural information should be integrated in all points of the curriculum for assistants. A mechanism for ASHA approval of the curriculum will be established.

Coursework pertaining to clinical populations, clinical management, or any of the duties to be assumed by the assistant should be taught by ASHA-certIfied speech-language pathologists (e.g., survey of disabilities, normal development, clinical methods, acquired disorders) or audiologists (e.g., introduction to audiology). Practicum supervision must be provided by ASHA-certified speech-language pathologists.

Suggested Course	*Suggested Number of Credit Hours*
English Composition/Grammar	6
Math	3
Psychology/Sociology/Multicultural Studies (some combination)	9
Phonetics	3
Human Anatomy and Physiology	6
Survey of Disabilities	3
Normal Speech, Language, and Hearing Development Across the Life Span	3
Articulation Disorders and Rehabilitation	3
Language Disorders and Rehabilitation	3
Clinical Methods/Procedures	3
Acquired Disorders and Rehabilitation	3

American Speech-Language Hearing Association. "Guidelines for the training, credentialing, use and supervision of speech-language pathology assistants. *ASHA*, 38 (Suppl.16) (1996): 21–34. Reprinted with permission.

Hagler, P., and McFarlane, L., Collaborative service delivery by assistants and professionals (Revised). Alberta Rehabilitation Coordinating Council. Edmonton, Alberta, Canada (1997). Reprinted with permission.

Practicum 1—Program-Based Observation	4*
Practicum 2—Public School (on-the-job-training)	4
Practicum 3—Hospital/Rehabilitation (on-the-job training)	4
Introduction to Audiology/Aural Rehabilitation	3
	60 hours plus electives**

Speech-Language Pathology Assistant Suggested Competencies (ASHA, 1996)

The functionally based proficiency evaluation may check competencies in the following areas:

I. **Interpersonal Skills (communicates honestly, clearly, accurately, coherently, and concisely.)**

1. Deals effectively with attitudes and behaviors of the patient/client
   a. Maintains appropriate patient/client relationships
   b. Communicates sensitivity to the needs of the patient/client and family
   c. Takes into proper consideration patient/client needs and cultural values
   d. Demonstrates an appropriate level of self-confidence when performing assigned tasks
   e. Establishes rapport with patient/client and family
   f. Demonstrates insight in patient/client attitudes and behaviors
   g. Directs patient/client, family, and professionals to supervisor for information regarding testing, treatment, and referral

2. Uses appropriate language (written and oral) in dealing with patient/client and others
   a. Uses language appropriate for patient/client and other's age and educational level
   b. Is courteous and respectful at all times
   c. Maintains appropriate pragmatic skills

3. Deals effectively with supervisor
   a. Is receptive to constructive criticism
   b. Requests assistance from supervisor as needed
   c. Actively participates in interaction with supervisor

II. **Personal Qualities**

1. Manages time effectively
   a. Arrives punctually and prepared for patient/client appointments
   b. Arrives punctually for work-related meetings (e.g., meetings with supervisor, staff, etc.)
   c. Turns in all documentation on time

*This practicum consists of extensive observation in at least two different sites selected by the training program.

**An elective in computer technology is strongly suggested.

2. Demonstrates Appropriate Conduct
   a. Respects/maintains confidentiality of patients/clients
   b. Maintains personal appearance appropriate for the work setting
   c. Uses appropriate language for the work setting
   d. Evaluates own performance
   e. Recognizes own professional limitations and performs within boundaries of training and job responsibilities

III. Technical-Assistant Skills

1. Maintains a facilitating environment for assigned tasks
   a. Adjusts lighting and controls noise level
   b. Organizes treatment space

2. Uses time effectively
   a. Performs assigned tasks with no unnecessary distractions
   b. Completes assigned tasks within designated treatment session

3. Selects, prepares, and presents materials effectively
   a. Prepares and selects treatment materials ahead of time
   b. Chooses appropriate materials based on treatment plan
   c. Prepares clinical setting to meet the needs of the client for obtaining optimal performance
   d. Selects materials that are age- and culturally appropriate as well as motivating

4. Maintains documentation
   a. Documents plans and protocols accurately and concisely for supervisor
   b. Documents and reports patient/client performance to supervisor
   c. Signs documents reviewed and cosigned by the supervisor
   d. Prepares and maintains patient/client charts, records, graphs for displaying data

5. Provides assistance to speech-language pathologist
   a. Assists speech-language pathologist during patient/client assessment
   b. Assists with informal documentation
   c. Schedules activities
   d. Participates with speech-language pathologist in research projects
   e. Participates in in-service training
   f. Participates in public relations programs

IV. Screening

1. Demonstrates knowledge and use of variety of screening tools and protocols
   a. Completed training on screening procedures
   b. Uses two to three screening instruments reliably

2. Demonstrates appropriate administration and scoring of screening tools
   a. Differentiates correct versus incorrect responses
   b. Completes (fills out) screening protocols accurately
   c. Scores screening instruments accurately

3. Manages screenings and documentation
   a. Reports any difficulty encountered in screening
   b. Schedules screenings
   c. Organizes screening materials

4. Communicates screening results and all supplemental information to supervisor
   a. Seeks supervisor's guidance should adaptation of screening tools and administration be in question
   b. Provides descriptive behavioral observations that contribute to screening results

V. Treatment

1. Performs tasks as outlined and instructed by the supervisor
   a. Accurately and efficiently implements activities using procedures planned by the supervisor
   b. Uses constructive feedback from supervisor for modifying interaction (interpersonal or otherwise) with patient/client

2. Demonstrates skills in managing behavior and treatment program
   a. Maintains on-task behavior
   b. Provides appropriate feedback as to the accuracy of patient/client response
   c. Uses feedback and reinforcement that are consistent, discriminating, and meaningful to the patient/client
   d. Gives directions and instructions that are clear, concise, and appropriate to the patient's/client's age level and level of understanding
   e. Applies knowledge of behavior modification during interaction with the patient/client
   f. Implements designated treatment objectives/goals in specified sequence

3. Demonstrates knowledge of treatment objectives and plan
   a. Demonstrates understanding of patient/client disorder and needs
   b. Identifies correct versus incorrect responses
   c. Describes behaviors demonstrating a knowledge of the patient's/client's overall level of progress
   d. Verbally reports and provides appropriate documentation of assigned activities

Approved Tasks for Communication Assistants (Hagler and McFarlane, 1997)

Provided that the assistant has appropriate training and that adequate supervision and documentation are provided, a supervising professional may assign the following duties to a Communication Assistant.

Evaluation Activities:

1. Administer and score standardized speech-language and hearing screenings (without interpreting results) following specific protocols directed by the supervising speech-language pathologist.
2. Assist the supervising speech-language pathologist with assessments.
2. Communicate information regarding the client (both oral and written) as assigned by the supervising speech-language pathologist.
3. Document client progress towards meeting goals assigned by the supervising speech-language pathologist.
4. Share client information with supervising speech-language pathologist.
5. Attend client care conferences.

[Adapted from Hagler et al. (1993) and the Communication Assistant Role Statement (The Formal Training of Rehabilitation Assistants in Alberta, 1994)]

Treatment Activities:

1. Provide direct individual and group treatment assistance to the supervising speech-language pathologist.
2. Follow documented client care plans developed, assigned and monitored by the supervising speech-language pathologist. These client care plans may include both group and individual treatment in the following areas:
   a. articulation/phonology
   b. auditory activities (awareness, discrimination, memory, etc.)
   c. voice
   d. fluency
   e. language (child and adult)
   f. augmentative communication
3. Plan communication and language stimulation activities according to the treatment plan developed by the supervising speech-language pathologist.

Program Support Activities

Assist or perform independently the following tasks:

   a. prepare room or materials
   b. check or maintain equipment
   c. order supplies, equipment or services
   d. inventory
   e. organize events
   f. loan or sell equipment
   g. operate audiovisual equipment
   h. clerical tasks (reception, phone, scheduling appointments, mail, photocopying, filing, bookkeeping, billing, statistics)
   i. assist with public education events
   j. laundry
   k. shopping
   l. attend staff meetings
   m. computer work

**Role Limitations (The Formal Training
of Rehabilitation Assistants in Alberta, 1994)**

Certain duties are beyond the scopes of practice of assistants. These duties include:

1. the initial interview;
2. independently administered diagnostic tests;
3. interpretation of referral, diagnosis or prognosis;
4. interpretation of assessment findings, treatment procedures, and goals of treatment or service;
5. determination of caseload;
6. counseling of clients, parents, primary care givers, or spouses;
7. decisions about initiation, duration or termination of treatment;
8. developing, planning, or modifying treatment programs, goals, or objectives;
9. referral of a client to other professionals or agencies; or
10. transmission of client information to any individual other than the professional under whose supervision the assistant is working.

A P P E N D I X   6 - B

1. Decision Matrix for Amount and Type of Monitoring
2. Assistant and Professional Planner
3. Client Review Table (Copyright 1995)

Decision Matrix for Amount and Type of Monitoring

The Decision Matrix for Amount and Type of Monitoring is designed to help assistants and professionals plan their observation and monitoring activities with optimal efficiency. A minimum of 20% of assistant-provided *direct patient/client care* should be monitored. Assistant-provided tasks that do *not* involve direct patient/client contact may require little or no monitoring. The Decision Matrix will help assistants and professionals differentiate between tasks requiring a high proportion of monitoring and tasks requiring a low proportion of monitoring. The Decision Matrix is intended to be used in conjunction with the *Assistant and Professional Planner.*

In the column labeled "Task Level" on the Planner, enter a task level (A–D) from the table below for each task delegated to the assistant. Then apportion the professional's monitoring time accordingly. For example, assistants and professionals will want to reserve a large proportion of the supervisor's time for monitoring Level A tasks which may require up to 80% direct observation. On the other hand, the supervisor will need little or no time for monitoring Level D tasks.

From Hagler, P., and McFarlane, L., Collaborative service delivery by assistants and professionals (Revised). Alberta Rehabilitation Coordinating Council. Edmonton, Alberta, Canada (1997). Reprinted with permission.

Task Level	A	B	C	D
Task Description	Tasks with extensive patient contact that are highly complex or highly technical or require high levels of interpersonal interaction.	Tasks with extensive patient contact that are minimally complex, minimally technical, and require minimal interpersonal interaction.	Tasks without extensive patient contact that are highly complex, highly technical, and require high levels of interpersonal interaction.	Tasks without extensive patient contact that are minimally complex, minimally technical, and require minimal interpersonal interaction.
Amount of Monitoring	20% to 80%	20% to 60%	10% to 40%	0% to 20%
Type of Monitoring	Direct ONLY	Direct (5% minimum) or a combination of direct and indirect	Direct (5% minimum) or a combination of direct and indirect	Indirect only or a combination of direct and indirect

N.B. The assistant's level of training and experience, as well as the type and complexity of patient/client disorder, will increase or decrease the amount of monitoring and the ratio of direct and indirect monitoring within a category. If the minimum amount of direct supervision required for an assistant to successfully carry out a Level A task exceeds 80%, that task probably should not be delegated to the assistant.

Source: Hagler and McFarlane (1997).

Assistant & Professional Planner

Speech-Language Pathology	Date: Date to review:		
Assigned Tasks	*Task level*	*Ass't* *hours/wk*	*Supervision Plan (type,* *amount, sched.)*
Evaluation Activities			
administer and score standardized screenings			
assist SLP with assessments			
communicate client information to others			
document client progress			
share client information with SLP			
attend client care conference			
Subtotals		hrs/wk	hrs/wk
Treatment Activities			
provide treatment assistance			
follow documented client care plans			
specify			
Subtotals		hrs/wk	hrs/wk
Program Support Activities			
specify			
Subtotals		hrs/wk	hrs/wk
Totals		hrs/wk	hrs/wk

Source: Hagler and McFarlane (1997).

Client Review Table

Client Information		Service Plan & Schedule		
Client name	Diagnosis & severity	Assistant/ professional* combined services	Professional alone	Assistant alone (with professional monitoring schedule)**

*The professional and assistant are concurrently providing services to the same patient/client.
**When the majority of services are provided by the assistant alone, the supervising professional must include a schedule of direct client contact to maintain accountability and quality of patient/client service.

Source: Hagler and McFarlane (1997).

7 Supervising in the Workplace

Clinical Supervision Tasks Relevant to Supervision in the Workplace

Task 1: Establishing and maintaining an effective working relationship with the supervisee;

Task 2: Assisting the supervisee in developing clinical goals and objectives;

Task 3: Assisting the supervisee in developing and refining assessment skills;

Task 4: Assisting the supervisee in developing and refining management skills;

Task 5: Demonstrating for and participating with the supervisee in the clinical process;

Task 6: Assisting the supervisee in observing and analyzing assessment and treatment sessions;

Task 7: Assisting the supervisee in the development and maintenance of clinical and supervisory records;

Task 8: Interacting with the supervisee in planning, executing, and analyzing supervisory conferences;

Task 9: Assisting the supervisee in the evaluation of clinical performance;

Task 10: Assisting the supervisee in developing skills of verbal reporting, writing, and editing;

Task 11: Sharing information regarding ethical, legal, regulatory, and reimbursement aspects of professional practice;

Task 12: Modeling and facilitating professional conduct;

Task 13: Demonstrating research skills in the clinical or supervisory processes.

Supervision in the workplace presents unique challenges and opportunities. In addition to the administrative aspects, the work setting is the site of service delivery with an accompanying charge to maximize clinical outcomes. Relationships with employees tend to be long-term, which provides a context for the implementation of effective supervision—an environment in which all participants grow. This chapter will touch on a variety of topics that will be helpful to the supervisor. Of prime importance is the role supervisors select and their job definitions. The hiring process is also critical. The supervisory models discussed in Chapter 5 continue to apply. The previously discussed data-collection strategies will also be valuable. Preparing supervisees for supervision, setting professional goals, using specific supervisory techniques, selecting conference strategies, communicating effectively, and incorporating performance evaluation are topics that impact the supervisory process. Organizational issues that affect the quality of work life and job satisfaction will also be prime factors in the supervision of the working professional. Finally, implementing the thirteen tasks of supervision continues to be the foundation for an effective working relationship with employees.

Several new ideas and challenges will be presented in the following material. Often, when one has been working in an environment for a period of time, a sense of an inability to change the system emerges. In reality, there are constraints related to specific jobs and workplaces, so some concepts will be directly applicable while others may not. It is hoped that the reader will select those that can be readily incorporated and then gradually work to add those that may require greater effort and persistence.

Supervision

It is important to note that working professionals are likely to vary in regard to levels of ability and overall competence. Ideally, marginal clinicians will have been weeded out prior to actual employment, leaving the average and outstanding supervisees to make up the workforce. Length of employment can also be a factor that affects performance levels, and a seasoned employee is typically expected to outperform the new hiree.

In the work setting, supervision has two primary goals: quality clinical service and the ongoing development of employees. The welfare of the patient comes first with secondary emphasis on the clinical personnel, supervisee, and supervisor.

Supervisor's Role Definition

Supervisors in work environments will have to decide how best to allocate their time: whether to function in a predominantly administrative role or one that encompasses active supervision of personnel. Many supervisors lean toward the administrative emphasis and incorporate only a limited amount of clinical supervision on the assumption that competent professionals have been hired, reducing the need for direct observation and conferencing. This may be a legitimate stance if all employees are certified speech-language pathologists or audiologists, but it does not optimize the quality of services provided or enhance employee job satisfaction. Theory suggests that skilled supervisees can use supervision creatively, resulting in innovative service and increased professional satisfaction (Cogan, 1973).

If a supervisor chooses an administrative orientation, his or her work effort will be directed primarily to budget preparation, monitoring the numbers and types of patients seen, justifying personnel needs, assigning caseloads, identifying program needs, creating value in the eyes of others for speech-language pathology services, arranging in-services, and engaging in marketing and fundraising. The job component related to observing and guiding supervisees is likely to be minimal, even though written evaluations of their work may be required once or twice a year. These assessments are likely to be based on quality of service as measured by several indirect parameters. A key consideration may be the number of patients that the clinician has successfully dismissed. Quality of report writing can also be a factor if the supervisor periodically reviews or signs off on this material. Evaluative information about someone's work can also be derived from feedback from patients and their families. While casual positive comments may be offered, it is more likely that it will be complaints that the supervisor will hear. In addition, input from other facility members who interact with the supervisee on a daily basis may come from peers, team members, receptionists, secretaries, and other providers such as teachers in the schools and physicians, nurses, and occupational and physical therapists in a hospital setting. Comments from facility members are likely to focus on the supervisee's cooperativeness, attitudes, promptness, attendance, and professional appearance. As a result, evaluation may be oriented to the peripheral aspects of performance rather than actual clinical competence.

To optimize people and services, a more active, clinically focused supervisory process is needed, but this type of interaction requires adequate staffing levels; there must be enough people to meet the demands of the job. Supervisors may also need to negotiate their job responsibilities and the division of time designated to administration and clinical, face-to-face, supervision (Anderson, 1988). This may be particularly true if the supervisor's emphasis on clinical supervision hasn't been the norm or if one is the first to be employed as a supervisor in that setting. As part of this same discussion, it will be particularly important for the supervisor to negotiate his or her involvement in the hiring and firing of staff members.

Once the supervisor's general orientation to the position has been defined, other aspects of the job can be considered. A major difference when contrasting the employment setting to the training environment is the length of the supervisor–supervisee affiliation. It is almost always longer in the work place. As a result, everything does not have to happen immediately, and there is time to let the relationship and process develop. In addition, expectations change. For example, employees want to have more autonomy, to be stimulated by their job, and to feel that they are competent professionals. The value of contingent reinforcers may also change over time. For example, early in a career, money may be a significant reward, while recognition and time off may become more important later (Shellenbarger, 2000).

There may other facets to the supervisor's role as well. Two in particular come to mind: regulatory and career counseling. Regarding the regulatory component, the goal will be to assist staff members in navigating reporting formats for a given setting and the funding maze. The protocols for assessments, treatment, and report writing vary across work settings. Even in the public schools, educational reform is likely to increase demands for accountability and documentation (Power-deFur, 1999). Requirements for obtaining reimbursement for services also vary. Johnson (1999) notes that the driving forces in medical settings are Medicare, managed care, and fee-for-service care. Thus, the supervisor will need to acclimate and guide employees in these areas to maximize outcomes.

A less happy but sometimes necessary role for the supervisor is assisting supervisees in finding alternate employment. Funding issues are having a far-reaching impact on speech-language pathology professionals, and many are being forced to leave health-care settings as revenues decrease. When necessary, a supervisor may need to take an active role in staff out-placement. This may include assistance in exploring other work settings and alternate career options.

Supervisee Interview

There is another ramification of the length of the relationship between supervisors and staff as well: An employee can be in a position for a long time. As a result, great care needs to be taken during the interviewing process to make sure that an individual will be a good fit with the facility if hired.

An underlying assumption is that supervisors will be involved in the hiring/firing of employees. If it is not explicitly in their job descriptions, it needs to be negotiated and incorporated as a routine function. This is critical because it enables the supervisor to optimize the staff by selecting competent, goal-oriented people and to eliminate those who do not have a desire to develop their own and others' abilities.

Once the hiring and firing function is established as part of the supervisor's role, specific strategies can be incorporated to optimize the quality of the professional staff. First, only those who meet the basic qualifications for the position—in terms of knowledge, skills, and past accomplishments—will be interviewed. Further, Heflich (1981) suggests that only those whose value systems match the work environment should be chosen, and Rodgers (1990) proposes having candidates complete a questionnaire. Questions he feels are important in assessing potential fit include:

> How is the morale in your company or department? Why? "What do you expect" this job "to offer you in the way of a work environment that your employer doesn't offer?" What would your boss say is your best attribute? What would the "needs improvement" section of your performance review address? Can you describe your personal experience with a difficult boss, peer, or subordinate (p. 88).

Interviewees might also be expected to participate in simulated situations that are likely to occur on the job in order to assess the applicant's ability to perform in a given circumstance (Thornton and Cleveland, 1990). An opportunity to view a sample of the candidate's diagnostic or therapy skills on videotape would also be an excellent addition to the preemployment evaluation process. A final topic during the actual interview may be the potential employee's experience with and expectations for supervision. Once obtained, this array of interview information will allow the supervisor to make an informed decision about hiring a given individual.

Job Initiation

The second phase begins when the individual has been hired. Early observations can assess the quality of the person's performance. As most employees will demonstrate average or above levels of skill, the supervisor can begin immediately to develop an optimal relationship that will foster the supervisee's professional growth. On the other hand, if there is a problem, in-depth supervision can be provided to resolve an area(s) of concern as quickly as possible. If the problem cannot be resolved, the person will still be in a probationary period during which appropriate due-process procedures can be implemented with an eye toward termination.

In all situations, but particularly when there is a problem, great care must be taken in regard to documentation and procedure because litigation is increasingly a possibility. Thus, documentation in regard to Equal Employment Opportunities (EEO) becomes important. Some school districts address this problem by working the employee's contract backward to determine the dates when each phase has to begin in order to fulfill every due-process requirement. As a result, they know when the observations have to take place and the necessary sequence for filing documentation.

At times, incompetent or minimally competent staff members may be permanent employees. Joyce and Showers (1988) refer to this type of person as the "reticent consumer" (p. 136). These individuals resent having to participate in staff development and do the bare minimum. They tend to distrust the system and its active participants. In rare instances, with creative supervision and peer support, this person will develop into a productive team member. In other cases, depending on the organization's policies and the situation, with adequate documentation and appropriate due-process procedures, it may be possible to encourage these employees to move out of the position. In other instances, these persons may choose not to leave. If all management options have been exhausted, the fallback position is to minimize the impact these people have on the quality of work in a facility and on the morale of other staff members.

A discussion between two friends reveals the attitudes some employees may bring to the supervisory process.

BRANDY: I'm glad my Clinical Fellowship Year is over. I benefited from having a supervisor but I'm anxious to finally be on my own.

JOE: I'm the only speech-language pathologist in the rehab settings I serve. I haven't had direct supervision for more than three years. There are times I'd really like to have someone to talk to. I have good ideas but I'd like someone else's perspective now and then.

> **BRANDY:** That's true. My supervisor was always helpful and did see things I hadn't thought about. I liked the way she encouraged me to set some goals. Getting feedback was really hard though.
>
> **JOE:** Yeah. Having someone evaluate your work is hard. I guess I'd like someone who was more focused on helping me grow than on judging me.
>
> **BRANDY:** I think we would all like that.

Working professionals' attitudes will vary in regard to the perceived need for professional growth and supervision. Yet, lifelong learning is the foundation for clinical excellence (Goldberg, 1995; Kamhi, 1995). In regard to supervision, Garett and Baretta-Herman (1995) note that social workers, once licensed, are not required to have further supervision as a condition of continuing licensure. Also, the availability of supervision is decreasing due to agency cutbacks and an emphasis on self-managed work groups. The same is true in speech-language pathology and audiology. In school psychology, Crespi (1997) too, notes that supervision is rare in the workplace in spite of the fact that quality supervision provides an unprecedented opportunity to enhance clinical services, a view shared by Anderson (1988) and Dowling (1992). Indeed, effective supervision is critical to the survival of the professions.

Supervision Implementation

Supervisee Preparation

Background. The new supervisor, or one who has made a decision to supervise actively, enhances this process by preparing employees. First, they need basic information about how they are expected to function on the job. Workers benefit from general introductions to others and an overview of the purpose and goals of the organization they are joining. They also need to acquire a sense of their role in the job setting and how it fits into the whole. In addition, they can benefit from specific training to perform their assigned function. Early identification of a role model or mentor will smooth the transition to the new employment setting (Bice-Stephens, 1987).

Second, they need to be prepared to actively participate in the supervisory process. Some, however, might wonder about the appropriateness of preparing employed professionals for supervision because it should have occurred as part of their academic training. Ideally, of course, it should have, but, in reality, it rarely does. Typically, supervisees have been trained to perform clinical work but they were given little or no direct guidance in participating effectively in supervision. As is always true, individual and program exceptions exist, but they remain few in number. Therefore, it is a safe assumption that the majority of staff members are not knowledgeable about the supervisory process. This is true even though they, as individuals, may have been supervised by a number of people or may even have monitored and guided the performance of others. For many, what was called "supervision" was just evaluation. They may, as a result, feel that supervision and evaluation are synonymous (Romero, 2000). Dowling and Wittkopp (1982) demonstrate that, without direct supervisory training, supervisees believe that what they personally experience is what the process should be, so it is likely that the majority of supervisees will only have a limited concept of what supervision can be.

In addition to the lack of specific supervisory training, the attitudes held by some supervisees can be an inhibiting factor. Staff members, particularly those who have been in a position for an extended period of time, may believe that the supervisor has a hidden agenda. This is more likely to be true if they have had negative experiences with a previous supervisor. Also, strong biases may exist among employees that can be constructive or cause interference. For example, some may feel that they are competent and won't benefit from supervision. Others may have stopped growing earlier in their career and have no desire for change or improvement, reflecting the adage that years of experience may be unrelated to competence. Some individuals, for example, may have had one year of experience just 10 different times (Anderson, 1988). In reality, all professionals need ongoing growth to maintain professional competence (Kamhi, 1995).

Implementation.   In preparation for implementation, the new supervisor without supervisory training should review the Anderson continuum of supervision model and the thirteen tasks of supervision. In general, once a decision has been made to engage in active supervision, a meeting with the supervisees as a group is helpful. It may begin with a general discussion of the supervisory process and the potential benefits. It is also important for supervisors to share their ideas and what they would like to see happen. In turn, it is critical to find out what the supervisees want from supervisors and the process. This is particularly true in relation to helping them grow professionally and increasing their job satisfaction.

Specifically, in preparing the supervisee, a discussion of supervision as an ongoing process and the Anderson continuum of supervision are good starting points. The participants need to understand that the supervisor's style will vary depending on their needs and behavior. Also, they, in conjunction with the supervisor, will select the approach that is most helpful to them at a given time. Then, objective setting and its relationship to continuing growth is an important part of the plan. Further, the anticipated increase in perceived professional self-worth, overall job satisfaction, and its potential relationship to performance evaluation are worthy of discussion. The value of data collection needs to be stressed. Finally, opportunities to practice selecting goals and gathering related information are worthwhile. In sum, this dialogue will pave the way for an effective working relationship.

Supervisee Goals

After the initial discussions of supervision and sufficient opportunity to observe supervisees, a good starting point in the process is for the supervisor to assist them in setting professional goals. It helps supervisees focus on the relevant aspects of the task and encourages persistence in obtaining the target (Locke, Shaw, Saari, and Latham, 1981). To be of value, objectives must be attainable and meaningful. Ideally, they should also be slightly out of reach to encourage individuals to stretch to their potential. According to Locke and Latham (1990) and Phillips and Gully (1997), specific, difficult goals lead to better performance. If goals are explicit, steady improvements in complex task performance occurs (DeShon and Alexander, 1996). Within this context it is important to remember that the difficulty of goals will be dependent on supervisees' levels of readiness. Anderson (1988) states that goals are of little value unless they are at the participants' levels of need, and Rodgers (1990) notes that an important part of goal-setting is the review of individual employees' successes at obtaining those that were previously identified. Finally, White, Kjelgaard, and Harkins (1995) feel that opportunities for supervisee self-evaluation allow employees to determine if they can achieve the goals set for them. Self-evaluation can also be used to increase their perceptions of self-efficacy (Phillips and Gully, 1997).

In developing goals, viewing workers from alternate perspectives increases the effectiveness of the process. First, work group and organizational needs are a consideration. Often, personal goals will arise from and contribute to those of the department (Hagan, 1990). Second, employees themselves are an important source. In this regard, an appropriate strategy is to have supervisees identify their own strengths and weaknesses. Once this is done they can discuss and compare their perceptions with those of the supervisor. Both strengths and weaknesses should be considered in selecting goals because it is as important to build a strength as it is to resolve an area needing growth. This, indeed, may even be the building of a strength the supervisee does not yet perceive (Borgen and Amundson, 1996). The final part of this dialogue, then, is for supervisees to identify and choose those goals perceived as most beneficial to their short- and long-term development and to define measures to assess their success in achieving them. Setting timelines for achievement will also assist employees in reaching their goals.

In the few cases when the above process is not successful, an alternate strategy may be needed. For those isolated employees who resist the idea of active supervision, the focus of goals may need to be related to peripheral issues such as work assignments, equipment procurement, and materials or facility brochure development. It may even be oriented to the overall improvement of the person's quality of work life. Once individuals begin to see that the process is in their best interest, they may feel more comfortable focusing directly on the work that they do. However, some employees may never become actively involved in self-development.

Examples of Potential Objectives

A variety of goals are appropriate to a work environment. For example, a clinician might agree to read three articles relating to cuing in aphasia therapy or learn more about dysphagia. An audiologist could aim to decrease the amount of time needed to complete a hearing test battery and to increase the effectiveness of the post-test conference with the patient as measured by the client's understanding of the identified hearing problem. In the public schools, enhancing one's ability to control client off-task times in group therapy would be appropriate. Another worthwhile goal would be to increase one's knowledge of varying professional roles and their unique contributions to the organization such as teacher, diagnostician, reading specialist, occupational therapist, physical therapist. In a hospital environment, speech pathologists might choose to improve the clarity of their directions or refine their control of task difficulty for patient activities, because the latter is often a critical factor in therapy effectiveness. In addition, Hagan (1990) suggests the following as relevant goals in a hospital setting: (1) doing research on coma protocols and producing a paper or presentation based on the findings; (2) developing a diagnosis or treatment-oriented computer program; (3) planning an in-service for nursing personnel on feeding in the presence of neurological involvement; (4) implementing a team (speech pathologist, physical therapist, occupational therapist, nurse) approach to augmentative communication; (5) increaseing communication effectiveness in family conferences by using nontechnical language and being concise; or (6) designing a facility orientation brochure for patients and families.

An important aspect of the objective setting process is an ongoing discussion of strategies the supervisee might use to work toward the goals. Similarly, decisions about the types of data to be collected, criteria for attainment, a time line, and related procedures are important. Romero (2000) suggests that employees might develop rating scales as a means to document progress toward their goals. So, objective setting will always include the who, what, and when aspects of data collection and assessment measures as well as the designation of specific targets.

After the initial practice with objective setting, working professionals will take primary responsibility for assessing their own growth and developing ongoing goals. As supervisees become increasingly independent, the supervisor can move into a facilitator or consultant role, although, with some individuals, hands-on supervisor involvement may continue for extended periods of time.

Supervisory Techniques

Once objectives have been set, the supervisor's attention can turn to specific techniques appropriate for use with working professionals. Several that are relevant to the average and outstanding supervisee in training apply equally well to those in the workforce. These include data collection, videotape, observation of others, and selective verbatim transcriptions. In addition, guiding employees to incorporate accountability into their daily practice and create perceived value for their services will be important supervisory strategies.

Data Collection.   Data collection is referred to here and in the preceding section as a way of selecting and monitoring professional objectives. Clinicians need to learn to collect data about their own performance. Data gathering, analysis, and problem-solving are the cornerstones of effective supervision. They are used to gathering client performance data but generally will not have done so in regard to their own clinical behavior. Their supervisor may demonstrate data collection by doing so during an observation and then sharing it with them. This will guide the employee to learn the process. The following are a few examples of data collection targets for the working professional: (1) closure of activities/procedures, (2) reinforcement, (3) efficiency of a bedside evaluation, (4) time spent per objective per client. For greater detail, the reader may wish to refer to the chapter on data collection with specific employees in mind.

Accountability and Value.   Employees, independently of their work setting, need to demonstrate that what they do makes a difference (Trulove and Fitch, 1998). This is and will continue to be critical in (1) justifying the provision of our services, (2) demonstrating that what we do works, and (3) obtaining reimbursement. The supervisor may need to provide in-services on how to collect meaningful group and single subject research data to document diagnostic and treatment effectiveness. Logemann (2000) refers to this as evidence-based practice. Moss (1999) suggests weaving research into our clinical practice. A related, but equally critical issue, is creating perceived value for speech-language pathology and audiology services in the eyes of consumers. Employees need to be guided to continually market and document the worth of their services to referral sources and to create awareness in clientele and their families of the benefit earned from each treatment session. After the supervisor provides a foundation for employees in measuring accountability and creating value for services, employee goals may be set in each of these areas.

Videotape.   Videotape is also extremely helpful if it is available. Its uses are diverse, ranging from an individually focused format to that for groups. As a personal tool, it is excellent for self-confrontation. People learn a tremendous amount about their performance by observing their own treatment and diagnosis. It helps them step out of themselves and see the events as others might. The supervisor and supervisee may also choose to jointly look at specific pieces of the tape to highlight the supervisee's strengths and/or discuss areas of concern.

Videotape is excellent for presenting a problem or unusual case to a group. Similarly, it may be used for in-services to demonstrate a new technique or client type being seen in a facility. Peers, as well as the supervisor and clinician, can collect data to talk about alternate strategies. This may be done in the context of a formal group format such as the Teaching Clinic or more informally.

Observation.   Observing a person proficient with a specific methodology may accelerate the learning of an individual who is less so. In facilities such as a school system, hospital, or large private practice, specific skills are likely to be used by a number of people. In most cases, some will be more adept than others. An opportunity to observe an individual implement a strategy masterfully typically assists observers in modifying their own performance.

Selected Verbatim.   Selected verbatim (Acheson and Gall, 1992; Anderson, 1988) is also effective for the working professional. Recall that this approach consists of a written transcription of a specified aspect of an interaction such as questions or reinforcements. For example, if a supervisee has set a goal to implement a certain type of verbal cue, a verbatim transcription may be made of the cues provided. The actual recordings may be done by the supervisor or supervisee depending on the decisions made during the supervisory conference. This technique focuses attention on a limited aspect of behavior in a concrete manner, making it a valuable growth tool for employees.

Conference Strategies

Conferencing will continue as an important tactic with the employed professional, either individually, in a group, or in combination. A one-to-one meeting allows for a more individualized focus and will be important in working toward specific professional goals. A group strategy is helpful for peer review, case staffings, team building, discussions of general issues, and for providing opportunities for skilled members to share their expertise. The format of multiperson exchanges may vary from informal to one like the structured teaching clinic method.

In planning the individual encounter, a basic decision needs to be made concerning the location of the conference. The site should be consciously considered depending on the needs of the persons involved. In that regard, Farmer (1989a) uses the terms *evaluator dominant, personnel dominant,* or *neutral* to describe the potential power balances generated by the setting. A basic question to be answered is whether the meeting will be on the supervisor's turf, the supervisee's, or neither. If a particular employee appears to be threatened by the supervisor, meeting in the clinician's workspace reduces the perception of a power imbalance and diffuses some of the anxiety. For this type of person, having to come to the supervisor's office will highlight the power discrepancy, increase his or her level of tension, and will impair communication. For others, the meeting can appropriately be in a neutral setting or in the supervisor's workspace.

Once the site for the meeting has been established, the conference orientation in regard to the Anderson continuum of supervision must be planned. Is it to be direct/telling, collaborative, or consultative? (Recall that this will be determined by the supervisor and supervisee's level of development as well as the specific task being considered.) Persons in their clinical fellowship year may need predominantly collaboration but, at times, direct telling and, in others, consultation. In contrast, highly skilled employees who are knowledgeable about the job may benefit most from consultation with limited telling and collaboration interspersed, as needed.

A typical conference using the Anderson collaborative style is earmarked by a planned agenda and colleagueship. It is clear that data has been collected, and the actual analysis of the data may have been done prior to the interaction or may be a focal point of the exchange. Joint problem-solving will ensue with increasing responsibility for this function shifting to the supervisee. Positive and negative feedback as well as questions will be generated by both participants. Finally, the two people are jointly responsible for the outcomes of the clinical and supervisory relationships.

Conference Issues

In the work environment, the frequency and length of conferences would be determined jointly by the supervisor and the supervisee. Meetings may be weekly or as infrequent as once a month or even every other month. The time spent in the exchange, whenever it occurs, is dependent on the topics under consideration. Some meetings may be brief and others lengthy. There is also an option to alternate individual and group conferences. The decisions regarding frequency, length, and conference type then, would be based on the supervisee's needs and those of the supervisor and facility.

Conferences are most likely to be effective if they are preplanned meetings. Anderson (1988), Farmer (1989b), and Dowling (1992) stress the critical nature of planning and having a strategy for meetings. Exchanges that are not predesigned tend to become "Well, what do we want to talk about today?" As a result, these scheduled but unplanned discussions often are not maximally productive.

Initially, the supervisor may find it helpful to prepare a written agenda by jotting down key points to be considered. Once this procedure has been established and routinely used, it may be done mentally without a formal written record. In all instances, it is critical that supervisees have input into the agenda. Indeed, after the initial phase of the relationship, the responsibility for the content of the meeting will become shared and then will shift almost exclusively to supervisees. In all cases, clinicians' input to the conference plan insures that their concerns are being addressed. The needs of both participants are best met, however, if the primary preparer opens the conference by asking the other member if there are items he or she would like to discuss that day.

As can be presumed, the nature of the agenda may be highly variable as the participants' needs change. A conference may be planned around data that was to be collected as an outcome of the last meeting. It may also be oriented to specific skills. And, in many cases, the focus may be supervisees' work toward their own professional goals.

Effective Communication

Once the agenda has been planned, there are five strategies to increase the effectiveness of the communication that occurs in the conference. The first is to look at the furniture arrangement in the room in which it is to be held. The second is to engage in active listening (Farmer, 1989b), and the third is to mirror the supervisee's verbal and nonverbal behavior (Brooks, 1989; Farmer, 1985–1986).

The fourth is to incorporate cognitive coaching (Costa and Garmston, 1994), which also includes verbal and nonverbal mirroring. It also focuses on guiding supervisee problem-solving and clarifying the supervisees' ideas. Fifth and finally, it is essential to provide a facilitative interpersonal climate (Caracciolo, Rigrodsky, and Morrison, 1978; Pickering, 1977). Each of these topics has been addressed in the chapter on conferencing. The reader may wish to review that material and extract the information relevant to communicating with the employed professional.

Conference Evaluation

A final facet of the conference is to evaluate it. It is a reflection on the content and effectiveness of the exchange. This examination is similar to that done in regard to treatment, and is based on data collection and analysis with an orientation toward problem-solving. The tools to gather information may be observation systems or informal data collection strategies.

Anderson (1988), Cogan (1973), and Dowling (1992) all suggest that both the supervisee and supervisor should be involved in the assessment of the conference. As supervisors grow in their roles, it helpful to ask the supervisee for input. Of particular value is determining whether employees perceive that the meetings are addressing their needs. It is also beneficial to find out which specific aspects of the conference are of value as well as those that are not, and whether there are other things the supervisor could do to assist the supervisee in performing his or her job. The working professional, more than any other group of supervisees, presents the potential for participating in a true collaborative/consultative relationship. Due to the maturity of the participants, the length of the affiliation, and increased discussion about the supervisory process, the outcomes are likely to be more effective.

Supervision Benefits

An audiologist and speech-language pathologist from a large medical facility are talking as they walk to the parking lot.

SAM: We dodged the bullet this time.

JOANN: Thank the stars for Margaret (supervisor). When they started on the budget cuts, she showed them exactly how we contribute. I resisted all this data collection at first. I thought it was a lot of busy work. Whew, am I glad I got on the band wagon.

SAM: If it hadn't been for her, one or both of us might have lost our jobs.

JOANN: I really like her most of the time. I'd never set professional goals before coming here. It's been a challenge, actually kind of fun.

> **SAM:**   I balked too. I like *my* way of doing things. But, yeah, I've grown too.
>
> **JOANN:**   See you tomorrow Sam.

Performance Evaluation

The topics addressed in this section, such as role definition, the continuum of supervision, supervisee preparation, goal-setting, supervisory strategies, and conferencing, constitute the heart of supervision. These are the components that actively foster supervisee growth. But supervision also has another part: evaluation. This latter aspect is important but should not be the only focus. If overemphasized, it may actually be destructive to the supervisory relationship. Ideally, the appraisal process will be growth-oriented and not just take the form of summative evaluation (Cousins, 1995). In particular, if supervisees are truly self-evaluating, they are aware of their levels of performance and assessment becomes a joint sharing of known information.

Bias

In evaluation, the supervisor must make every effort to be objective and fair, but personal biases can unconsciously impact this process. According to Lowe (1986), the following prejudices may interfere:

1. Some workers may excel in an area that the supervisor feels is important but not do well in others. As a consequence, there may be a tendency to see only the strength while overlooking deficit areas—the "halo effect."

2. A worker may exhibit a behavior that the superior perceives very negatively. This specific weakness may color the evaluation, causing the person to be seen as an overall poor performer. This is true even though, in reality, there may be only one aspect that is a problem.

3. Some individuals have a tendency to rate everyone as average on all items.

4. Other people tend to focus on recent events and forget strengths or areas of difficulty in the past. To avoid this problem, Lowe (1986) suggests regular documentation of performance.

5. Sometimes length of service may also bias ratings. If an employee has consistently performed well in the past, the assumption is made that the same quality of work will continue. As a result, sufficient scrutiny may not occur with seasoned performers.

6. Employers who personally have trouble dealing with conflict are more likely to gloss over problems to avoid having to confront the individual. As a result, they inflate all ratings.

7. In contrast, supervisors with high personal expectations for performance may never give superior ratings. They justify this stance by indicating there is always room for improvement.

8. Some superiors may inadvertently tie their performance to their perception of the supervisee. If the boss is not doing well, it may be viewed as the employee's fault.

Other problems exist in evaluation as well. Cousins (1995) notes that, in the public schools, evaluation is often ritualistic, superficial, and benign in nature. Manatt and Benway (1998) note five persistent problems when the supervisor is the only evaluator: (1) self-serving "like-me-ness" expectations; (2) scant data; (3) refusal to confront marginal performance; and varying degrees of rigor in making evaluation ratings (p. 18). To minimize these problems and those of bias, a conscious awareness of the potential for distortion needs to remain foremost in the supervisor's mind. The collection and use of data as the foundation for evaluation will also decrease the degree and numbers of misinterpretations. Lowe (1986) also suggests listing the behaviors to be judged and rank-ordering all employees on each factor. He feels this forces the rater to recognize variations in performance. Rodgers (1990) suggests a similar strategy but on a global level. He urges a pair-by-pair comparison of persons within a job class, identifying in each case the better performer. The end result is a rank-ordering of all workers in a given job class. He, too, feels that this forces managers and supervisors to make fine differentiations among subordinates.

Three-Sixty Evaluation

Evaluations may stem from a variety of sources. The most common are those done by the employee or the supervisor. Input from peers may also play an important role. A more formal structure, team or three-sixty evaluation, as described by Manatt (1997), may also be implemented to obtain quality feedback from critical individuals who interact with the employee. Manatt describes such a process in the public schools. In this setting, students provide feedback by answering twenty questions relating to teaching, instructional delivery, and their related interests. A peer selected by the teacher provides feedback after visiting the classroom while focusing on the same criteria as the students and principal. The teacher self-evaluates by answering the same, although slightly modified, twenty questions that were provided to the students. The principal evaluates through observations, interviews, review of work samples, and by looking at the progress the teacher is making toward professional goals. Parents also contribute to the evaluation process by completing a five-question report card after each conference with the teacher. The final component of this three-sixty evaluation is student achievement. This process results in a high degree of teacher accountability.

In other settings, three-sixty evaluation takes the form of employees sending out information about their goals and working projects to those who deal with the individual (Agan, 1999). Performance feedback is then obtained from multiple perspectives. In medicine, as a result of feedback from several sources, 66 percent of physicians change at least one aspect of their practice (Fidler, Lockyer, Toews, and Violato, 1999). In addition, Makiney and Levy (1998) found that supervisors who value having input about an employee from more than one source are more likely to incorporate discrepant ratings from peers than from the supervisee's own self-evaluation in arriving at a final determination.

Portfolio Assessment

Portfolio assessment is being used in schools and medical settings (Snadden and Thomas, 1998) for professional growth and as an alternative evaluation strategy. A highly structured portfolio is implemented in the Teach for America program (Oakley, 1998). The teacher builds documentation relative to student learning and teaching effectiveness. The packet consists of student goals, a statement of one's personal teaching philosophy, student performance results, lesson plans, teaching videotapes, and evaluations from the principal, a peer, parents, and students. The completed packet is then reviewed for the purpose of evaluation.

Smith and Tillema (1998) see portfolios as a professional growth tool. Employees collect evidence about their own performance to demonstrate ongoing growth and competence. They have the opportunity to select not only the goals but also the strategies for attainment and documentation. Smith and Tillema do note that it is difficult to stimulate employees' self-reflection about performance and the data they have gathered. In addition, they find that portfolio quality tends to increase over time. Portfolios, in general, provide a flexible, personalized, systematic method to assess professional development (Ashelman, Dorsey-Gaines, Glover-Dorsey, 1997). A key advantage of portfolios is their ability to track clinical performance over an extended period of time (Snadden and Thomas, 1998).

Supervisor-Driven Evaluation

In instances when the supervisor is assuming the primary role of evaluator, the form of evaluation may be formal or informal and is typically presented in a verbal or written format. In general, care must be taken to give both positive and negative feedback. Realistically, each person has areas of strength and those that would benefit from growth, but there is a human tendency to assume that evaluation and punishment are synonymous. Individual supervisors often emphasize the negative and assume that the supervisee knows about the positive. In reality, affirmative input is of equal if not greater importance. In fact, Cogan (1978) suggests focusing only on strengths because, as areas of asset grow, weaker ones will improve as well.

In contrast, Manatt (1997) says the valleys of performance rather than the peaks should be used for goal-setting. Barlow (1990) further indicates that poor individual performance needs to be punished. If it is not, it tends to have a negative impact on morale because more competent employees resent having to "take up the slack" for those not doing their job. Rodgers (1990) also feels that good performers need to be paid more than those who are weak.

Research in speech-language pathology shows that feedback from a superior is perceived more positively and constructively if the supervisee is first asked to self-evaluate (Brown and Block, 1975). It appears that once a person has considered his/her own behavior and has acknowledged both strengths and weaknesses, similar observations by another are seen as accurate and fair. This same self-evaluation also contributes to higher employee performance levels (White, Kjelgaard, and Harkins, 1995).

Format and Content

Some facilities have set forms and evaluations scheduled at specific times of the year—quarterly, biannually, or annually. The best circumstance occurs when an organization designs or adapts evaluation tools to fit job definitions and responsibilities. The worst is when a facility-wide tool is used for everyone independently of their role or assigned task. The latter situation often happens in work settings. In school systems, the classroom teacher, diagnostician, speech pathologist, and audiologist are all rated with the same document and factors independent of their relevance. Similarly, hospitals may apply the same instrument to all employees ranging from housekeeping staff to skilled professionals. In this circumstance, broad descriptors such as quality and quantity are used. The negative aspects of a generalized form are compounded if the person completing it is not knowledgeable about individual job functions. For example, building principals and hospital administrators often are only minimally aware of the unique functions of specialists within a facility. These global evaluative tools, particularly when they are completed by an uninformed individual, create a serious morale problem. Supervisors, if they are not involved in the evaluation process, are going to have to work extremely hard to compensate for and overcome this barrier to job satisfaction.

The timing of evaluations is also a factor. As mentioned earlier, many are scheduled at fixed intervals. It was noted earlier that simultaneous ratings may be used to decrease supervisor bias in the evaluation of individuals (Lowe, 1986), but it can also have a negative effect, particularly if salary increments are also awarded at that time. If everyone is judged in the same timespan, competitiveness among staff members is likely to increase. If only a certain number or percentage of individuals may earn a certain rating and the related dollar amount, workers become increasingly aware that they are directly competing with each other for those slots. Further, discussion among employees of differential salary increases are also likely to contribute to feelings of elation or frustration. An alternative in some settings is to schedule formal appraisals on one's employment anniversary date. This staggers the process over time and, as a result, minimizes the employees' opportunities for direct comparison. Also, a policy restricting discussion of relative salaries among staff members is also constructive.

In the ideal world, the direct supervisor will be completing personnel evaluations. The items on the form will parallel job descriptions and will be designed to fit individual positions. The supervisees will be involved in decisions regarding what is to be assessed and how, and they will be encouraged to self-evaluate using the same instrument before receiving the completed tool from the superior. There will also be a direct relationship between evaluation and the provisions of rewards, whether they be salary increments, recognition, or continuing education opportunities. Evaluation, both in terms of preparation and distribution, should occur on a timely basis.

The ideal circumstance as described above, however, tends to be the exception rather than the rule. Given the constraints of the particular environment, the supervisor must work to optimize the process. The perceived productiveness of evaluation in all settings is increased if it is coupled with the development of objectives for continued development. In the conference regarding the evaluation, the supervisee's strengths and areas needing improvement are identified. Objectives to increase strengths and resolve average or lower areas would be a logical step. In essence, one is saying "You had trouble in this area this year, but let's plan and work on a specific skill so that you will rate higher next time." In this context, formal evaluation becomes an important part of the ongoing development of the employee. In essence, it can become the foundation for supervisee growth plans.

Organizational Effectiveness

There are a variety of factors that directly impact job satisfaction, in addition to those already presented, factors that play a significant role in determining whether a person will accept a job, be happy in the position, and remain as an employee. These are widely used in successful corporations but are rarely considered in the service delivery environment.

Successful Workplaces

Peters and Waterman (1982) identify eight characteristics of highly successful organizations: (1) a *bias for action,* a tendency to move forward with a best effort and then make modifications as needed; (2) is a *customer orientation,* with strong efforts to work with and for the consumer; (3) *innovativeness is rewarded and entrepreneurship* is encouraged; (4) *productivity is based in individual employees* and each is treated as a valuable member of the team; (5) successful organizations are guided by *corporate values* and management is directly involved at all levels of the organization; (6) excellent companies *do what they do best* and don't branch out in areas where they lack sufficient expertise; (7) strong companies have fewer levels between top management and workers; (8) successful companies combine *centralized and decentralized structure* and have sufficient flexibility to shift the composition as needed. Fisher (1989), describing high commitment workplaces, adds four additional traits to this list of components for excellence: the *institutionalization of continuous improvement;* a focus on *developing people;* the *elimination of barriers* to success, and the belief that work is an essential part of life.

These ideas drive successful corporate environments. Logically, these same ideas should apply in the human service delivery workplace. If incorporated, they have the potential to increase the health and productivity of the organization as well as enhancing worker satisfaction. Several of the characteristics of excellent corporations appear to have direct applicability to the supervision of the working professional.

Bias for Action.   The focus here is to move forward with one's best effort. If it doesn't work, modifications are then made. This type of orientation reduces stagnancy and encourages employees to take educated risks. Most importantly, it reduces complacency with the status quo. In speech-language pathology and audiology, it sets the stage for creativity and innovation in the delivery of clinical services.

Working with and for the Consumer.   Our consumers are the people we serve. For example, in the schools the customers are parents, students, and other professional personnel (Manatt, 1997). In private practice, clients, families, team members, and referral sources are our consumers. Thus, it is important that we, as professionals, continually remember that our customers are our reason to be. The pressure of daily work life has a tendency to make employees lose sight of the importance of the individuals who make up and contribute to our case loads. To keep customers foremost, each departmental decision must be weighed in regard to its impact on clientele.

Rewarding Innovativeness and Encourage Entrepreneurship.   The idea here is to foster innovation by encouraging working professionals to move forward with new ideas. If a staff member has a novel idea that is logical, is theoretically sound, and capable of working, implementation should be supported. Even if the intent is not accomplished, something will be learned. This rewarding of "successful failures" fosters experimentation and growth. Important innovations often emerge from this type of testing. Examples in this realm might be a new scheduling strategy, an alternate treatment approach, or the application of methods successful with one client type to a markedly different group.

Valuing Individual Team Members.   In any work unit, each and every participant is a valued member of the team. This includes receptionists, secretaries, professional staff, janitorial members, administrators, and others. Each has an extremely important role in making a facility function on a day-to-day basis. Independently of the position or the persons filling the job, each needs to feel a sense of esteem and perceive the worth of their contribution. This is true even if a given supervisor's job is primarily focused on a subset of the group. Constructive interactions with everyone in an organization will improve the quality of the total work environment. Similarly, individual workers need to be reinforced for displaying productive attitudes toward each other. They need to get along with and support each other. Team members do not need to be personal friends but must respect each other professionally. Back-stabbing and pettiness need to be left outside the work environment.

Eisenberger, Fasolo, and Davis-LaMastro (1990) report that organizational caring about workers has a widespread impact. First, workers who perceive they are respected are more conscientious in carrying out routine job responsibilities. Second, they verbalize greater commitment to the company. Third, they are likely to contribute to corporate innovations even when they will not receive rewards or personal recognition. In sum, respect for and the valuing of employees improves satisfaction and contributes to an optimal work environment.

Effective Values. A successful work environment is guided by a vision. Effective values have a minimum of six characteristics: "imaginable, desirable, feasible, focused, flexible, and communicable" (Kotter, 1997, p. 15). The identified creed drives the system. Thus, for a decision to be considered or money allocated, the idea being considered must be consistent with the long-range objective of the facility. The overriding motto typically comes from the top and filters down, but it is possible to develop one within a department with the intent of having it move from the bottom up. To date, most companies, universities, hospitals, schools, and private facilities do not incorporate this extremely important idea. As a result, most workplaces have not identified an organizational motto or focus. Thus, an important supervisory goal will be the fostering of this ideal. The intent will be to demonstrate its success at the unit level with hopes for broader acceptance by the rest of the organization. Some of the following would be good mottoes for service delivery facilities.

> Excellence through Knowledge, Commitment, and Effort
> The Communication Disorders Family
> Providing Services on the Cutting Edge
> Quality Service from Those Who Care
> Excellence by and for People
> Quality, Service, Human Dignity

The critical issue is insuring that, once this creed is selected, it will be implemented as an ongoing direction for the unit. When decisions are made or money allocated, the first consideration will be whether they are compatible with organizational values. Further, supervisors and other members of management should continually model and incorporate these ideas and work to instill them at all levels of the institution. Finally, behaviors consistent with these goals should be rewarded when practiced by any member of the team or company.

Doing What One Does Best. After outlining the resources, staff, skills, and mission of a unit, effort must be made to channel organizational energies effectively. Most facilities do this. In essence, they do not try to be all things to all people. A specific setting might want to build a reputation of excellence in one area. For example, a clinic may strive to specialize in pediatric audiology, laryngectomy patients, or preschool age children rather than attempting to provide services for all disorders. Specialization tends to enhance the quality of assessment and treatment because personnel can be trained and necessary equipment and materials obtained. In contrast, attempting to serve all clientele, independent of disorder, may stretch both staff and resources so thin that nothing is done well.

Flatter Organizations, Centralization, and Decentralization. Typically, supervisors will not have the opportunity to address this issue unless their positions are placed high enough administratively. Supervisors may impact their own area by selecting issues to be handled directly by the administration and filtering those that are more appropriate for staff consideration and implementation. In addition, the maintenance of an open-door policy for the professional and support staff as well as clients and their families will increase access and foster decentralization.

On the company level, ready access to administrators fosters the sense of a flatter organization. Open meetings in which employees may initiate discussion of issues obstructing development or job satisfaction are valuable. Smaller exchanges involving a department and the chief operating officer and administrators are also helpful. In each instance, employees feel they are heard an that they have an opportunity to impact the system. The likely result is an increase in job satisfaction.

Continuous Improvement. Drucker (1998) and Deming (1986) indicate a continuous improvement attitude is fundamental to productivity in the workplace. The organization as a whole—departmental units, natural work groups, and individuals—strives to evaluate and improve performance on an ongoing basis. The focus is a cooperative consideration of each aspect that contributes to the performance of the organization. Then constant effort is expended to improve individual components as a means to increase overall organizational outcomes. Bruce (Dowling and Bruce, 1996) discusses continuous quality improvement as a elemental strategy to improve diagnostic and treatment outcomes in clinical practice.

In this regard, natural work groups consisting of the supervisor and all reporting speech-language pathologists and audiologists or a team consisting of a leader and a rehabilitation unit may meet on a regular basis in order to identify opportunities for improvement, solve problems, and plan and assess the effects of implementation. Bruce (Dowling and Bruce, 1996) refers to this as the plan, do, study, and act cycle. The underlying goal is to select a desired outcome, plan a strategy for its achievement, review the results, and prepare again for continuous improvement.

Further, it is the author's opinion that professional burnout is linked, at least in part, to the absence of individual, ongoing professional goals. When learning and striving to improve ceases, complacency ensues. Boredom and frustration typically follow. Similar feelings may also be linked to a specific job. For example, this may happen when workloads are excessive, routine, and individuals have little control over their work lives. Leiter (1989) identifies burnout as a cognitive–emotional reaction to chronic stress in human service settings. The contributing factors appear to be work demands accompanied by insufficient organizational support from coworkers and immediate supervisors, an underutilization of the employee's abilities, and the tactics an individual uses to cope with stress. In addition to the above, Lubinski (1994) notes that a lack of autonomy and sufficient opportunities for self-actualization are contributing factors to burnout in speech-language pathology.

Burnout and turnover can be reduced in the workplace. To achieve this end, several events need to occur. First, an attitude of continuous improvement for all employees, independent of job function, and the organization, as well, is essential. Second, ongoing efforts to improve job parameters, such as optimizing caseloads and enhancing teamwork are necessary. Third, striving for quality individual, unit, and organizational products will serve as a constant impetus for change. Fourth, workers need to be given as much control over their work and the assessment of outcomes of their efforts as possible. In sum, goal-setting and the rewarding of efforts in each of these areas will provide continuing professional stimulation and a sense of achievement. The result is an increase in productivity, job satisfaction, and stability of the workforce.

Eliminating Barriers to Success. The supervisor is the individual who is best situated to insuring employees' success. Removing barriers may range from scheduling and procuring room assignments and adequate supplies to providing training for the supervisee. For example, a clinician may be having a major difficulty dealing with patients with dysphagia. The problem, once identified, may stem from a lack of knowledge rather than a deficit in ability. Accordingly, funding must be identified to remove this hurdle by providing an in-service or by sending the person for the appropriate training. In another case, streamlining paperwork may give an employee more time to do the things that are important. The goal here is to eliminate or minimize those factors that negatively impact work performance and/or job satisfaction.

Barriers can also be entrenched in an organization. Examples are a lack of diversity in the workforce or workspaces with limited accessibility for the handicapped. An expectation that everyone work and act like the supervisor is also a barrier, although less overt. The supervisor needs to look at the work setting from the viewpoint of a neutral, diverse observer and eliminate anything that does not welcome all employees. Encouraging workers to celebrate their individuality within the context of the workplace will also increase the supervisor's effectiveness (Miller, 1998).

Developing People. Working to help people grow is highly compatible with continuous institutional improvement, because people are the most valuable resource in any organization. On a day-to-day basis, though, how can people be developed? Objective setting, as previously discussed, is an excellent starting point. Sharing expertise among staff members, in-service training, continuing education, mentoring, and career ladders are others. In particular, sharing one's special skills encourages and rewards people working collaboratively, gives needed information to others, furnishes an opportunity for recognition for the speaker, and builds leadership skills. Further, in-services and continuing education foster growth in a structured manner. Mentors provide encouragement, assist supervisees as they adjust to a position, and model strategies for success in an organization (Freedman, 1990). Career ladders may also be used to afford opportunities for growth. In addition, they provide guidelines for achievement and represent future occasions for promotion. In general, career plateauing, which will be presented in relation to job-related rewards, does not occur until the above options are exhausted.

Career ladders are also used in nursing (French, 1988), in the public schools and for supervisors at some universities. For example, a Georgia State Department of Education (1988) document describes three different types of career ladders: teacher's career ladder program, instructional leader's career ladder program, and nonteaching certified personnel career ladder program. Each type has five levels with stated criteria for each. Similar approaches are in place in a variety of states.

A hospital facility has a defined career ladder for speech-language pathologists. According to Hagan (1990), there are five potential levels: student traineeship, clinical fellowship year, staff speech pathologist, senior I speech pathologist, and senior II speech pathologist. Each tier has specified criteria for inclusion. In this system, a person earning a specified grade, for example Senior I speech pathologist, during one time period must maintain that level of performance to keep the designation during the next interval. In addition, relative to developing people, this organization also continually works to improve the recognition given to workers and to increase compensation. Hagan also (1990) reports that they were able to award bonuses varying in dollar amount depending on one's level on the career ladder.

Thompson, Baker, and Smallwood (1986) indicate career discussions with supervisees are a critical component in developing people. They further feel supervisees themselves must take an active hand in developing a long-term career plan because supervisors vary throughout a work span. Workers need to verbalize their professional aspirations and the ways in which they anticipate increasing their own value within the organization. From these authors' point of view, developing people begins within the individual employee and is not the sole responsibility of the supervisor.

In reality, supervisors do have a wide variety of opportunities to enhance supervisees' professional self-esteem. For example, guiding them in setting and achieving goals is helpful. Designing a long-term career plan also fosters a feeling of perceived potential. Data collection works, as well, because it provides concrete documentation of growth. Teaching the supervisees analysis and problem-solving skills also assists them in accurately assessing their own behavior, a significant source of reinforcement. Positive feedback and recognition regarding work performance and contributions to organizational goals are also helpful.

Job Satisfaction

Herzberg (1966) indicates there are motivators and demotivators that impact job satisfaction, those that promote self-esteem, recognition, and self-actualization

(Maslow, 1954). The dissatisfiers are similar to the first three levels of the Maslow hierarchy relating to survival, safety, and social needs. These hygienic factors include basic issues such as insurance/pension plans, working conditions, colleagues who get along, salary, and vacation time (Bittel, 1985). The key point is that the dissatisfiers need to be neutralized to avoid employee discontent. Once this is achieved, enhancement of factors perceived as motivators will increase employee productivity and their sense of job fulfillment.

There are specific strategies that may be implemented to increase employee job satisfaction. These are, in general, factors that make people proud of themselves and their jobs. Ladany, Ellis, and Friedlander (1999) say strengthening the emotional bond between the supervisor and employee will increase job satisfaction. Also, enhancing those aspects of the job that facilitate feelings of self-esteem and stimulate self-actualization are helpful (Maslow, 1954). Relative to self-actualization, a good beginning point is to show supervisees how they fit in and then assist them in seeing the importance of their contribution to the organization. Treating employees as the valued, skilled professionals that they are is also important. This is also true of giving credit where it is due as is providing opportunities to earn recognition and to demonstrate leadership. Hagan (1990) suggests a method that conveys confidence in a personnel member's ability to perform. This is to delegate tasks employees find rewarding, such as orienting new employees or giving tours for other professionals visiting a facility, scheduling patients for the various disciplines represented within a team, organizing rounds for a patient and insuring that the paperwork from all involved is in place, representing the facility at a health fair, being selected to present an in-service, and rotating the leadership for group meetings. In addition, to enhance contentment in the workplace, rewards should be dependent on an individual's position in the worklife cycle, workers should have as much control within the context of their job as possible, and supervisees should be assisted in setting and working toward professional objectives.

One note of caution needs to be added in regard to giving employees increased control over their work life. Roberts and Foti (1998) find that individuals' general personal orientations impact the degree of worker autonomy desired. Individuals who are self-directed thrive in environments with little structure. In contrast, persons low in self-leadership do better if their role is clearly defined and the environment is highly organized. In response, as part of the diagnosis process, the supervisor will need to determine the level of the supervisee's independence to select an appropriate supervisory style and to provide the degree of organizational structure needed for the worker. Roberts and Foti say employees are most satisfied with their work when job structure matches their personal needs.

Rewards.   A variety of rewards may be built into the system. Bonuses or salary increments are always appreciated (Lewis, 1997). Cole-Holliday, McNichol, and Pietranton (1999) note salary levels contribute to the perceived value of the services provided by a profession. But money tends to be a hygienic factor rather than a motivator (Herzberg, 1966). In fact, Frase (1989) reports the receipt of professional travel, as a reward, fosters job enrichment while cash does not. In the nonmonetary realm, a day off from work or release time is an excellent prize. General recognition on a smaller scale is important, too, as it contributes to feelings of self-esteem. Examples of such awards are: (1) acknowledgement of the staff member of the month; (2) informal social events to recognize employees for special efforts; (3) a personal thank-you note on company stationary; (4) a reserved parking space for a set amount of time; (5) a plaque with the employee's name; (6) lunch or dinner with a superior; (7) a lapel flower; (8) selection for participation in a conference; 9) a special seat in the cafeteria; (10) an announcement in the organization's newsletter; (11) growth ladders; (12) a promotion; (13) incentive systems such as earning a bonus or continuing education opportunities. Barlow (1999) says that rewards with zero cost have the most impact on productivity; these include: personal notes from supervisors, public recognition, and morale-building meetings to celebrate success. In fact, Nelson (1996) reports that personal congratulations from a manager was ranked first of sixty-seven potential incentives by employees. Second was a personal note of thanks. Occasions for recognition abound in the workplace and need only be sought out by the creative supervisor.

Without a doubt, acknowledgment enriches work life, although it is important to note that what is perceived as rewarding may change as individuals move through their job-related life cycle. Gavett (1987), in discussing the work of Hall (1976), describes the four typical stages of career development: exploration, growth, stability, and decline/withdrawal from work. In the first stage, employees are in a period of acclimating to a position and are seeking a sense of belonging, safety, and recognition. According to Earley, Lee, and Hanson (1990), entry-level employees must sort through a variety of relevant and irrelevant data generated by the job and its environment. In essence, they are trying to define their position and role and determine where they fit. During the growth period, they strive for achievement in the organization by doing those things necessary to move upward within the system. Once mobility goals are achieved and opportunities for further promotions cease, workers tend to move into a stability stage. In this phase, performance has a tendency to level off although individual employees may continue to grow while others stagnate. At this level, personal interests other than work become increasingly important for these persons as general commitment to the organization decreases (Stout, Slocum, and Cron, 1988). The final period, decline, often leads to disengagement from the employment setting or retirement.

Accordingly, that which is perceived as rewarding may vary depending on an individual's stage in his or her work life cycle. Hall (1976) indicates that this is not an age-related issue but rather is strictly linked to career development. For the worker in the first stage of exploration, salary increments, recognition, job clarification, and assurance of continuing employment may be highly rewarding. For the person in the growth stage, evidence of achievement, personal objective obtainment, and promotions may be more important. For the individual in the stability stage, someone who is exhibiting a plateauing or declining level of commitment and interest in career issues (Stout, Slocum and Cron, 1988), time off and opportunities to explore new interests may be motivating. Further, recognition and nonmonetary rewards may encourage continuing strong performance in spite of the fact that career advancement is no longer available. Job-sharing options, released time for special projects, and/or the development of a new specialization may also be beneficial (Evans, 1989). Finally, for the employee in the decline stage, stimulating productivity may be difficult as this individual is beginning the disengagement process.

There also appears to be an age-related life cycle. Glickman (1985) discusses the pioneer work of Buhler (1956), who divided adult life into three stages. The first is from eighteen to twenty-five, a period in which adults are preoccupied with life and occupational dreams. The years from twenty-five to forty-five are directed to creative growth and the realization of goals related to occupation, marriage, and home. Forty-five to sixty-five is a time of inner reflection and the establishing of an inner order. As a result, these chronological issues are likely to affect performance within the work cycle described above and increase the complexity of determining appropriate awards. Nelson (1997) feels it wise to ask employees what is rewarding to them and then adapt incentives to individuals in a way that is meaningful to them.

Control. A major factor impacting job satisfaction is the amount of work-related control and autonomy one has (Orphen, 1984). A lack of perceived authority on the job can result in decreases in performance (Bazmerman, 1982). Dominion over one's work life is an important issue. According to Greenberger and Strasser (1986), personal control is "an individual's beliefs, at a given point in time, in his or her ability to effect a change, in a desired direction, on the environment." Thus, it is important to consider supervisees' positions and give them as much power as possible. An easy way to do this is to identify the tasks and the deadlines for which they are responsible, and then let them decide how and when they will achieve the objectives. Setting one's work schedule is an important part of the sense of "being in charge." Another alternative, being responsible for a larger portion of the work process and job enrichment, is of even greater value. In implementation, the supervisee will plan how to do a job, implement it, assess the outcomes, and then engage in future planning. Thus, the employee's scope of responsibility and control increases. A collaborative supervisory relationship also heightens this sense because the process is adapted to and is responsive to supervisee needs. Finally, having the opportunity to provide input into decisions that affect one's job also increases this sense of command.

Goals. Goal-setting is a fundamental factor in job satisfaction. Cousins (1995) notes that it is critical to growth-oriented professional appraisal and development. Feedback, followed by the development of objectives, is directly related to increases in contentment and organizational commitment (Tziner and Latham, 1989). Similarly, Roberson (1990) indicates that job satisfaction is strengthened by four factors: increasing commitment to goals, enhancing the probability of success in meeting those objectives, providing the supervisee with information on how to achieve targets, and setting specific deadlines for attainment of each. Manatt (1997) suggests that goal achievement is more likely if performance is linked to feedback data, a specific measurement of success is used, adequate time is allowed for goal achievement, and deadlines are enforced.

Outcomes.   Three clinicians are walking down the hall after a team meeting in which the value of a strong organizational culture became evident.

JOLENE: When I interviewed and Bob (supervisor) mentioned the value QUALITY, SERVICE, HUMAN DIGNITY, I thought it probably was window dressing, lip-service material.

FRAN: It sure came through in today's meeting. I thought John would croak when Bob rejected his plan to move all treatment into open areas to cut costs and maximize space utilization.

CARLOS: I agree with Bob though. The added noise would hurt quality of service and talk about violation of privacy. That does impact a client's feeling of dignity.

JOLENE: The creed has helped us decide what is important. I like having a direction.

FRAN: See, I think the quality improvement focus has helped, too. There are a lot of little things, when planned and monitored, that really make a difference.

CARLOS: Being part of such a good company makes me feel good about myself too.

Relationship of Supervising in the Workplace and the Specified Supervision Tasks

As indicated at the outset of the chapter, each of the thirteen tasks of supervision is relevant to involvement with the working professional. Employee selection through the interview process, acculturation of the person to the organization, preparation of the individual for the supervisory process, and the selection of the appropriate conference style all contribute to the establishment and maintenance of an effective working relationship. Further, assisting the supervisee in setting clinical and professional goals, fostering assessment, management, observation and the related analysis skills, enhancing professional writing, facilitating professional conduct, and stimulating independence through self-evaluation and active involvement in the supervisory process are at the heart of working with employees. The topics of goal-setting, supervisory techniques, conference strategies, collaborative interactions, performance evaluation, developing people, and job satisfaction directly address these tasks. The development and maintenance of records, and information regarding ethical, legal, regulatory and reimbursement aspects of professional practice tend to fall more in the administrative domain. They are typically addressed as a part of the initial and then ongoing acculturation of employees. Finally, the task of demonstrating and encouraging research skills in both the clinical and supervisory process is relevant to several topics presented in this chapter. Fostering continuous improvement for both individuals and the organization, improving service to consumers, earning recognition, and furthering professional development are all related to data collection and the implementation of research methods. In sum, the thirteen tasks of supervision are integral to the development of an optimal working relationship with employees.

Summary

This chapter deals with a variety of topics relating to the supervision of the working professional. It is a complex issue incorporating all of the components of the basic supervisory relationship and then adding those linked to long-term job involvement. The role adopted by the supervisor in job settings is critical as is the preparation of the supervisee for effective participation in supervision. The unique characteristics of the employed professional are also examined and specific supervisory strategies suggested. The conference is touched on, as is effective communication. Performance evaluation is explored extensively as is the organizational acculturation of the supervisee. Factors that contribute to employee job satisfaction are also considered at length. The final topic addresses the relevance of the thirteen tasks of supervision in supervising the employed professional.

REFERENCES

Acheson, K., and Gall, M. *Techniques in the Clinical Supervision of Teachers: Preservice and Inservice Applications.* New York: Longman, 1980.

Agan, J. Personal communication, 1999.

Anderson, J. *The Supervisory Process in Speech-Language Pathology and Audiology.* Austin, TX: Pro-Ed, 1988.

Ashelman, P., Dorsey-Gaines, C., and Glover-Dorsey, G. "Application of portfolio assessment in a teaching and nursing program." Collected papers: China–U.S. Conference on Education. Beijing, People's Republic of China, July, 1997.

Barlow, J. "Goof-offs, gains and graduates." *Houston Chronicle,* April 10, 1990.

Barlow, J. "How to motivate without much cash." *Houston Chronicle,* May 11, 1999,: C1.

Bazmerman, M. "Impact of personal control on performance: Is added control always benefi-

cial?" *Journal of Applied Psychology, 67* (1982): 472–479.

Bice-Stephens, N. "Easing the way." *The Journal of Practical Nursing,* March (1987): 44–45.

Bittel, L. *What Every Supervisor Should Know.* (5th ed.) New York: McGraw-Hill, 1985.

Borgen, W. and Amundson, N. "Strength challenge as a process for supervision." *Counselor Education and Supervision, 36* (1996): 159–169.

Brooks, M. *Instant Rapport.* New York: Warner Books, 1989.

Brown, E., and Block, F. "Evaluating supervision." Paper presented at the Annual Convention of the American Speech-Language and Hearing Association, Washington, DC, 1975.

Buhler, C. *From Childhood to Maturity.* London, England: Routledge and K, Paul, 1956.

Caracciolo, G., Rigrodsky, S., and Morrison, E. "A Rogerian orientation to the speech-language pathology supervisory relationship." *American Speech Hearing Association, 20* (1978): 286–290.

Cogan, M. *Clinical Supervision.* Boston, MA: Houghton-Mifflin, 1973.

Cogan, M. "Clinical supervision and exploration." Paper presented in the conference Supervision of Students in Communication Disorders. University of Wisconsin, Madison, Wisconsin, 1978.

Cole-Holliday, P., McNichol, J., and Pietranton, A. "Getting what you are worth: Valuable lessons." *American Speech-Language Hearing Association, 41* (4) (1999): 26–32.

Costa, A., and Garmston, R. *Cognitive coaching: A foundation for renaissance schools.* Norwood, MA: Christopher Gordon Publishers, 1994.

Cousins, J. "Using collaborative performance appraisal to enhance teachers' professional growth: A review of what we know." *Journal of Personnel Evaluation in Education, 9* (1995): 199–222.

Crespi, T. "The clinical supervisor in school psychology: Continuing education and professional development for the schools." *The Clinical Supervisor, 16* (1) (1997): 191–201.

Deming, W. *Out of Crisis.* Cambridge, MA: Massachusetts Institute of Technology, Center for Advanced Engineering Study, 1986.

DeShon, R., and Alexander, R. "Goal setting effects on implicit and explicit learning of complex tasks." *Organizational Behavior and Human Decision Processes, 65* (1) (1996): 18–36.

Dowling, S. *Implementing the Supervisory Process: Theory and Practice.* Englewood Cliffs, NJ: Prentice-Hall, 1992.

Dowling, S., & Bruce, M. "Improving Clinical Training through continuous quality improvement and critical thinking." In B. Wagner, (Ed.), *Proceedings: Partnerships in Supervision: Innovate and Effective Practices.* Grand Forks, ND: University of North Dakota, 1996: 66–72.

Dowling, S., and Wittkopp, J. "Student's perceived supervisory needs." *Journal of Communication Disorders, 15* (1982): 319–328.

Drucker, P. "Management's new paradigms." *Forbes, 162* (7) (1998): 52–177.

Earley, P., Lee, C., and Hanson, L. "Joint moderating effects of job experience and task component complexity: Relations among goal setting, task strategies, and performance." *Journal of Organizational Behavior, 11* (1990): 3–15.

Eisenberger, R., Fasolo, P., and Davis-LaMastro, V. "Perceived organizational support and employee diligence, commitment and innova-tion." *Journal of Applied Psychology, 75* (1) (1990): 51–59.

Evans, R. "The faculty in midcareer: Implications for school improvement." *Educational Leadership, 46* (8) (1989): 10–15.

Farmer, S. "Relationship development in supervisory conferences: A tripartite view of the process." *The Clinical Supervisor, 3* (4) (1985–1986): 5–21.

Farmer, S. "Assessment in supervision." In S. Farmer and J. Farmer, *Supervision in communication disorders.* Columbus, OH: Merrill Publishing, 1989a.

Farmer. S. "Communication competence." In S. Farmer and J. Farmer, *Supervision in communication disorders.* Columbus, OH: Merrill Publishing, 1989b.

Fidler, H., Lockyer, J., Toews, J., and Violato, C. "Changing physicians' practices: The effect of individual feedback." *Academic Medicine, (74)* (6) (1999): 702–714.

Fisher, K. "Managing in the high-commitment workplace." *Organizational Dynamics.* Winter (1989): 31–50.

Frase, L. "Effects of teacher rewards on recognition and job enrichment." *The Journal of Educational Research, 8* (1) (1989): 52–57.

Freedman, S. "The veteran and the beginner." *Teacher Magazine, 1* (7) (1990): 60–65, 68–69.

French, E. "Clinical ladders for nurses: Expect a resurgence of interest but there will be changes." *Nursing Management, 19* (2) (1988): 52–55.

Garett, K., and Baretta-Herman, A. "Moving from supervision to professional development." *The Clinical Supervisor, 13* (2) (1995): 97–109.

Gavett, E. "Career development: An issue for the master's degree supervisor." In M. Crago and M. Pickering, (Eds.), *Supervision in Human Communication Disorders: Perspectives on a Process.* San Diego, CA: Singular Publishing Group, 1987: 55–78.

Georgia State Department of Education. Career ladder for public elementary and secondary school professional personnel: Program description. Atlanta, GA: Georgia State Department of Education, 1988, p. 103.

Glickman, C. *Supervision of Instruction: A Developmental Approach.* Boston, MA: Allyn and Bacon, 1985.

Goldberg, B. "The transformation age: The sky's the limit." *American Speech Hearing Association 37* (1995): 44–50.

Greenberger, D., and Strasser, S. "The development and application of a model of personal control in organizations." *Academy of Management Review, 11* (1986): 164–177.

Hagan, E. Team Supervisor-Head Injury Program, Del Oro Institute for Rehabilitation, Houston, TX. Personal Communication, 1990.

Hall, D. *Careers in Organizations.* Pacific Palisades, CA: Goodyear, 1976.

Heflich, D. "Matching people and jobs: Value systems and employee selection." *Personnel Administrator, 26* (3) (1981): 77–85.

Herzberg, F. *Work and the Nature of Man.* Cleveland, OH: Work Publishing, 1966.

Johnson, A. "Speech-language pathology in health settings: A view of the future." In S. Cornett, (Ed.), *Clinical Practice Management for Speech-Language Pathologists.* Gaithersburg, MD: Aspen Publishers, 1999: 219–241.

Joyce, B., and Showers, B. *Student Achievement through Staff Development.* New York: Longman, 1988.

Kamhi, A. "Research to Practice: Defining, developing and maintaining clinical expertise." *Language, Speech and Hearing Services in Schools, 26* (4) (1995): 353–356.

Kotter, J. "Leading by vision and strategy." *Executive Excellence, 14* (10) (1997): 15–16.

Ladany, N., Ellis, M., and Friedlander, M. "The supervisory working alliance, trainee self-efficacy, and satisfaction." *Journal of Counseling and Development, 77* (1999): 447–455.

Leiter, M. "Conceptual implications of two models of burnout": A response to Golembiewski." *Group and Organizational Studies 14* (1989): 15–22.

Lewis, B. "Used strategically, money can really talk to motivate and reward employees." *Infoworld, 19* (41) (1997): 104.

Locke, E., and Latham, G. *A Theory of Goal Setting and Task Performance.* Englewood Cliffs, NJ: Prentice-Hall, 1990.

Locke, E., Shaw, K., Saari, L., and Latham, G. "Goal-setting and task performance." *Psychological Bulletin, 90* (1981): 125–152.

Logemann, J. "What is evidence-based practice and why should we care?" *ASHA Leader, 5* (5) (2000):3.

Lowe, T. "Eight ways to ruin a performance review." *Personnel Journal, 65* (1986): 60–62.

Lubinski, R. "Burnout." In R. Lubinski and C. Frattali, (Eds.), *Professional Issues in Speech-Language Pathology and Audiology: A Textbook.* San Diego, CA: Singular Publishing Group, 1994,: 345–358.

Makiney, J., and Levy, P. "The influence of self-ratings versus peer ratings on supervisors' performance judgments." *Organizational Behavior and Human Decision Processes, 74* (3) (1998): 212–228.

Manatt, R. "Feedback from 360 degrees: Client-driven evaluation of school personnel." *The School Administrator, 54* (3) (1997): 8–13.

Manatt, R., and Benway, M. "Teacher and administrator performance evaluation: Benefits of 360-degree feedback." *ERS Spectrum,* (1998): 18–23.

Maslow, A. *Motivation and Personality.* New York: Harper and Brothers, 1954.

Miller, F. "Strategic culture change: The door to achieving high performance and inclusion." *Public Personnel Management, 27* (2) (1998): 151–160.

Moss, S. "Weaving research into your clinical speech-language pathology practice." *American Speech-Language Hearing Association, 41* (4) (1999): 40–44.

Nelson, B. "Rewarding employees: Asset appreciation produces best results." *Canadian Manager, 21* (4) (1996): 24.

Nelson, B. "Motivating people." *Executive Excellence, 14* (9) (1997): 17–18.

Oakley, K. "The performance assessment system: A portfolio assessment model for evaluating beginning teachers." *Journal of Personnel Evaluation in Education, 11* (1998): 323–341.

Orphen, C. "The effects of job tenure on the relationship between perceived task attributes and job satisfaction." *Journal of Social Psychology, 124* (1) (1984): 135–136.

Peters, T., and Waterman, R. *In Search of Excellence: Lessons from America's Best-Run Companies.* New York: Harper and Row, 1982.

Phillips, J., and Gully, S. "Role of goal orientation, ability, need for achievement, and locus of control in the self-efficacy and goal-setting process." *Journal of Applied Psychology, 82* (5) (1997): 792–802.

Pickering, M. "An examination of concepts operative in the supervisory process and relationship." *American Speech Hearing Association, 19* (1977): 607–610.

Power-deFur, L. "Predicting the future of speech-language pathology in public schools." In S. Cornett, (Ed.), *Clinical Practice Management for Speech-Language Pathologists.* Gaithersburg, MD: Aspen Publishers, 1999: 243–257.

Roberson, L. "Prediction of job satisfaction from characteristics of personal work goals." *Journal of Organizational Behavior, 11* (1990): 29–41.

Roberts, H., and Foti, R. "Evaluating the interaction between self-leadership and work structure in predicting job satisfaction." *Journal of Business and Psychology6, 12* (3) Spring (1998): 257–267.

Rodgers, T. "No excuses management." *Harvard Business Review, 68* (4) (1990): 84–98.

Romero, D., Personal communication, 2000.

Shellenbarger, S. "Work-vs.-nonwork equation seems likely to keep changing." *Houston Chronicle,* Jan. 2, 2000: 8D.

Smith, K., and Tillema, H. "Evaluating portfolio use as a learning tool for professionals." *Scandinavian Journal of Educational Research, 42* (2) (1998): 193–205.

Snadden, D., and Thomas, M. "The use of portfolio learning in medical education." *Medical Teacher, 20* (3) (1998): 192–199.

Stout, S., Slocum, J., and Cron, W. "Dynamics of the career plateauing process." *Journal of Vocational Behavior, 32*(1) (1988): 74–91.

Thompson, P., Baker, R., and Smallwood, N. "Improving professional development by applying the four-stage career model." *Organizational Dynamics, 15* (2) (1986): 49–62.

Thornton, G., and Cleveland, J. "Developing managerial talent through simulation." *American Psychologist, 45* (2)(1990): 190–199.

Truelove, B., and Fitch, J. "Accountability measures employed by speech-language pathologists in private practice." *American Speech-Language Hearing Association, 7* (1) (1998): 75–80.

Tziner, A., and Latham, G. "The effects of appraisal instrument, feedback and goal-setting on worker satisfaction and commitment." *Journal of Organizational Behavior, 10* (1989): 145–153.

White, P., Kjelgaard, M., and Harkins, S. "Testing the contribution of self-evaluation to goal-setting effects." *Journal of Personality and Social Psychology, 69* (1) (1995): 69–79.

PART FOUR

Training Participants

8 Preparing Supervisees for the Supervisory Process

Clinical Supervision Tasks Relevant to Preparing Supervisees for the Supervisory Process

Task 1: Establishing and maintaining an effective working relationship with the supervisee;

Task 2: Assisting the supervisee in developing clinical goals and objectives;

Task 3: Assisting the supervisee in developing and refining assessment skills;

Task 4: Assisting the supervisee in developing and refining clinical management skills;

Task 5: Demonstrating for and participating with the supervisee in the clinical process;

Task 6: Assisting the supervisee in observing and analyzing assessment and treatment sessions;

Task 7: Assisting the supervisee in the development and maintenance of clinical and supervisory records;

Task 8: Interacting with the supervisee in planning, executing, and analyzing supervisory conferences;

Task 9: Assisting the supervisee in evaluation of clinical performance;

Task 10: Assisting the supervisee in developing skills of verbal reporting, writing, and editing;

Task 11: Sharing information regarding ethical, legal, regulatory and reimbursement aspects of professional practice;

Task 12: Modeling and facilitating professional conduct;

Task 13: Demonstrating research skills in the clinical or supervisory process.

The focus of this chapter is the introduction of the supervisee to the supervisory process. The content is directed to the preprofessional in the training setting who is about to begin clinical work. For persons in the workplace, such as public schools, hospitals, or private practice, the basic ideas continue to apply but the content will need to be adapted and ideas from those environments substituted.

The discussion of the preparation of the supervisee for the supervisory process begins with a review of pertinent literature. The continuum of supervision and expectations for active supervisee involvement will be presented. The specific aspects of the practicum experience such as reviewing the case file and implementing therapy will then be addressed. In regard to each of the components of the practicum experience, three topics will be considered: supervisee behaviors expected by the supervisor, the division of responsibility between the supervisor and supervisee, and strategies supervisees may use to enhance their performance. Finally, a significant portion of this chapter will be devoted to the importance of a long-term commitment to professional growth, supervisee assessment, goal development, and approaches clinicians might use to independently further their own professional development.

Context for Supervisee Preparation

Numerous studies indicate that supervisees tend to be passive participants in the supervisory conference (Culatta and Seltzer, 1976; Roberts and Smith, 1982; Smith and Anderson, 1982). But, if the goal of supervision is to foster supervisee independence and ultimately an ability to self-supervise, this dependent style of interaction is not effective. Strategies to increase supervisee participation focus largely on the training of supervisors so that they can engage in behaviors that facilitate supervisee interaction, but supervisees must also be trained to enhance the outcomes of the supervisory process (McCrea, 1985; Anderson, 1988; Casey, Smith, and Ulrich, 1988; Dowling, 1988).

Speech-language pathologists and audiologists in training, if asked to state their expectations for the supervisory process, are often vague and will frequently say something like "the supervisor will tell me what I need to do." Cogan (1978) says that children below the age of five have expectations for the behaviors a teacher will exhibit as a function of having been parented. In essence, they learn what teaching behavior is by observing their mothers' interactions with them. Similarly, life experiences with superiors, whether a teacher, organizational leader, or employer, shape beginning clinicians' expectations for supervision. As a result, without training, they begin clinical work with a nebulous idea of what is expected of them and generally anticipate functioning in a passive role. The employed professional is likely to expect supervision to be similar to what he or she has experienced in the past.

Training Supervisees for the Supervisory Process

Supervisees' performances will be enhanced if they have prior knowledge of the process and what is expected; if, that is, they are acculturated to being supervised. This is particularly true if clinicians come to understand that they are ultimately responsible for their own professional growth and need to take an active role in that development. The issues to be addressed, then, are: What should be included in a curriculum for supervisee growth, and when might it be taught?

The "what" component will be considered first and then the "when." Both are discussed at length by the American Speech-Language and Hearing Association Committee on Supervision, a group that has now ceased to function, in its report, "Preparation models for the supervisory process in speech-language pathology and audiology" (ASHA, 1989). Among other suggestions contained within the report, a supervisory process training component for a course in clinical management or procedures is outlined, showing the parallels between the clinical and supervisory process.

Because the time available for learning about the supervisory process at this level is limited, it may be most efficient to highlight the interactive and complementary nature of the clinical and supervisory processes. Each component of the clinical process has a counterpart in the supervisory process and the two may be developed in tandem. To illustrate this overlap, a sequence of topics might include:

The clinical process:	*The supervisory process:*
An overview	An overview
Assessment	Generating a clinical skill baseline
Goal-setting for the client	Goal-setting for the clinical development of the supervisee
Treatment strategies	Supervisory strategies
Reinforcement	Reinforcement
Observation of client behavior	Observation of supervisee clinical behavior
Data collection in the clinical process	Data collection in the supervisory process
Data analysis	Data analysis
The clinical conference	The supervisory conference
1. Purpose	1. Purpose
2. Dynamics	2. Dynamics
3. Client/family anxiety/concerns	3. Supervisee anxiety/concerns
Evaluation	Evaluation (p. 99)

Harris, Ludington, Ringwalt, Ballard, Hooper, Buoyer, and Price (1991–1992) also compare the complementary processes, identifying distinctions as well.

In regard to the "when" component of the equation, supervisee training for the supervisory process will probably fit best as part of a clinical procedures/management course as is suggested by the ASHA Committee on Supervision (ASHA, 1989). The practicum meeting, which often accompanies the first clinical experience, is also suggested as an appropriate point of dissemination. If the information is not presented in one of the above formats, individual supervisors may need to take the responsibility for discussing this important subject. Those in an employment setting also benefit from preparation for supervision. This remains true even if they have been previously supervised by a variety of people.

Supervisee Preparation

Two clinicians beginning their first practicum are talking. All of their preclinic coursework is complete, but they have not had a clinical procedures course or specific training about the supervisory process.

> **CAROL:**   I'm supposed to meet with my supervisor for the first time tomorrow. I've gone through the case file and I've tried to write a plan. There is so much and I don't know what Ms. Tran expects. I feel like I'm getting off on the wrong foot.
>
> **JERRY:**   Me, too! I feel the same about my meeting with Johnson (supervisor). I guess she will tell me what to do next. You know, it's her job to point me in the right direction.
>
> **CAROL:**   I suppose. I want to do well. I wish I had a sense of where I was going.
>
> **JERRY:**   You and me both.

The confusion and uncertainty Carol and Jerry express underscore the importance of preparing supervisees to participate actively in the supervisory process.

The place to begin, whether the material is presented in a course or individually, is with an overview of supervision and an explanation of the joint nature of the supervisory and clinical process (ASHA, 1989). A point to be stressed, as noted above, is that many aspects of clinical practice have a parallel component in the supervisory domain (McCrea, 1985). Later, at each stage of the clinical and supervisory process, it is helpful to share the supervisor's perspective on that topic. In essence, supervisors state what they are looking for as well as describe strategies supervisees can use to enhance their performances. A discussion of the appropriate division of responsibilities between supervisor and clinician at each juncture is also helpful. An opportunity for supervisees to share their perceptions and to provide their input into each of these issues sets the stage for joint supervisor–supervisee interaction. In addition, supervisees will be guided to give input to supervisors about behaviors that would be helpful to the supervisee (McLeod, 1997). Thus, supervisee training will often begin with a general explanation of the supervisory process.

Supervision Continuum

Supervision occurs on a continuum ranging from direct to indirect. The supervisor who is purely direct in style is likely to tell the clinician how to proceed, analyze the behaviors reported by the clinician, problem-solve and generate strategies for the supervisee's future sessions, ask numerous closed questions, and give both positive and negative feedback. The conference in this style is likely to have a superior–subordinate orientation with the supervisee functioning as a passive participant (Anderson, 1988; Culatta and Seltzer, 1976; Smith and Anderson, 1982). In most instances, there will be no evidence of data collection or of a preplanned agenda.

At the other end of the continuum is the indirect style. In general, the term *indirect* is used to describe a style that often emerges if a supervisor embraces the philosophy of the Cogan (1973) clinical supervision model or the collaborative phase of the Anderson (1988) continuum of supervision but does not incorporate planned agendas or use collected data as the basis for conferences. Supervisees dominate talk time and are encouraged to reflect on their clinical experiences. In theory, a Socratic approach, which is even more indirect, exists. In the latter, the supervisor does not provide a direct response but rather redirects all statements to the clinician. The supervisee is led, through questioning, to a solution. Given the time frame of supervision, the Socratic method is probably impractical, although it may be used by certain individuals as a preferred style.

In Cogan's (1973) clinical supervision approach, a method more centrally located on the direct/indirect continuum, the following would be noted in the conference: (1) collegiality, (2) equal participation by the supervisor and supervisee, (3) evidence of data collection and analysis, (4) joint analysis and problem-solving, (5) indications of a preplanned agenda, and (6) positive feedback from the supervisor.

A major contribution to supervisory models in speech language pathology and audiology is the work of Anderson (1988). She feels that a supervisor's conference style may range at various points along the direct to indirect continuum depending on the supervisee's level of readiness. Her model stresses the fluid nature of supervision. A beginning clinician, another who is more experienced but working with an unfamiliar client type, or the marginal clinician may need very direct guidance or a telling style from the supervisor. As the supervisee grows professionally and is guided into the transitional stage of supervision, increasing amounts of collaboration between the supervisor and supervisee become appropriate. As the supervisee moves through the transitional phase, the collaborative style itself will vary as the supervisee assumes increasing responsibility for the clinical and supervisory interaction. This shift will be evidenced by more extensive clinician conference talk time, data analysis, problem-solving, and strategy development. With increasing supervisee independence, growth into the self-supervision phase of supervision occurs. In this stage, the supervisor functions in a consultant role as the supervisee assumes responsibility for his or her own behavior. A unique aspect of the Anderson model is the idea that both the supervisor and supervisee are equally responsible for not only the outcomes of the clinical interaction but also for that of the supervisory process.

Cognitive coaching (Costa and Garmston, 1994) is also a viable supervisory conference style. The goal in this approach is to guide supervisees as they gain increasingly accurate problem-solving skills. The supervisees are assisted in clearing defining concerns and then are directed to develop their own solutions. Key supervisor behaviors are pushing for precision and active listening. The supervisor using this style will also mirror the supervisees' verbal and nonverbal behaviors to increase communicative effectiveness and to create trust.

The potential range of supervisor behavior that can be expected by the supervisee then, ranges along a continuum from direct to indirect (Figure 8.1). If the supervisor and supervisee have not had specific supervisory training, the style of supervision that is most probable is direct. As Anderson (1988) and Harris, Ludington, Ringwalt, Ballard, Hooper, Buoyer, and Price (1991–1992) predict, the supervisor probably became a supervisor without specific preparation for the role and has developed a supervisory approach that combines all the styles of that individual's previous supervisors. The supervisor's basic personality will also be a factor in his or her chosen style. Rarely does an indirect, cognitive or coaching continuum of supervision style emerge without supervisory training.

Figure 8.1 reflects the author's view of the placement of the different supervisory approaches on a continuum of supervision ranging in style from direct to indirect.

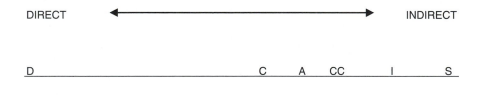

D = Direct
C = Cogan
A = Anderson Collaboration
CC = Cognitive Coaching
I = Indirect
S = Socratic

FIGURE 8.1 Supervision Models on a Direct to Indirect Continum

In particular, supervision is likely to be direct in style and static regardless of the clinician's level of training or the specific site (Culatta and Seltzer, 1976; Roberts and Smith, 1982; Smith and Anderson, 1982). Two studies demonstrate that supervisors provide interpersonal conditions that are essentially nonfacilitative (McCrea, 1980; Pickering, 1984). Each of these investigations assesses supervisors who have had little or no supervisory training. In contrast, a limited number of studies document that trained supervisors perform differently (Caracciolo, Rigrodsky, and Morrison, 1978; Dowling, 1986; Strike-Roussos, 1988). Thus, the statement regarding the anticipated directness of conferences in which untrained supervisors are involved must be understood within the context of available research.

The directness often occurring in conferences may be further confounded by the untrained supervisee who enters the relationship confused about expectations. Most likely the supervisor will assume a directive, unchanging stance and the supervisee will slip into a passive role. If a trained clinician interacts with an untrained supervisor, a more optimal supervisory mode may emerge if the supervisee engages in behaviors likely to encourage and/or trigger indirectness on the part of the supervisor. That is, the supervisee who collects and analyzes data, has a personal agenda, and actively participates in the conference may cause the supervisor to interact in a manner more facilitative to the supervisee's growth (Dowling, 1998).

In summary, the supervisee's introduction to the supervisory process begins with a discussion of the continuum of supervision and its effect on his or her development. A discussion of the impact the supervisee's behavior may have on a supervisor and the conference interaction is also helpful. In addition, supervisees need to understand that they are as responsible for the outcomes of supervision as supervisors are. For example, if they come to the conference unprepared and have not identified issues to be resolved, the likelihood is that the supervisor will tell them how to proceed, nudging them into passive participation. Similarly, if a supervisee reacts to discussions defensively, the quality of the exchange with the supervisor is likely to be compromised. On the other hand, supervisees who have prepared and come to the conference with an agenda are more likely to be active participants in the conference and leave the exchange feeling satisfied. Therefore, the impact of supervisor style on clinician growth and an awareness of the impact of one's own behavior, not only on clients but on the supervisor, are critical concepts to be conveyed to supervisees as they are being prepared for the supervisory process.

In reference to the Anderson continuum of supervision, most beginning supervisees and the marginal clinician in training and the workplace are likely to want/need, at least initially, a direct style of supervision. This will assist them in getting their feet on the ground and assure them that they are on the right track clinically. But, as the supervisees grow, the desired style of supervision should begin to change in the direction of collaboration and ultimately become consultation. Some more advanced supervisees may benefit from varying degrees of collaboration almost from the outset. All supervisees benefit from supervision that is adapted to their needs, moves them toward clinical independence, and guides them to become active participants in their own growth.

Supervisory Process

Supervisees are expected to become active participants in the supervisory conference. Brasseur (1989) suggests that concrete planning will increase supervisee involvement. In general, as clinicians develop, they should expect to assume expanding responsibility for contributing agenda items for the meeting, collecting data, problem-solving, developing strategies and, according to Brasseur (1989), defining the roles of the conference participants. They may also enhance their involvement by giving feedback and actively discussing the supervisory process. These behaviors are critical to their professional development and movement toward self-supervision. The reader may wish to review the chapters on data collection and conferencing for strategies that will enhance supervisees' participation.

Shapiro and Moses (1989) further suggest that supervisees should expect and work toward increasing their level of problem-solving ability. This is reflected outwardly by changes in perspective. The shift is from seeing an event and potential resolutions from one's own point of view to being able to consider it from that of others as well. It includes growth toward perceiving behavior as multidimensional instead of unidimensional. The supervisee is also likely to learn to generate multiple alternatives in dealing with a problem rather than just one (Moses and Shapiro, 1996). The final yardstick in problem-solving development is noted in a supervisee who is not only able to implement alternate strategies but can also see the cause and effect relationship (Shapiro and Moses, 1989). In sum, increases in problem-solving ability relative to both the clinical and supervisory process are anticipated as supervisees mature clinically.

On a more basic supervisory level, supervisees must plan to interact with supervisors on a professional level. A fundamental aspect is to learn how to "get along" with people (Deal, 1990). Receiving and giving feedback, both positive and negative, is difficult at times, but supervisees must learn to do so in a constructive manner. Similarly, it is important to sense when it is appropriate to press a point and when to back off. Also, the intensity of early clinical experiences may be so great that participants may not be aware, at the time, of what they are learning. Indeed, it may not become apparent until after the experience is complete. Thus, patience and tolerance are constructive attitudes. Similarly, the desire to learn as much as possible from the experience is a valued supervisee trait (Deal, 1990).

By engaging in the behaviors described above, the supervisor's perceptions of supervisees may also be influenced. In particular, conveying a desire to learn, putting your "best foot" forward, making an effort to "get along" and giving positive feedback to the supervisor are forms of impression management. Wayne and Kacmar (1991) state that a supervisor is likely to rate supervisees higher and provide less criticism of performance, if they have previously managed the impression they give. These behaviors, then, are ones supervisees might choose to incorporate in their repertoires as they begin to interact with supervisors.

Practicum Components

As a part of discussing the supervisory process and supervisees' roles, it is first helpful to share information about the beliefs and values of the profession. According to Taylor and Horney (1997), this assists beginning clinicians in engaging behaviors consistent with views of best practice. It is also appropriate to address the specific segments of the practicum experience. As mentioned earlier, as supervisees are introduced to each aspect of the clinical process, it is helpful to identify the supervisee behaviors expected by supervisors, the division of responsibility at each juncture, and strategies for enhancing clinician performance. Supervisees also need to anticipate some variability among supervisors in priorities assigned to specific aspects of the clinical components. For example, some supervisors may attach greater value to skillful report writing than others. Thus, it is important for supervisees to actively engage individual supervisors in discussions regarding the perceived importance of the elements occurring during the clinical experience. Perkins and Mercaitis (1995) suggest providing supervisees with a concrete practicum guide specifically outlining the competencies that are to be gained on a weekly basis (see Appendix 3-B). The latter reduces confusion and is likely to enhance growth as targets are clearly stated. Mercaitis (1993) further recommends a prepracticum assessment of core supervisee skills and the implementation of remediation as needed.

Case File. Because a clinical procedures/methods course generally follows the progression of experiences typically encountered during practicum, an early topic is the review of the case file and preparation for client assessment. In regard to the case file, the supervisee's task is to review the material with a focus on four aspects: (1) the most recent case summary, (2) the original diagnostic report, (3) the case history form filled out by the client or family members, and (4) reports from related professionals such as a physician, audiologist, and psychologist. The supervisee's job is to be thorough, to review the material in a comprehensive manner, and to identify key information necessary for further assessment. The supervisor's responsibility is to ensure that the supervisee has identified the relevant information and has interpreted it in a logical manner. The clinician's performance is enhanced by thoroughness and accuracy and by demonstrating this competence verbally or in writing. The supervisee may wish to state the key points in the file or prepare a written outline.

Client Assessment. Typically, clients assigned to the beginning clinician exhibit the more common language and phonology disorders. Assessment is generally limited to a hearing screening, an oral peripheral examination, and formal and informal testing in the areas of language, articulation, phonological awareness, and, at times, problem-solving. The supervisor expects the supervisee to do the following: (1) to select an array of comprehensive but nonredundant measures, (2) to administer protocols in an appropriate, organized fashion, and (3) to score, interpret, and summarize the results accurately. It is the supervisee's responsibility to meet these expectations while the supervisor's obligation has a twofold focus: supervisee and client. The supervisor's charge is quality clinical training while safeguarding the integrity of clinical services. The supervisor's role, therefore, is one of support and the provision of information/assistance to assist the performance of supervisees.

Supervisees may enhance their performance by considering the available assessment tools and then selecting only those appropriate to the case, allowing for nonredundant, albeit complete, measurement. Once the measures have been selected, the next step is a thorough review of the tests to be administered, focusing on basals, ceilings, and the prompts that may or may not be given. Practicing with the test is also a good strategy so that the actual administration goes smoothly with no surprises. In addition, coming to the testing session with the necessary tests, materials, and reinforcers and allowing adequate organization time facilitates successful performance. Following testing, the supervisee needs to take great care to score, interpret, and summarize the measures accurately. The quality of the written test summary will be enhanced if the supervisee not only determines if the client is within normal limits but also identifies strengths and deficits in each area assessed. Of import is the supervisee's awareness that, throughout the testing process, the greater the degree of competence and independence exhibited by the supervisee the more positively he or she will be viewed by the supervisor.

Client Objectives.   Following testing, the logical clinical progression is the development of a treatment program. This often begins with the writing of behavioral objectives, both long- and short-term, and the projection of treatment outcomes. Often the trainee will not have had previous experience with the preparation of objectives, considering the prognosis of patients, or the formal writing format. A formal lecture, written material on the preparation of long- and short-term objectives, and an opportunity for practice are often needed to convey this information. It may be noted that the structure or actual wording of objectives will vary from site to site.

Objective Setting.   In terms of planning for the clinical process and writing objectives, the supervisor expects the supervisee to prioritize and select from the test results those areas most appropriate for treatment, meet with the family and make sure their views are reflected in objective planning, generate long-term and short-term objectives for the areas to be treated, and write them up in a behavioral format. It is the supervisee's responsibility to select treatment targets that will benefit clients and make a maximum contribution to their speech and language and to them and their families. It is the supervisor's job to insure that the clinician has been thorough and accurate and that the objectives are logical and as comprehensive as possible. The supervisor's task is to assist the supervisee in thinking through the test data, gaining insight into client behavior, and translating that information into concrete planning. The supervisor will also insure objectives are consistent with the needs stated by the family. The supervisor may also identify areas that may have been overlooked or were misinterpreted. The supervisor will also provide feedback in relation to writing style.

Supervisees may enhance their performance in this area several ways. They may begin by being thorough, literally going through the data with a fine-tooth comb. The findings and their implications for the client's development should be considered and discussed with the client and family prior to writing down the first goal. Once the objectives are under way, care should be taken to make sure that each is a reasonable and a logical extension of the test findings. The writer also needs to take care that each objective is solidly based on collected data and is written in an appropriate behavioral format.

Lesson Plan Preparation. Following the preparation of objectives, the supervisee's thoughts are likely to shift to lesson-plan writing. Variations in the format, style, and formality of lesson plans are usual when comparing various sites. In training, behavioral writing is generally expected with a formal objective, procedure, criterion and a place reserved for the results and interpretations. The supervisor expects the blueprint for therapy to contain as many objectives as can be appropriately treated within the intended timespan, for the procedures to be appropriate and a logical extension of the objectives, to see evidence of a good control of task difficulty within and across plans, and an indication that previous treatment results have been considered in developing the current goals and procedures. It is the supervisee's responsibility to meet the above expectations and the supervisor's role to provide feedback in regard to both the content and form of the plan. The supervisor needs to continually monitor (1) the appropriateness of the strategies and the likelihood that objectives will be attained, (2) the control of task difficulty, and (3) the clinical insight reflected in the written material. The supervisor's most critical role in lesson-plan preparation is stimulating supervisee thought, problem-solving, and strategy development while, at the same time, increasing supervisee independence.

Supervisees may enhance their performance in lesson-plan writing by being thorough and making sure that a sufficient quantity of procedures have been incorporated for the period to be covered. Great care should be taken to make sure that the underlying logic is sound. Similarly, the lesson plan should be written in a manner that reflects thought and individualization to the client's identified needs and previous performance. Evidence of creativity also strengthens the quality of the submitted material. A final area, although superficial on the surface, is neatness and readability. In that regard, care should be taken to avoid spelling or grammar errors and the final product should be written so that it looks like it was carefully prepared. Supervisees may find the book *Survival Guide for Beginning Speech-language Clinicians* (Meyer, 1998) to be helpful for lesson-plan and report writing.

Treatment Data Collection. Prior to therapy sessions, the clinician is expected to devise a strategy for collecting client performance data as an accountability measure.

Charting may take the form of a simple tally or more complex as in sequentially gathered information. For example, one might count the number of times a client used a specific language structure or assess in order, the types of models provided, the accuracy of a response, and the precision of the client's self-evaluation. The supervisee benefits from viewing each treatment session from a research perspective (Moss, 1999) in that hypotheses are generated in the form of goals and data are collected to determine the success of the session.

In the area of charting, the supervisor has expectations for a method that allows for accurate data collection but does not interfere with the flow of treatment. The supervisee's task is to review the client's objectives and devise a method to document progress in each area. The supervisor's duty is to insure that a comprehensive, efficient method of data accumulation is developed and then implemented.

Supervisees can enhance their performance by being thorough and selecting methods that facilitate clinical problem-solving but do not interfere with the progression of therapy. Similarly, the strategy selected should minimize the amount of time the supervisee devotes to amassing statistics. For example, listening to a tape of treatment following the therapy session in order to gather information is not efficient due to the extra time involved. A chip in a can or a check on a piece of paper during activities may make for better time management. Supervisee innovativeness in the planning and implementation of charting is critical to the successful completion of this task.

Therapy Implementation. Once diagnostic testing is completed and the lesson plans and the related charting formats are written, treatment begins. Although the supervisee brings a variety of experiences to the clinical process such as academic coursework, preclinical observations, and relevant personal experiences, excellence in the execution of treatment is challenging. Due to the complexities and ambiguities of the clinical process, the definitive components of good and bad therapy remain elusive. This may change as "best practice protocols" emerge from evidence-based practice (Logemann, 1999). The diversity of views about therapy is apparent in the variation of items included on clinical evaluation tools. As a result, a certain set of skills may be stressed to a greater degree in one environment while other settings may focus on different aspects. In addition, supervisors using an identical evaluation format may have varying criteria or interpretations that influence their perceptions of what constitutes good therapy (Schalk and Peroff, 1972). Due to the intricacies and varying perceptions of the clinical process, it is therefore in the supervisee's best interest to discuss the characteristics of "good therapy" with each supervisor so that differences in perception between the supervisee and supervisor can be clarified and resolved.

In general, the following core of supervisee behaviors are envisioned by supervisors: providing clear, meaningful directions; communicating objectives to patients when relevant; employing procedures appropriate to the objectives; giving correct verbal/visual models; using time effectively and achieving a corresponding high response rate; exhibiting a sensitivity to clients' needs; evaluating responses accurately and reinforcing accordingly; collecting appropriate data, adapting task difficulty as needed, and implementing closure at the end of activities; instituting productive behavior management; being prepared and having materials well organized; exhibiting professional conduct; and demonstrating personal flexibility and creativity.

It is the responsibility of supervisees to implement therapy to the best of their ability. It is the supervisor's charge to guide and assist clinicians in achieving their potential. Therefore, the supervisor is expected to read lesson plans, observe therapy, and conference with the supervisee.

Supervisees may enhance their performance during and after the provision of therapy in a variety of ways. Effective planning prior to the session is critical for successful implementation. Exhibiting core behaviors expected by supervisors also markedly impacts the supervisor's perception of the supervisee. Enthusiasm and the demonstration of a willingness and even eagerness to go the extra mile in order to excel is often the earmark of the exceptional clinician. Following treatment, thoughtful reflection on the events occurring during therapy and the related affective impact is a strong first step. Similarly, a written or verbal reflection of the long-term projected treatment progression for a patient, such as the client's current level of performance, goals, and a general outline of the steps needed to achieve the end product, is characteristic of the stronger emerging professional. In addition, solid clinicians actively strive to broaden their perspectives and increase the complexity of their problem-solving skills. Shapiro (1998) suggests that the goals are to see a situation from the perspective of the client, clinician, and supervisor, to see that events are complex, and to have many potential solutions. Trainees should feel comfortable asking questions and requesting assistance as long as they clearly demonstrate effort and previous thought about the issues. Although diverse in scope, each of the above gives the impression that the trainee has the potential for excellence. As such, it is to the benefit of supervisees to incorporate as many of these attributes as possible.

Report Writing.   As supervisees move through the clinical experience, report writing will be required. The format of written summaries and the timing of due dates will vary across facilities. Some divide the client report into segments submitted at various points during the term while others require the bulk of the writing at the end. In reference to report writing or the completion of the case summary, the supervisor expects the supervisee to do the following: adhere to the facilities format, be accurate, complete, and concise, and use a professional writing style that incorporates appropriate terminology, grammar, and spelling.

It is the supervisee's responsibility to meet these expectations while it is the supervisor's job to read submissions promptly and to give feedback that assists the supervisee in completing the task efficiently and successfully. The supervisor also needs to strive for consistency to minimize the rewrites required of the supervisee. Demonstration of support and a reasonable amount of supervisor flexibility increases the productivity of this process.

Supervisees may enhance their report-writing performance by showing a desire to do the best job possible. A lack of defensiveness and a willingness to complete rewrites is also helpful. Promptness and careful proofreading for typographic errors further strengthen performance.

Family Interaction.   Conferencing with clients and their families occurs at various points during the treatment process. Typically, the first contact supervisees have with clients and/or their families is the phone call made to confirm the appointment and to determine, if appropriate, the types of reinforcers likely to be most effective. A more formal conference will soon be held to insure that families' needs and their desires for client development are incorporated into treatment planning. This makes families critical partners in client growth (Bruce, DiVenere, and Gergeron, 1998). Test results will also be discussed with families and objectives for treatment will be jointly selected for the treatment period. These meetings build the foundation for ongoing interactions with the family. Brief interactions are also likely to occur prior to and following individual sessions. The last exchange between the clinician and family typically occurs at the end of the treatment term when progress, results, and recommendations are discussed during the final conference.

Supervisors have several expectations for supervisee performance in regard to familial contact. Professionalism is of prime importance. That is, supervisees must insure that all contacts with the clients and their families stay within the confines defined by the American Speech-Language and Hearing Association's code of ethics (ASHA, 1994). In addition, it is anticipated that the supervisee will convey information accurately and succinctly. Clinicians will also take care that the nature of their communication is value-neutral and their use of language is sensitive and respectful to families (Bruce et al., 1998). Finally, the supervisee is expected to foster two-way communication that reinforces families as partners in the treatment process. It is the supervisee's responsibility to meet these expectations while it is the supervisor's task to protect the integrity of the interactions between the clinicians, the clients, and their families.

Supervisees may enhance their performance in this area in numerous ways. A first consideration in preparing for interactions with parents and/or significant others is a consideration of appearance both in terms of dress and grooming. The supervisee needs to insure that the image portrayed is one that conveys confidence and professionalism. Similarly, supervisees may wish to monitor their speech and language to eliminate slang, fillers, and cultural/regional sayings. Utterances should also be checked to confirm that word endings such as *-ing* and appropriate grammar are included.

In the informal interactions that occur on the phone and in the encounters throughout therapy, the exhibition of professional appearance and behavior remains critical. In addition, it is important to recognize the limits of one's competence. If information is requested that one does not have, it is appropriate to acknowledge the lack of an answer and then find out the particulars for later transmission to the family. Similarly, it may be important to clarify the limits of the role of the speech-language pathologist and audiologist as families may be unclear about the boundaries between this profession and, for example, clinical psychology and social work.

Several tactics may be used to enhance formal, prearranged conferences with clients and/or their families. Preplanning of the content as well as the room arrangement is critical to success in this area. An outline, graph, or written summary may be helpful in presenting information as a means to stimulate active on-task communication. Clinicians must remember that their role is to share information while, at the same time, gathering input through active listening. Once the ideas to be discussed are outlined, seating arrangements need to be considered. They should be comfortable with no barriers between the clinician and the other conference participants. Finally, in organizing the meeting, the clinician may plan to use a communication strategy—pacing—to increase rapport (Farmer, 1989; Costa and Garmston, 1994). If this option is selected, supervisees will match both the verbal and nonverbal behaviors of those with whom they are communicating. This tends to put participants at ease and encourages them to talk. This topic and active listening is addressed more fully in the chapter on conferencing. In summary, a consideration of each of the above facets for implementation will markedly enhance the quality of communication that occurs between clinicians and families.

Supervisee Professional Growth

The sequence of the therapy process and supervisee involvement is considered in the preceding material. The growth of the supervisee is addressed both directly and indirectly in regard to those topics. But the specific idea of clinician professional development will now be isolated and addressed more thoroughly.

From the outset, it is essential for supervisees to embrace a long-term commitment to their own personal and professional development. Shapiro (1998) suggests that it is a lifelong endeavor to be and remain the best one can be. This view is echoed by Kamhi (1995) and Goldberg (1995). The overt purpose of clinical training is professional growth, but client improvement is also a prime consideration. Clinicians will discover that, on a day-to-day basis, supervision is likely to be client-oriented. To safeguard supervisees, targets for their professional growth should also be specified in addition to those for clientele. Supervisors and supervisees both need to step back and assess the latter's level of development and then write goals to foster continued growth.

In essence, clinicians need to be the overseer of their own professional development. Even if supervisees are fortunate enough to have supervisors who encourage the generation of professional objectives, these particular supervisor–supervisee interactions are unlikely to last more than one term. The next supervisor may not use this approach or might have a markedly different philosophy. Even if all supervisors actively encourage objective setting for supervisees, the overall continuity needs to be guided by the supervisees themselves.

Clinicians need to take an active responsibility for their own professional maturation throughout their career and not leave it to chance. Professional development,
then, begins in training but remains critical throughout an individual's career
(Goldberg, 1995; Kamhi, 1995; McLeod, 1997).

As pointed out earlier, the degree of emphasis on supervisee growth may
vary markedly among supervisors. This will depend on their philosophical orientation and the amount and type of supervisory training they have received.
Indeed, many supervisors will not directly address this issue at all. Therefore, the
trainee needs to be prepared for variability in this area as some supervisors will
expect data collection and the writing of formal objectives while others will not.

Given that both ends of the continuum of supervisor involvement in supervisee growth exist, each will be discussed here. First, consider the situation in
which supervisors are predominantly client-focused and do not engage in objective setting for supervisees. In this circumstance, supervisees must take the primary responsibility for their own development. The first task for the supervisee is
to carry out a self-assessment in the clinical/professional realm with an eye to
identifying areas of strength and those needing growth. Supervisees should then
collect baseline information in regard to these behaviors as a foundation for writing personal objectives. Once the initial assessment process is complete, supervisees will select objectives in both the strength and weakness domains for
development during that term, as enhancing an asset may be equally as important
as resolving a deficit (Juhnke, 1996). Supervisees will also need to determine a
method for collecting data to guide progress toward their individual objectives.
Throughout the term, the clinicians will gather information, monitor growth, and
update and add objectives when appropriate. Supervisees may further enhance
their performance in this area by making a firm commitment to the concept of
growth and insuring that time is devoted each week to this end.

In more ideal circumstances, supervisors will be actively involved in fostering the growth of supervisees. In this event, supervisors will request supervisees to
consider their level of development and to identify a list of strengths and weaknesses. McLeod (1997) describes a supervisee self-appraisal procedure that provides a structure for such a discussion. The supervisors will also engage in a similar
thought process so that, together, they can develop reasonable objectives that will
make a maximal contribution to the growth of supervisees. Individual supervisor
and supervisee pairs will then jointly determine strategies for and take part in data
collection to assess the supervisee's progress toward stated ends. In this scenario,
supervisors' expectations for supervisee performance will be for supervisees to
honestly and openly assess assets and deficits, identify potential targets, consider
alternate points generated by the supervisor, select a reasonable number of goals,
contribute to the data-collection process, thoughtfully reflect on the findings, and
make a concentrated effort to achieve the stated objectives.

Self-Directed Growth

In regard to taking control of one's own growth, there are several additional
strategies supervisees might employ, independently of the supervisor: (1) self-

analysis through the observation of taped therapy sessions, (2) data collection, (3) self-evaluation, (4) knowledge tree generation, (5) observation of others, (6) peer supervision, and (7) independent goal-setting. Each has the potential to enhance supervisee performance.

Videotape/Audiotape. A videotape or audiotape of a therapy session used for self-analysis assists the supervisee in a variety of ways. Audiotapes may be least desirable, as nonverbal behaviors are lost and it may be more difficult for listeners to attend to the auditory signal alone for extended periods of time. This may be particularly true for visually oriented learners. Independently of modality selected, self-observation provides the opportunity to learn about oneself and one's impact on client performance. The goal is to identify aspects of the session that went well and those that were less successful. Observing self enables clinicians to step out of themselves and view the behaviors as others might.

The productivity of videotape or audiotape self-confrontation will be enhanced even further by data collection. Data focuses the viewer on smaller aspects of the process and, thereby, increases objectivity. It also tends to reduce or eliminate gut reactions, which are often judgmental in nature and are frequently difficult to translate into change. In addition, data gathered in response to a specific question generally establishes a foundation for modifying future behavior.

Videotape analysis may also be used advantageously by inviting a peer or supervisor to periodically observe with the supervisee providing alternate points of view. Feedback also provides an excellent opportunity for supervisees to increase the accuracy of their observation skills (Dowling, 1998) by comparing their impressions with others. Thus, videotape usage as described above has the potential to be an important ally for the developing professional.

Data Collection. Data collection is a critical professional growth tool for clinicians. It is an objective way to gather data about clinical performance, both verbal and nonverbal (Dowling, 1992; Shapiro, 1998). It may take the form of the data-gathering strategies described in Chapter 2 or a formal observation system. Interest in observation systems in speech-language pathology has waned, yet they are a wonderful tool for self-analysis with or independently of a supervisor. For the developing clinician, a useful observation system is the Boone and Prescott (1972) "Content and sequence analysis of speech and hearing therapy." Ideally, exposure to the ideas behind observation systems and their use will be introduced as part of a clinical methods course or in conjunction with the clinical practicum. If formal training is not provided, the supervisee may begin by reading the Boone and Prescott (1972) article. In addition, several observation systems are reviewed in the Casey, Smith, and Ulrich (1988) guide to self-supervision and in Shapiro (1998).

The Boone and Prescott system consists of ten categories, five clinician and five client. The clinician categories are: Explain/describe, model/instruction, good evaluation, bad evaluation, neutral/social. The client categories are as follows: correct response, incorrect response, inappropriate/social, good self-evaluative, and bad self-evaluative. The behaviors are scored sequentially, by category, as they occur. The end product is a visual representation of the treatment interaction. Boone and Prescott suggest recording the middle twenty minutes of treatment and then randomly selecting a five-minute segment for analysis. They indicate that coding of the segment will take approximately seven to eight minutes. Then, a variety of ratios may be calculated to assist in interpreting the scored data.

The collected data from the Boone and Prescott system may be analyzed for the occurrence of critical incidents and the relationships among the categories and the overall incidence of individual behaviors. When using an observation system, clinicians may consider whether or not the events that are occurring parallel those they would like to see. As an observation tool condenses and organizes information, it provides supervisees with a powerful method of self-analysis.

The data-collection strategies described in Chapter 2 and/or a formal observation system objectify clinical behavior. They form the basis for logical problem-solving and are a primary tool for the enhancement of clinical performance. Thus, training beginning clinicians in these strategies will be an important part of their preparation.

Self-Evaluation.   Another strategy for supervisee self-development is to consider the behaviors appearing on the clinical evaluation forms used by their own facilities. Prior to treatment, the checklist may be used in planning therapy to affirm that the various areas are adequately addressed. Following clinical sessions, supervisees may self-evaluate by completing the evaluation tool in regard to their own behavior. This strategy helps supervisees focus on the specific subcomponents of therapy and stimulates thought in regard to the clinical process. On the basis of this self-analysis, supervisees may choose to continue in the same vein or make modifications for the next session. Donnelly and Weinrich (1996) incorporate the strategy of supervisee self-ratings on a clinical evaluation instrument into clinical training to foster self-supervision. Their approach is computer-based and tracks supervisee performance during the clinical training process. In education, Anderson and Freiberg (1995) advocate self-assessment in conjunction with audiotapes as a tool for self-reflection.

If clinicians self-evaluate and their supervisors have observed and rated the same sessions, it is helpful for supervisees to compare the two pieces of data. This technique is most effective when the supervisees complete the self-critique before receiving or considering feedback from supervisors, as prior input may interrupt or distort the self-analysis process. The comparison of the two sets of information provides insight into the accuracy of the supervisees' perceptions. As this process continues, the ratings on the two sets of evaluations should converge. Mercaitis and Peaper (1989) indicate this type of procedure is highly effective in teaching accurate self-evaluation skills.

Another component of self-evaluation is self-reflection. The supervisee might consider either valuative or objective data. Thought about the affective aspects of interactions with clients is also constructive. Taylor and Horney (1997) suggest this type of reflection assists supervisees in making sense of the clinical experience and helps them understand why events occurred as they did.

Knowledge Trees.   Knowledge tree construction is a potent method for supervisees to use when assessing and building their own clinical skills (Dowling and Bruce, 1996, 1997). Think of a knowledge tree as a tree trunk with branches. Initially, the tree will have a limited number of branches with a goal at the top. An example is the goal of competent clinical performance. The supervisee then thinks about the factors as branches needed to achieve this goal, for example: (1) clinical knowledge and experience, (2) assessment procedures, (3) clinician personal attributes, (4) knowledge of the profession, (5) related personal experiences contributing to clinical performance such as past work, and (6) interpersonal skills relating to clinical interaction. Kamhi (1995) states that four basic areas underlie clinical expertise: self-monitoring skills, knowledge base, procedural and problem-solving skills, and interpersonal skills and attitudes. Each of these would be an appropriate branch for the tree. The named branches will be individualized to meet the needs of the person striving for growth. One side of each branch will be used to note what the clinician already knows in this domain. The other side of the branch will be used to identify additional knowledge needed and will guide the supervisee in seeking out that information. The self-guided clinician will add to this tree with each clinical experience. The branches will grow in number and definition with an awareness of the nuances of clinical practice and increases in clinical expertise. Knowledge trees are intended to guide clinical growth. They also reassure clinicians by giving them an insight into the volume of what is known and give them the confidence to conquer the challenges that lie ahead. An example of a therapy skills knowledge tree (Dowling and Bruce, 1997) appears in Figure 8.2.

Dowling uses knowledge trees as a tool in a clinical procedures course and Bruce in diagnostics (Dowling and Bruce, 1996, 1997). Bruce also views knowledge trees as a quality improvement strategy. Her diagnostic teams add and subtract from the group and their own individual knowledge trees after each diagnostic evaluation. The trees, in this context, are used to enhance and guide clinical growth.

Therapy Observation.   The observation of therapy carried out by peers, staff, and faculty is also a self-development strategy for supervisees as it increases the depth and scope of one's experience. It also has the potential to enhance clinical flexibility through the discovery of a variety of options for achieving a specific goal. This process is particularly helpful if supervisees have the opportunity to observe someone who excels in an area in which they are having difficulty. Extensive treatment observation also has a broader benefit in that it helps supervisees build an internal concept of good as compared to less successful therapy. On the basis of that standard, supervisees may gain a relative sense of their ability, an aspect of the development of the professional self-concept.

Peer Supervision.   To foster professional growth independently of the supervisor, supervisees may also wish to participate in formal peer group supervision such as the Teaching Clinic presented in Chapter 10. An alternative is meeting informally with peers to discuss therapy. The discussions may be oriented to an issue or directed to the observation of a therapy session. In the latter case, strengths and

Desired Outcome: Effective Clinical Management

Perceived Current Knowledge

Additional Knowledge Needed

1. Transcribe speech phonetically
2. Knowledge of how sounds are made i.e. place, manner, voicing
3. Knowledge of normal speech mechanism and how it works
4. Knowledge normal language development and disorders
5. Knowledge of neurology and neuropathologies i.e. aphasia, dysarthria, dysphagia
6. Knowledge of developmental milestones
7. Knowledge of different types of scores i.e. Z scores, T scores, Percentile etc.
8. Knowledge of learning disabled population
9. Knowledge of scientific method
10. Knowledge of physiology and aerodynamics of fluency and stuttering and factors relating to the onset and development of stuttering

1. Good charting skills
2. Oral-Peripheral-Know normal and how to look for abnormal
3. Knowledge of developmental mile stones
4. Knowledge of some diagnostic test/screenings
5. Knowledge of what to includes in a standard assessment battery
6. Knowledge of how to consider a test's efficiency—reliability/validity
7. Knowledge that there will be variability
8. Knowledge of what to look for in a case history
9. Knowledge of how to make prognostic and severity statements

Therapy Skills

Academic

1. Voice assessment and treatment methodologies
2. Stuttering assessment and treatment methodologies
3. Phonological processing
4. Auditory discrimination and central auditory processing

1. Administration of diagnostic test
2. Scoring of diagnostic test
3. Interpretation of diagnostic test
4. Treatment planning
5. Report writing
6. VISI pitch
7. Macintosh computer skills

1. Patience
2. Good interviewing skills i.e. developing rapport, adapting behavior accordingly to the client
3. Open minded—I try not to have preconceptions
4. Goal setting skills
5. Provide release and support i.e. acknowledge feelings and praise efforts

1. Presently observing repaired cleft-palate patient—working on articulation and pitch
2. Learning reinforcement techniques

Personal Experience

Personal/Interpersonal

1. Decrease in anxiety
2. Knowledge in cultural differences
3. Behavior management

1. Experience interacting with patients
2. Insight into behaviors with children and to know what to realistically expect

FIGURE 8.2   Clinical Management Knowledge Tree

areas for growth may be identified and strategies for future intervention generated. In these interactions, the collection of data and an identified purpose will increase the productivity for participants.

Goal Setting.   The setting and striving toward ongoing professional goals is a key to self-development. At fixed intervals, the supervisee is wise to review professional goals. Like client assessment, data is reviewed to see if stated personal objectives have been met. It is also a time to reflect on what has and has not been learned. Then, it is time to turn thoughts to renewed objective setting for continuing growth. Often behaviors previously out of reach become possible as the individual develops. This process of regular reassessment provides the professional with opportunities to celebrate goal achievement and to plan for future growth.

In summary, the supervisee eager for professional growth has a variety of alternatives for independent development. Several have been presented in the preceding material. The successful clinician will discover others as well.

Outcomes

The impact of supervisee preparation for the clinical and supervisory process is reflected in a discussion between three classmates, Simone, Ana, and Sue, as they prepare to begin their first practicum.

SIMONE: I'm scared but I think I will be able to pull it off. I feel a lot better knowing about the therapy process and the continuum of supervision.

ANA: Yeah. I like knowing about supervision and what I need to do to make sure I get the most out of it. Feeling like I am the captain of my own ship is a little frightening but pretty cool.

SUE: I like knowing about ways to improve therapy on my own. If my supervisor is busy, I can do a lot of it myself.

SIMONE: What I like best is knowing what's expected of me in therapy and when I go to meet with my supervisor. I'm not going to have to worry about overstepping my bounds or not doing enough.

SUE: Hey, the clinical assignments are just being posted. Let's wish each other luck.

Relationship of the Thirteen Tasks of Supervision to Preparing the Supervisee for the Supervisory Process

The thirteen tasks are highly relevant to the preparation of the supervisee for the supervisory process. Because the implementation of these concepts constitutes good supervision, it is appropriate for supervisees to anticipate and plan for their incorporation. The supervisee should expect a constructive working relationship with the supervisor. Indeed, the clinician may enhance this process by being prepared for the different aspects of the clinical and supervisory process and by being open on an interpersonal level. Trainees may foresee assistance from the supervisor in developing clinical goals and objectives, assessment and clinical management skills, accurate observation and data collection skills, and professional writing competencies. The development of proficiency in data collection and analysis procedures will lead supervisees to demonstrate basic clinical research skills. They are also the foundations for accurate self-evaluation skills. A by-product of data-gathering will be the accurate maintenance of clinical and possible supervisory records. In all cases, growth is fostered by those clinicians who take active responsibility for learning and evolving these skills in conjunction with their supervisors. In addition to these fundamental abilities, supervisees may expect that their supervisors will demonstrate professional conduct for them. Also, as a component of the supervisory relationship, supervisees may envision opportunities to learn about the ethical, legal, regulatory, and reimbursements aspects of professional practice. Then, as time goes on, the supervisee will be encouraged to take an increasing role in planning and actively participating in the supervisory conference. In practice, supervisees will discover that each of the thirteen tasks is important for fostering their own professional growth.

Summary

This chapter addresses the training of the supervisee for the supervisory process from a variety of prospectives. It begins with a consideration of the relevant supervisory tasks adopted by the American Speech, Language and Hearing Association (1985). The continuum of supervision and its relationship to supervisee initiation is then outlined and the importance of active involvement in the supervisory process is stressed. The sequence of events likely to occur in the clinical practicum experience are then presented with a three-pronged focus: the supervisee behaviors expected by the supervisor, the related division of supervisor–supervisee responsibilities, and strategies supervisees might use to enhance their performance. This is followed by a section on approaches supervisees may employ for independent self-growth. In the last segment, the thirteen tasks of supervision are linked to the preparation of supervisees for involvement in the supervisory process.

REFERENCES

American Speech, Language and Hearing Association. "Clinical supervision in speech-language pathology and audiology." *American Speech Hearing Association, 27* (1985): 57–60.

American Speech, Language and Hearing Association. "Code of ethics of the American Speech-Language-Hearing Association." *American Speech Hearing Association, 36* (Supplement 13) (1994): 1–2.

American Speech and Hearing Association. "Preparation models for the supervisory process in Speech-Language Pathology and Audiology."

American Speech Hearing Association, 31 (1989): 97–106.

Anderson, J. *The Supervisory Process in Speech-Language Pathology and Audiology.* Austin, TX: Pro-Ed, 1988.

Anderson, J., and Freiberg, J. "Using self-assessment as a reflective tool to enhance the student teaching experience." *Teacher Education Quarterly.* Winter (1995): 77–91.

Boone, D., and Prescott, T. "Content and sequence analysis of speech and hearing therapy." *American Speech Hearing Association, 14* (1972): 58–62.

Brasseur, J. "The supervisory process: A continuum perspective." *Language, Speech and Hearing Services in the Schools, 20* (1989): 274–295.

Bruce, M., DiVenere, N., and Gergeron, C. "Preparing students to understand and honor families as partners." *American Journal of Speech-Language Pathology, 7* (3) (1998): 85–94.

Caracciolo, G., Rigrodsky, S., and Morrison, E. "Perceived interpersonal conditions and professional growth of master's level speech-language pathology students during the supervisory process. *American Speech Hearing Association, 20* (1978): 467–477.

Casey, P., Smith, K., and Ulrich, S. *Self-Supervision: A Career Tool for Audiologists and Speech-Language Pathologists.* Rockville, MD: National Student Speech Language Hearing Association, 1988.

Cogan, M. *Clinical Supervision.* Boston, MA: Houghton-Mifflin, 1973.

Cogan, M. "Clinical supervision and exploration." Paper presented in the conference Supervision of Students in Communication Disorders. University of Wisconsin, Madison, Wisconsin, 1978.

Costa, A., and Garmston, R. *Cognitive Coaching: A Foundation for Renaissance Schools.* Norwood, MA: Christopher Gordon Publishers, 1994.

Culatta, R., and Seltzer, H. "Content and sequence analyses of the supervisory session." *American Speech Hearing Association, 18* (1976): 8–12.

Deal, T. Personal communication, 1990.

Donnelly, C., and Weinrich, B. "The development of a computer program designed to teach self-supervision." In B. Wagner, (Ed.), *Proceedings: Partnerships in Supervision: Innovative and Effective Practices.* Grand Forks, ND: University of North Dakota, (1996): 224–228.

Dowling, S. "Supervisory training: Impetus for clinical supervision. *Clinical Supervisor, 4* (4) (1986): 27–34.

Dowling, S. "Impact of preclinical supervisory process training." Paper presented at the Annual Convention of the American Speech-Language and Hearing Association. Boston, MA, 1988.

Dowling, S. *Implementing the Supervisory Process: Theory and Practice.* Englewood Cliffs, NJ: Prentice-Hall, 1992.

Dowling, S. "Facilitating Clinical Training: Issues for Supervisees and their Supervisors." *Contemporary Issues in Communication Science and Disorders, 25* (1998): 5–11.

Dowling, S., and Bruce, M. "Improving Clinical Training through Continuous Quality Improvement and Critical Thinking." In B. Wagner, (Ed.), *Proceedings: Partnerships in Supervision: Innovative and Effective Practices.* Grand Forks, ND: University of North Dakota, (1996): 66–72.

Dowling, S., and Bruce, M. "Clinical Training: Enhancing Clinical Thought and Independence." Seminar presented at the Annual Convention of the American Speech, Language and Hearing Association, Boston, MA, Nov., 1997.

Farmer, S. "Communication competence." In S. Farmer and J. Farmer (Eds.), *Supervision in Communication Disorders.* Columbus, OH: Merrill, 1989: 94–153.

Goldberg, B. "The transformation age: The sky's the limit." *American Speech Hearing Association, 37* (1995): 44–50.

Harris, H., Ludington, J., Ringwalt, S., Ballard, D., Hooper, C., Buoyer, F., and Price, K. "Involving the student in the supervisory process." *National Student Speech Language Hearing Association Journal, 19* (1991–1992): 109–118.

Juhnke, G. "Solution-focused supervision: Promoting supervisee skills and confidence through successful solutions." *Counselor Education and Supervision, 36* (1996): 48–57.

Kamhi, A. G. "Research to practice: Defining, developing and maintaining clinical expertise." *Language, Speech and Hearing Services in Schools, 26* (4) (1995): 353–356.

Logemann, J. "The state of our professions." University of Houston, Houston, TX, Jan., 1999.

McCrea, E. *Supervisee Ability to Self-Explore and Four Facilitative Dimensions of Supervisory Behavior in Individual Conferences in Speech-Language Pathology.* (Doctoral Dissertation, Indiana University, Bloomington, IN. 1980.) *Dissertation Abstracts International, 41,* 2134B. (University Microfilms No. 80-29, 239).

McCrea, E. "Supervision component in undergraduate clinical management class." In K. Smith (moderator), "Preparation and training models for the supervisory process." Short Course presented at the Annual Convention of the American Speech-Language and Hearing Association, Washington, D.C., 1985.

McLeod, S. "Student self-appraisal: Facilitating mutual planning in clinical education." *The Clinical Supervisor, 15* (1) (1997): 87–101.

Meyer, S. *Survival Guide for the Beginning Speech-Language Clinician.* Gaithersburg, MD: Aspen Publishers, 1998.

Mercaitis, P. "Supervisor method for prepracticum skill development." *Clinical Supervisor, 11*(1) (1993): 179–187.

Mercaitis, P., and Peaper, R. "Strategies for helping supervisees to participate actively in the supervisory process." In D. Shapiro, (Ed.), *Supervision: Innovations: A National Conference on Supervision* held in Sonoma County, California, July, 1989. Cullowhee, NC: Western Carolina University, 1989.

Moses, N., and Shapiro, D. "A developmental conceptualization of clinical problem solving." *Journal of Communication Disorders, 29* (1996): 199–221.

Moss, S. "Weaving research into your clinical speech-language pathology practice." *American Speech-Language Hearing Association, 41* (4) (1999): 40–44.

Perkins, J., and Mercaitis, P. "A guide for supervisors and students in clinical practicum." *The Clinical Supervisor, 13* (2) (1995): 67–78.

Pickering, M. "Interpersonal communication in speech-language pathology supervisory conferences: A qualitative study." *Journal of Speech and Hearing Disorders, 49* (1984): 189–195.

Roberts, J., and Smith, K. "Supervisor–supervisee role differences and consistency of behavior in supervisory conferences." *Journal of Speech and Hearing Research, 25* (1982): 428–434.

Schalk, M., and Peroff, L. "Consistency and reliability of supervisory evaluations at university training centers." Paper presented at the Annual Convention of the American Speech-Language and Hearing Association, San Francisco, CA, 1972.

Shapiro, D. "Professional preparation and lifelong learning: The making of a clinician." In D. Shapiro, (Ed.), *Stuttering Intervention: A Collaborative Journey to Fluency Freedom.* Austin, TX: Pro-Ed, 1998: 474–571.

Shapiro, D., and Moses, N. "Creative problem solving in public school supervision. *"Language, Speech, and Hearing Services in the Schools,"* 20 (1989): 320–332.

Smith, K., and Anderson, J. "Relationship of perceived effectiveness to content in supervisory conferences in speech-language pathology." *Journal of Speech and Hearing Research, 25* (1982): 243–251.

Strike-Roussos, C. *Supervisors' Implementation of Trained Information Regarding Broad Questioning and Discussion of Supervision during their Supervisory Conferences in Speech-Language Pathology.* Doctoral Dissertation, Indiana University, Bloomington, Indiana, 1988.

Taylor, C., and Horney, M. "A phenomenographic investigation of students' approaches to self-evaluation of their clinical practice." *The Clinical Supervisor, 16* (2) (1997): 105–123.

Wayne, S. and Kacmar, M. "The effects of impression management on the performance appraisal process." *Organizational Behavior and Human Decision Processes 48* (1991): 70–88.

9 Creating Solutions: Supervisor Professional Growth

Clinical Supervision Tasks Relevant to the Professional Growth of the Supervisor

Task 1: Establishing and maintaining an effective working relationship with the supervisee;

Task 2: Assisting the supervisee in developing clinical goals and objectives;

Task 3: Assisting the supervisee in developing and refining assessment skills;

Task 4: Assisting the supervisee in developing and refining clinical management skills;

Task 5: Demonstrating for and participating with the supervisee in the clinical process;

Task 6: Assisting the supervisee in observing and analyzing assessment and treatment sessions;

Task 7: Assisting the supervisee in the development and maintenance of clinical and supervisory records;

Task 8: Interacting with the supervisee in planning, executing, and analyzing supervisory conferences;

Task 9: Assisting the supervisee in evaluation of clinical performance;

Task 10: Assisting the supervisee in developing skills of verbal reporting, writing, and editing;

Task 11: Sharing information regarding ethical, legal, regulatory, and reimbursement aspects of professional practice;

Task 12: Modeling and facilitating professional conduct;

Task 13: Demonstrating research skills in the clinical or supervisory processes.

The topic of this chapter is the professional growth of the supervisor. Numerous authors suggest a parallel between the clinical and supervisory processes (McCrea, 1985; Brasseur, 1989; Harris, Ludington, Ringwalt, Ballard, Hooper, Buoyer, and Price, 1991–1992). Because supervisees are expected to grow as they move through clinical training, it seems fitting that supervisors should do so as well. In particular, supervisors are expected to implement the thirteen tasks of supervision. This means they will not only carry out these tasks but will also exhibit the underlying competencies as described in the ASHA position statement on supervision. Through training and ongoing professional growth, supervisors become increasingly accomplished in their role, and will be able to foster the development of supervisees as they move toward clinical independence, identify the supervisee's developmental level so that supervision can be adapted accordingly, improve the quality of clinical services to clientele by optimizing the performance of supervisees, make cases for establishing and maintaining professional staffing in work settings, increase the perceived value of speech-language pathology and audiology services throughout a facility, and enhance the supervisor's own job satisfaction.

This chapter begins with a review of the literature pertinent to the professional growth of the supervisor. It includes work from a variety of disciplines. Ideas regarding training and its effects will be noted. This is followed by information concerning the conditions surrounding supervisor growth in typical environments and those that exist in certain settings. The focus then shifts to the specifics of supervisor development. A variety of options for self-guided and formal training are presented.

Literature

Speech-Language Pathology and Audiology

Although this committee has sunsetted, the American Speech-Language and Hearing Association Committee on Supervision (1985) states "The major goal of training in supervision is mastery of the "Competencies for Effective Clinical Supervision." These are the skills underlying competent implementation of the thirteen tasks of supervision. The committee suggests gaining these abilities through coursework, continuing education, and involvement in research with an emphasis on supervision. A supervisory focus in speech-language pathology and audiology is at the heart of the training. Once this is obtained, additional work in the speech-language pathology and audiology discipline and/or a study of the common aspects of supervision across the disciplines of "teaching, counseling, social work, business and health care professions" are thought to be of benefit.

Training: Its Nature and Effects.   Anderson (1981) describes a training program for supervisors. She notes the value of an array of training alternatives. She feels that in-service training for staff supervisors enhances the supervision provided in a facility. Persons external to the training program are thought to benefit from summer coursework designed to meet state supervision certificate requirements. She also indicates that master's degree candidates will profit from an introductory course in supervision as it provides them with insights about the process, facilitates their own clinical work, and makes them better supervisors when they assume this responsibility, as most speech-language pathologists and audiologists do at some point in their career.

The major thrust of the training that Anderson discusses is at the doctoral level. It consists of several components. The first is a basic introductory course in supervision. This provides an overview of the process and an in-depth consideration and application of the clinical (Cogan, 1973) and continuum of supervision models (Anderson, 1988). The second aspect is active participation in a variety of supervisory practicums. Third, an advanced seminar in supervision is included, one designed to explore available research across disciplines. Fourth, an immersion in the study of the research process in theory and application is incorporated as the core around which the training sequence is designed.

Brasseur (1989) also describes a regimen of training for persons with a master's degree. The program consists of nine credit hours completed over a three-semester period. It begins with an introductory course in supervision in speech-language pathology. This is followed by a practicum and then a more advanced didactic course in supervision. The persons taking the courses are off-campus practicum supervisors. Their supervision practicum experience is also off-site as they supervise student teachers in the public schools. The instructor of the course conferences regularly with the "supervisors" about the supervision that they are providing. In addition, they meet each month as a group to analyze their video-tapes, discuss issues, and plan strategies for achieving the competencies underlying the thirteen tasks of supervision. Brasseur reports that this process allows participants to add behaviors that were previously not in their repertoires. In particular, their conference styles become collaborative and move steadily in the direction of consultation as the term progresses. The supervisor trainees also feel that their interpersonal skills improve, which facilitates their effectiveness in the conference.

Strike-Roussos (1988) also describes a training program for supervisors. Her program is designed to teach two specific supervisor behaviors: increasing the time spent discussing supervision during conferences, and asking broad questions as contrasted to narrow during dialogues. Training consists of three phases for each of the variables. Each session lasts approximately one hour. The first hour for each variable is designed to teach participants to distinguish between the behavior under consideration: clinical and supervisory process or broad and narrow questions. Phases two and three are implemented if the supervisor does not engage in the behavior at a criterion level following the training session. Strike-Roussos finds that training does make a difference. Discussions of supervision within conferences and an increase in broad question usage does occur.

Barrow and Domingo (1997) provide ten hours of supervisory training to one group of supervisors while the remainder serve as a control group. The curriculum consists of (1) research on the supervisory process, (2) models of supervision, (3) the supervisory conference, (4) and the ASHA (1985) competencies for supervisors. The Individual Supervisory Conference Rating Scale (Brasseur and Anderson, 1983; Smith and Anderson, 1982) is used pre and post to assess the supervisory process. Differences are found between the trained and untrained supervisors. Trained supervisors exhibit an increase in indirect conference behaviors, are more supportive interpersonally, and are more effective in helping supervisees set realistic client goals. Supervisees of trained supervisors verbalize more needs, receive fewer value judgments from the supervisor, and perceive less of a superior–subordinate relationship, with their supervisors.

The North Carolina Association for supervisors in speech-language pathology and audiology (NCASSPA) uses a series of training workshops for persons supervising speech-language pathology assistants. McCready (1999) reports that these training sessions make the participants feel more comfortable supervising assistants and reduces their anxiety about the role these persons will play in the work setting. Hagler and McFarlane (1998), too, are actively working to train supervisors of SLP assistants in Canada.

Dowling (1993, 1994) studies the impact of graduate student supervisory training. The training consists of a three-credit-hour academic course consisting of over thirty-five hours of lecture, role-play, and participation in a three-part simulation game. Trainee conference behavior at the outset of the course is assessed and three goals for professional growth are set. At the end of the course, conferencing skills are again measured. Supervisor trainees achieve their goals, are able to modify their conference talk, and move toward a more effective conference style. These findings document the value of preprofessional training in supervision.

Qualifications and Competencies.   A note of history is in order. In 1980, the ASHA Committee on Supervision presented proposed minimum qualifications for supervisors to the ASHA membership (VanDemark, Borton, Dowling, Nelson, Rassi, Ulrich, and Vallon, 1980). They consisted of the following: (1) master's degree in speech pathology or audiology, (2) three years of experience beyond the Clinical Fellowship Year, (3) Certificate of Clinical Competence in the area to be supervised, and (4) six semester hours of academic coursework or its equivalent in continuing education credits. At least three of these hours were to be in supervision in speech-language pathology and/or audiology. The remaining hours could pertain to the common body of knowledge in supervision but be in a related discipline such as counseling, business, or social work. The final requirement, number five, was fifty hours of practicum in supervision. At the time these were presented, the ASHA membership felt strongly about any proposal that might lead to specialty certification. The outcry from the membership was strong and the proposal was withdrawn. In response, the ASHA Committee on Supervision turned its efforts to defining the supervisor competencies needed to implement effective supervision. These competencies were approved as an official position of the American Speech-Language Hearing Association. The competencies cited at the beginning of this chapter are from that position statement. The intent is to foster quality supervision in a variety of settings by enhancing the skills of supervisors.

Education

In-service supervisory training for educational administrators is described by Killion and Harrison (1985). Three levels of training are made available. The first consists of thirty hours of work designed to teach the clinical supervision process and to identify desirable on-the-job teaching and administrative behaviors. For example, tasks such as conducting meetings, motivating personnel, creating a vision for the facility, and managing resources are recognized as preferred administrative behaviors. Level two consists of an additional twenty hours devoted to application of the skills learned and new information about adapting supervision to the needs of supervisees and effective conferencing. In level three, ten additional hours are devoted to the practice of earlier learned information.

Killion and Harrison report that individuals who completed only stage one of the training rarely use the skills taught. If any aspects are employed, they are only implemented for a brief time and in a fragmented manner. Those participating in both parts one and two perform better but need ongoing support and encouragement to continue applying their new skills. In contrast, those who finish each of the three levels of training tend to utilize their new abilities on a regular basis.

In contrast, Jensen, Parsons, and Reid (1998) report that a combination of a limited amount of formal teaching and then on-the-job monitoring and feedback are an effective form of training. Seven teachers supervising assistants learn to accurately observe and provide feedback to their assistants about their data collection and teaching performance. Improvements in teaching behaviors are noted and maintained for more than seventeen months.

Counseling

In psychotherapy, several authors propose levels of supervisor development. Stoltenberg, McNeill, and Delworth (1998) describe a three-stage model followed by a fourth, integrative. The accompanying range of supervisor behaviors are from naive or anxious to that of a master supervisor. Supervisory training is viewed as critical to the development of a supervisor. Watkins (1990), according to Blair and Peake (1995), describes four stages of supervisor development. The four levels are: (1) role shock, (2) recovery and transition, (3) role consolidation, and (4) role mastery. During role shock, supervisors struggle with the boundaries of supervision and have limited confidence. As a result, they tend to be rigid about rules and basic procedures and have a low tolerance for ambiguity. During recovery and transition, they begin to develop their identity as a supervisor, become more assertive, and are able to tolerate limited ambiguity. As supervisors move into role consolidation, they gain a broader and more informed perspective of supervision and increase the consistency of their behavior. With role mastery, the supervisors' identity strengthens. They are able to deal consistently with issues emerging in supervision, are less threatened by supervisory mistakes, and are able to provide supervision that is useful to the supervisee.

Stevens, Goodyear, and Robertson (1997) study supervisory behavior, relating it to several factors: (1) prior supervisory training, (2) level of experience, (3) theoretical orientation, (4) type of criticism used, (5) supervisee supportiveness, and (6) personal effectiveness. Participants range from novice supervisors to those with more than ten years of experience. Sixty-one percent of the supervisors have a doctoral degree. Participant supervisory training prior to the study ranges from none to three or more structured experiences such as a course or workshop. The participants view a videotape excerpt of a counseling session implemented by a supervisee. The supervisors complete several paper-and-pencil instruments about themselves and the types of information they would provide to the supervisee. The results of the study indicate that supervisors' perceptions of their own effectiveness does increase with experience. In addition, the more formal supervisory training a supervisor obtains, the greater the feeling of self-efficacy. With training, supervisors also become more flexible, supportive, and less dogmatic. The latter does not occur without supervisory training. Watkin (1995) also notes that supervisory experience alone does not improve the quality of supervision provided.

Business

Key supervisory skills in business are identified by Green, Knippen, and Vincelette (1985). They list the following: "motivating, delegating, evaluating performance of subordinates, setting goals with subordinates, interviewing, giving directions and instructions, disciplining, coaching, counseling, terminating subordinates, planning, clarifying communications, listening actively, building self-confidence, handling conflict, giving positive reinforcement, taking initiative, coping with stress, problem-solving, and managing time." They further suggest a strategy for teaching each of these skills. Each is presented in a separate four-hour training module consisting of three components: teaching, demonstration, and practice–feedback. After the content is introduced in a lecture format, the participants observe the tactic used correctly in a variety of videotaped situations. They then implement the skill in a role-play format. After critiquing their own and others' performances, the participants reimplement the technique to demonstrate mastery. Green and colleagues feel that this methodology not only teaches a skill but instills confidence in participants' abilities to use it successfully in their own work environments.

Further, Marx (1986) suggests the incorporation of a relapse prevention strategy to increase the carryover of skills learned during management development training to the work setting. He indicates that only 40 percent of material presented is typically applied immediately after training. In fact, the average participant is only using 15 percent of it a year later. Thus, he suggests a method to increase the transfer of information to the job. A seven-step procedure is recommended: (1) Choosing a competency to retain; (2) Setting a goal; (3) Making a commitment to retain the skill; (4) Applying the relapse prevention strategies; (5) Predicting the circumstances of the first relapse; (6) Practicing tactics necessary to cope with difficult situations; and (7) Monitoring the target behavior following training. He further suggests that a minimum of three to four hours be devoted to teaching persons how to retain the behaviors being taught.

Phillips (1986) points out that not all supervisory training need occur in a classroom environment. He suggests that in business environments, job rotation, self-study, mentor relationships, special assignments, and memberships in professional organizations are also effective. Temporary job rotation or cross-training allows supervisors to learn new skills demanded by alternate positions. This movement presents a challenge to the individual and eliminates stagnation due to the potential redundancy in a given position. Self-study also generates new skills. This often takes the form of reading lists provided by the organization or programmed learning. Establishing a relationship with an experienced, influential mentor is also thought to stimulate supervisor growth. In addition, special assignments to complete a task or study a problem serve as a basis for individual development. Finally, membership in professional organizations functions as a source for technical knowledge. Phillips notes that the job environment provides significant opportunities for growth.

A management training program at Human Synergistics, Inc. results in a significant improvement in fifty-five different behaviors (Lafferty and Colletti, 1985). The three-year program begins with an extensive diagnostic evaluation of participants. The ensuing training consists of interaction with a clinical psychologist, lectures, computer-based games, and experiential simulations requiring decision making in both work and nonjob-related situations. The participants develop goals for both personal and professional growth. They each receive follow-up information such as readings and self-instructional materials. They are also periodically reminded of the objectives they had set.

The results indicate effective behaviors increase while those that are less so fade (Lafferty and Colletti, 1985). Scores reflecting healthy and productive thinking increase as do those concerning self-actualization. Managements' humanistic tendencies, defined as the desire to help others, are also enhanced. Time usage improves as do feelings of self-esteem. Further, others in the organization perceive that participants improve their decision-making abilities, delegate more responsibility, develop subordinates, and handle stress with greater proficiency.

Curtis and Zins (1988) also find that classroom training in consultation does improve certain participant skills. Instruction consists of classroom lectures focusing on collaborative consultation, observation of the course instructor engaging in counseling, videotape observations and critiques, and role-play exercises. A subset of the subjects also receives individual feedback regarding their videotaped role-plays from a second instructor. All subjects significantly improve their level of questioning and the quality of their utterances. In addition, the members receiving input regarding their performance are also able to modify their statements by making them more concrete and behaviorally specific. This study demonstrates consultation improves with training.

Summary

Supervisory training is recommended as a strategy in a variety of disciplines. Research in business environments demonstrates that instruction does make a difference in the behavior of those who participate (Lafferty and Colletti, 1985; Curtis and Zins, 1988). Work in speech-language pathology and audiology also shows that training does alter supervisors' behavior. Caracciolo, Rigrodsky, and Morrison (1978) find that trained supervisors provide facilitative interpersonal conditions in the conference resulting in a decrease in the gap between the clinician's real and ideal professional self, and an increase in supervisee self-esteem. Strike-Roussos (1988) documents that two supervisor talk behaviors, broad questions and the discussion of supervision during conferences, may be increased through training. Brasseur (1989) reports that supervisors are able to add new behaviors to their repertoire as a result of training. Dowling (1993, 1994) indicates supervisor trainees are able to achieve set goals and modify their conference talk in the direction of increased collaboration. Finally, Barrow and Domingo (1997) report that trained supervisors increase indirect behaviors in the conference, are more supportive interpersonally, and are more effective in helping supervisees set realistic client goals.

An array of literature regarding supervisory training is presented in the preceding material. Training does make a difference. Given this background it seems appropriate to turn thoughts to a description of the environments surrounding supervisory positions and the related options for professional development.

State of the Art

A variety of forces impact the character of supervision in a given setting. Public schools are proving to be a stable work environment, although the availability and the number of supervisors varies from district to district. The inclusion of speech-language pathology assistants has markedly increased the demand for supervision in the schools. Many individuals without previous supervisory experience are now being asked to supervise an assistant.

The fallout from managed care is reducing the number of speech-language pathologists in many hospital and rehabilitation settings. Some facilities have only "on-call" staff. Thus, the number of persons in roles with supervision as a formal part of their job description is declining in some medical settings. Supervisors are also seeing a broadening of their role to include occupational and physical therapy.

In training programs, the primary providers of supervision are likely to be in staff positions, both full and part-time. As documented by Gavett (1987), the majority do not hold academic positions. In practice, those hired on partial assignments, such as a quarter or half-time, are often assigned adjunct status. Frequently the appointments are on a year-by-year basis. Position availability is dependent on student enrollments and/or the presence of funds. As a result, many supervisory positions in universities are unstable and do not offer opportunities for career advancement or even predictable employment. In addition, Gavett chronicles the status gap that frequently exists between academic faculty and clinical staff members.

Currently, in most work settings, the prerequisites for being hired as a supervisor are personal clinical competence and the ASHA Certificate of Clinical Competence in the area to be supervised, speech-language pathology or audiology. To supervise an assistant, the supervisor must have two years of experience beyond certification and a one-hour course or ten hours of continuing education in supervision. The skills underlying the thirteen tasks of supervision should also be in evidence. However, compliance with the ASHA position statement on supervision remains voluntary as an enforcement mechanism does not exist. Of note though, the ASHA (1999) standards for Accreditation of Graduate Education Programs in Audiology and Speech-Language Pathology do stipulate that "the nature, amount, and accessibility of clinical supervision are" to be "commensurate with the clinical knowledge and skills of each student."

Growth Opportunities

Opportunities for professional growth may or may not be built in to given positions. In facilitative environments, career ladders for professional staff will exist. For example, Jones-McNamara (McCrea, Jones-McNamara, and Ringwalt, 1989) describes a career ladder for supervisors in a large private practice organization. In addition, one training program has the following levels for both full and part-time supervisory staff members: clinical instructor, clinical assistant professor, clinical associate professor, and clinical professor (Ringwalt, 1989–1990). To be promoted, staff members must demonstrate excellence in one of four areas: teaching, including clinical teaching (supervision), clinical activity, scholarship and research, and/or administration. Appointments are from one to five years and reappointment and promotions range in the same time span. The procedure is similar to standard academic appointments in that a document is prepared and moved thorough the committee structure of the university. The prime differences being that it is not a tenure-track position and excellence is expected in only one of four areas.

Another training facility has similar ranks for clinical faculty: clinical lecturer, clinical assistant professor, clinical associate professor, and clinical professor (McCrea, Jones-McNamara, and Ringwalt, 1989). Each rank has unique characteristics plus all of those included in the lower levels. For example, the clinical associate professor is described as follows:

> The rank for clinical faculty who have excelled in the performance of their clinical specialty as indicated in periodic evaluations and who:
>   a. Participate in classroom teaching by serving as the instructor of record for clinical courses or teaching clinical-procedures sections of academic courses.
>   b. Participate in applied research (optional) in collaboration with academic or clinical faculty members.
>   c. Serve on departmental committees, represent the Department to governmental agencies, work with philanthropic support groups and other extra-University organizations.
>   d. Contribute to the vigor of the Department and the profession by conducting clinical training workshops at regional and national meetings and through other continuing education activities (Department of Speech and Hearing Sciences, IU, 1989). (The full text is reprinted with permission in Appendix A.)

The promotion procedure parallels that for academic faculty in that it is first reviewed by a committee made up of members holding higher ranks. It then makes its way through the university committee structure. The key differences are that it is not a tenure track and the focus is clinical and/or teaching rather than scholarship.

The examples cited above tend to be exceptions rather than the rule. Supervisors will often find themselves in environments in which they are valued as competent individuals. But, they will not be actively encouraged to continue to grow as a professional. As a result, persons in supervisory positions are likely to hold a master's degree and have a certificate of clinical competence in the area in which they supervise. They will strive to do the best job possible but may not have opportunities provided or be rewarded for ongoing professional growth and/or studying the supervisory process.

Growth Decision

The real question then becomes "Why should I strive to improve the supervision I provide?" The reasons are similar to those discussed in relation to supervisees. They relate to job satisfaction, self-fulfillment, burnout prevention, and ethical behavior. Striving toward goals increases job satisfaction, a sense of self-control, and makes people feel better about themselves. It increases work-related stimulation and, as a result, minimizes burnout. It may also impact the perceived status of the supervisor. In all cases, it will result in improved clinical services to patients and increased supervisee independence. Heid (1997) suggests that focusing on growth, both as a person and as a professional, is valuable. Goldberg (1995) and Kamhi (1995) underscore the importance of lifelong learning for all professionals. Therefore, even though a position may neither require nor reward continuing development, it is in the best interest of supervisors to engage in these behaviors on their own. The discussion that follows is between two supervisors. They highlight concerns that emerge in supervisors' work lives relating to the issue of professional growth.

Problem Identification

Two supervisors are talking after a local professional meeting.

> **CHANDRA:**   I have been supervising for four years now. It isn't as much fun as it used to be. I feel like I'm getting in a rut.
>
> **AMILIO:**   I felt that way about two years ago. Then, I attended several workshops on supervision. The presenters encouraged everyone to audiotape a conference and analyze it. My style surprised me. Since then, every three months, I sit down, analyze one of my conferences and then set a goal to improve my supervision. It has made me feel challenged and excited again. Those workshops were a real shot in the arm.
>
> **CHANDRA:**   Hmmm. I need to do something like that.

Growth Commitment

Once a decision has been made to devote time and effort to professional growth, available opportunities will need to be explored. At this time, a body of supervisory literature has grown in speech-language pathology and audiology and is readily available. This includes both books and articles. Also, a variety of opportunities for exploring supervisory theory and practice exists. Courses are available from select universities and supervision is a frequent topic at national conventions and workshops throughout the country.

For most supervisors, the most common avenues for growth are workshops, reviewing the literature, self-development, networking, formal coursework, and involvement in supervisory research. The best option for a given individual may vary depending on time available, strength of commitment, the point in one's development, and accessible resources. To begin, most persons need some basic exposure to supervisory theory. An understanding of the value and use of the Anderson continuum of supervision, clinical supervision, cognitive coaching, or other models of supervision is fundamental to the building of a plan for supervisor enhancement.

Then, mastering the competencies underlying the thirteen tasks of supervision becomes the overall goal. A key factor in meeting this objective and the ASHA (1999) mandate of providing supervision at the level of supervisee need, is to effectively diagnose a given supervisee and then, adapt supervision accordingly. In practice, the supervisor, in conjunction with the supervisee, needs to determine the supervisee's readiness in relation to the Anderson Continuum of Supervision. The question is whether the supervisee is in the direct/active stage with a need to have concrete guidance from the supervisor or is this person ready, on a given day, to shift into the transitional stage with increasing amounts of collaboration. Following the assessment of the supervisee's level in general and more specifically, relative to that day and the issues to be addressed, the supervisor needs to be able to adapt his or her supervision accordingly. This is a very complex task requiring on-going supervisor thought and effort. Thus, diagnosis, self-assessment, and the ability to adapt supervision as needed, are key skills to be developed when planning for supervisor growth.

Self-Guided Growth

Reading

Supervisory training may be obtained in a variety of ways and need not always be in a classroom. Therefore, the discussion will begin here with those strategies supervisors might use in the workplace to foster their own development. A good beginning point is to read material presented in this text, articles on supervision, and other available books. In regard to the latter, the works of Anderson (1988), Farmer and Farmer (1989), Crago and Pickering (1987), Rassi (1978), Dowling (1992), and Rassi and McElroy (1992) may be helpful. Initially, theory and the related practice are likely to be most valuable. At a later point, specific research that may be found in a variety of journals will be beneficial. The purpose of this dabbling in the literature is to foster a supervisory philosophy on which to build specific skills. In particular, the continuum of supervision, the clinical supervision model, and cognitive coaching provide such a foundation. Key points to be abstracted are: (1) supervision is best when it is adapted to the individual supervisee's level of need, (2) analysis of the supervisory conference is the foundation for growth, (3) the goal of supervision is to optimize treatment and foster supervisee independence, and (4) job satisfaction is enhanced through ongoing professional development.

Reflecting

Another strategy for personal growth is self-reflection. Once basic reading has been done with a focus on supervisory models and conference styles, reflection on one's own supervisor behaviors and conference style is helpful. The goal is to identify the conference style being used and compare it to a desirable theoretical model. Identifying perceived conference strengths and weaknesses is of value. Listening to a tape of a conference and collecting data will also assist in forming these impressions. Recall that using data-based self-evaluation was thought to help supervisees see their performances more objectively. It should have a similar impact on supervisors' observations of their own work. In addition to a specific focus on the conference, the supervisor is wise to reflect on other aspects of his or her supervision as well. Examples would be examinations of feedback tools and strategies, interpersonal relationships with supervisees, and levels of participant satisfaction. Reflection may thus be specific or broad in scope.

Data-Collecting

The gathering of objective information, as described in the chapter on data collection, is an invaluable tool for the supervisor. Either formal observation systems may be used to obtain a global picture of the conference or informal methods applied to specific aspects of behavior. These strategies enhance goal-setting by providing a concrete foundation. They also assist in the achievement of goals by providing a method to monitor change. For the use of formal observation systems, good resources are the work of Casey, Smith, and Ulrich (1988) and Shapiro (1994, 1998). See Appendix B for a guide developed by Dowling (2000) to analyze the conference. This tool is used as part of a supervision course to assist trainees in analyzing their conferences. On the basis of the data collected, it is possible to determine conference style and to set goals for growth.

Modifying

Once this is done, a supervisor might select one or two behaviors for modification, for example, strengthening an asset, building an area of deficit, or learning a new skill. It is important to begin small with a specific focus. Examples may be to decrease supervisor talk time, increase active listening, increase the frequency of open-ended questions, or enhance the interpersonal climate. Attempts to modify multiple behaviors simultaneously can lead to frustration and discouragement as it increases task difficulty too quickly and is likely to overwhelm the supervisor. This same individual may think there is so much to change that it is impossible to succeed and then may decide to do nothing at all. In contrast, tackling a specific behavior makes the task difficulty manageable, sets the stage for success, and increases self-confidence in one's ability to change.

Goal-Setting

Translating targets into behavioral objectives increases the probability that they will be obtained. Goals may come from a variety of sources. Self-reflection may be the origin of some while others may come from theory or be based in collected data. Another alternative is to use the rating scale developed by Casey (1988) to assess levels of proficiency in implementing each of the thirteen tasks of supervision. Feedback from supervisees or peers might yet be another stimulus. The concepts presented in this text may also be a beginning point. Remember that the ultimate intent is to build the competencies underlying the thirteen tasks of supervision. Consistently setting goals and working toward achievement will foster supervisor professional growth. Making the goals explicit and achievable will also aid this effort (DeShon and Alexander, 1996).

Gathering Feedback

Feedback from a variety of sources is also an excellent growth tool. Valuative information from supervisees at the end of a clinical experience is helpful. In a work environment, data may be solicited as needed or on a regular basis. Glaser and Donnelly (1994) describe a formal evaluation tool that assesses implementation of the thirteen tasks of supervision that would provide valuable information to supervisors (see Appendix C). Three-sixty degree evaluation (Manatt and Benway, 1998) may also be useful. In this approach, the supervisor self-evaluates in addition to soliciting feedback from a superior, peer, supervisee, and/or clients, and their families. Thus, feedback is requested from everyone interacting with the supervisor on a regular basis.

In considering this feedback, the overall patterns are most useful. For example, if all supervisees feel they are not actively involved in the conference, supervisors need to consider the quantity and types of verbal behavior they are using. If peers note a consistent effective or ineffective behavior, the supervisor will want to take this into account in goal-setting. The supervisor may also wish to solicit formal and informal feedback from the supervisee regarding specific supervisor behaviors that are helpful versus those that are not.

Collaborating

An extension of the idea of obtaining feedback from supervisees is to actively involve them in a collaborative relationship. Sharing the Anderson continuum of supervision with supervisees and guiding them to understand their role in their own professional development will assist them in becoming active participants in the process (Dowling, 1998). Supervisees may then prompt the supervisor to provide the types of supervision that will optimally foster their own growth. In addition, they may help the supervisor identify valued supervisory strategies. This partnership with supervisees and their feedback optimizes the supervisory process and participant growth.

Taping

Audiotape and videotape are excellent mediums for feedback. Similarly, data collection and monitoring of goals while viewing or listening to tapes is a valuable source for self-learning. In addition, working with colleagues, a mentor, or a supervisee in analyzing the content of taped conferences may lead to insights that benefit the developing supervisor.

Networking

Networking and group discussion of supervisory procedures are also helpful. Interaction with experienced supervisors often eases the confusion felt by the novice. Dialogues in relation to what works also appear to be beneficial. Supervisors who find themselves in an isolated environment may need to seek out others in a similar position to form a support or growth team. This may even extend to involvement in state and national supervisors' groups. These assist the growing supervisor by providing encouragement and identifying potential resources.

Meetings

Small groups are an excellent resource for growth. This is particularly true if meetings are used as a format for conference observation, data-gathering, analysis, and problem-solving. A formal peer group mechanism, the teaching clinic (presented in a later chapter) may also be used as a mechanism for supervisor development. As will be noted later, McCrea (1994) incorporates teaching clinics into formal supervisory training.

As groups evolve, the supervisors' analysis, problem-solving, and strategy development skills will flourish. Shapiro and Moses (1989) note that improvement in problem-solving is reflected in the ability to take varying perspectives, to see behavior as multidimensional, to generate several alternatives, and to understand the cause and effect relationships linked to the implementation of varying strategies. As development occurs, supervisory goals may also increase in difficulty. The participants may gather data relative to conferences and develop strategies for increasing the productivity of the meetings. In general, as supervisors grow, they will be better able to adapt supervision to the needs of the supervisee. Supervisors are also likely to feel a sense of accomplishment. In addition, they will often realize that their interest in and satisfaction with the supervisory process is growing.

Formal Supervisor Training

In addition to or more likely as a result of self-development, supervisors will often seek out continuing education opportunities. This may take the form of a series of workshops or formal enrollment in a survey course of supervision in speech-language pathology and audiology. It is important to note that what persons in the field perceive as constituting supervisory training is highly variable. Anderson (1972) reports that individuals in supervisory positions feel business management, school administration, research techniques, additional coursework in communication disorders as well as specific work in supervision were all within the realm of this type of training. As a result, the consumer will need to take care in selecting educational offerings to insure that training truly is in supervision.

Coursework

Ideally, the first endeavor is enrollment in a survey supervision course in speech-language pathology and audiology. This will provide the foundation for further course selection. If structured courses are not available, workshops and continuing education opportunities focusing on models of supervision and their implementation are good starting points.

The potential contents of a beginning course in supervision are described by the ASHA Committee on Supervision (1989):

- role of supervisor;
- professional/political issues in supervision in speech-language pathology and audiology;
- phases of the supervisory process;
- supervisory techniques;

- interpersonal components of the supervisory process;
- leadership styles and management approaches;
- variations in the process across settings;
- adaptation of supervisory style to meet the needs, expectations, and clinical competence of supervisees;
- accountability and evaluation of the supervisory process;
- preparation of supervisors, research in supervision; and
- incorporating the tasks and competencies from the ASHA position statement into practice (p. 98).

Problem-Solving

The supervisors we met early in the chapter share their impressions of supervisory training.

AMILIO: Hi Chandra. It's been a while since we talked.

CHANDRA: I've been looking forward to seeing you. Remember, we were talking about how frustrated I was. I felt I was in a rut as a supervisor.

Amilio nods.

CHANDRA: After we talked, I started to do some reading in supervision. Then, I found a course to take on supervision. It was really exciting. One of the things I discovered that I was doing was supervising everybody the same way. I hadn't thought about how much I was telling people how to do their jobs. No wonder I was getting bored. Well, I started working on one thing at time. The clinicians have been happier and I am enjoying supervising again. Thanks for giving me something to think about.

AMILIO: That's great. Maybe we can get together once a month or so and talk about the way we supervise. I'd like to have someone to look at my conferences with me and collect some data.

CHANDRA: I'd like to do that and share my conferences too. Let's plan to meet within the next couple of weeks.

The author teaches a course in supervision. It consists of an exposure to the literature, lecture material, role-play, and simulation. Course topics include supervisory models, the role of the supervisor, data collection and analysis, the supervisory conference, group supervision, interpersonal effectiveness, productive communication, feedback, organizational behavior and acculturation, preparing the supervisee for participation in the process, supervising supervisees at differing levels of professional development, and supervisor qualifications. Enrollees also analyze their own conferences with a role-played supervisee and set professional conference goals for the term. They then participate in role-plays and conference with a peer to practice the behaviors they are tying to modify in their conferences. This gives them experience and a background for dealing with actual conference situations. In addition, a simulation game is incorporated at three points in the course. (This simulation is included in the chapter on roleplay and simulation.) For this component, they assume the identity of a supervisor who has accepted a new supervisory position. The participants select two of three settings in which this person is employed: a university training program, a public school system, and/or a hospital/rehabilitation facility. They then deal with the issues confronted by this supervisor on the job. They first respond in writing as individuals and then bring the completed work to class for group discussion. By the end of the course, they have a working understanding of the supervisory process. An ideal follow-up to a beginning course such as this is a practicum in supervision. A second didactic course delving extensively into the literature would also be beneficial.

McCrea (1994) also offers supervisory training at the level of the master's degree. The introductory course in supervision emphasizes the literature in supervision, the Anderson model of supervision, data collection, conference variables, and the observation and analysis of supervisory conferences. A second component in the training is a second semester of participation in teaching clinics (Dowling, 1992). The latter focuses on participant supervisory behavior. McCrea feels involvement in the teaching clinics allows students to practice what they have learned in the didactic course.

Practicum

A practicum experience in supervision is recommended by Anderson (1981) and the ASHA Committee on Supervision (1989). It assists individuals in translating theory learned in a workshop or classroom to implementation. Green, Knippen, and Vincelette (1985) indicate these experiences increase the participants' confidence in applying these new skills in other environments. Under optimum conditions, a trained supervisor serves as the enrollee's mentor. The supervisor-in-training is actively supervising a supervisee while receiving feedback from a trained supervisor. Active efforts to implement an effective supervisory style and then collecting data and analyzing the outcomes are the basis of this process. This experience may be completed in either a training or work environment as a trained supervisor is able to provide feedback in either of these settings. As described earlier, Anderson (1981) implements such an approach in doctoral training and Brasseur (1989) describes its use in a public school setting.

Advanced

Doctoral level training in the supervisory process is also an excellent alternative. The components as described by Anderson (1981) earlier in this chapter constitute an outstanding program for the person interested in studying the process in depth. Anderson feels doctoral level training is best thought of as having a two-pronged purpose: "(a) to prepare personnel who can teach other supervisors, and (b) to prepare researchers in the supervisory process" (Anderson, 1988, p. 236). Clearly, a doctoral degree is not necessary to provide quality supervision. But it does provide additional credibility and may open doors typically unavailable to the master's level supervisor. In particular, opportunities for tenure-track appointments at universities increase. In addition, as stated by Anderson (1988), persons who opt for doctoral training will be in a position to make significant contributions to the body of knowledge in supervision through research. This is true because critical research skills pertaining to design and statistical analysis are developed during this advanced training.

Research-Directed Development

Involvement in supervisory research is another potent strategy for ongoing professional development. This is true for the master's level supervisor as well as the those with advanced training. It is beneficial in at least four ways. First, as concepts are assessed through a review of literature, a hypothesis and research design is developed, and the resulting data is collected and analyzed, new ideas emerge. Supervision practice is refined as novel information is gained. Second, research is stimulating and increases one's desire to know. Third, it opens the door for presentations and publication. Fourth, it increases the perceived status of supervisors.

Persons with doctoral level training will have a substantial background in experimental design and statistical analysis. With an extensive exposure to the supervision literature, they are well prepared to begin their own investigations. It is important to note that doctoral level training is not a prerequisite for quality research, although such a background facilitates the process. Others, with less training in statistics and/or supervision, may benefit from an alliance with an established researcher. Ideally, the more experienced serves as a mentor assisting the novice in the design, analysis, and interpretation of studies. The mentor removes barriers that might prove insurmountable for the beginning researcher. Without this assistance, excellent questions may fail to be answered even though extensive effort is expended.

Research may also begin on a smaller scale, particularly for the person with limited or no background in statistics and research design. The posing and answering of questions relating to personal growth are good strategies with which to begin. An informal single-subject design with a supervisors as their own subject is useful when examining one's own behavior. The findings, when applied, will enhance the quality of supervision provided on a daily basis. As a result of several of these experiences, supervisors may then wish to expand their endeavors by becoming involved in more formal, rigorously designed research. The point being that experiments for personal growth are worthwhile and an excellent place to start.

Involvement in research has the potential to impact the status of supervisors in the workplace. The issue of perceived status is an important consideration. Major concerns cited by supervisors, particularly in university environments, are low status, low salaries, and lack of job security. This is documented in the American Speech-Language Hearing Association Supervision Committee statement (ASHA, 1978). Further, Dowling (1989) indicates recognition and involvement in research are inextricably entwined:

For supervisors to have status and to be perceived as having equal status in an academic environment in the eyes of administrators and those who primarily teach and do research, the supervisor must also engage in scholarly activity (p. 338).

These statements are true even though job descriptions may not include or reward scholarly efforts. Long-term, to impact status, job security, and salary, supervisors must demonstrate the ability to function as equals in valued behaviors; that is, in giving presentations, contributing to and producing publishable work. Research provides the key to these opportunities.

Relevance of the Thirteen Tasks of Supervision to Supervisor Professional Growth

The tasks define the components of effective supervision. Professional growth that enhances supervisors' abilities to implement these tasks will, therefore, improve the quality of supervision provided. As supervisors develop, they will become increasingly able to establish and maintain effective working relationships with supervisees. An awareness of a continuum of supervision will assist supervisors in selecting a facilitative style to assist supervisees in developing clinical goals and developing and refining clinical assessment and management skills. Incremental uses of data collection and analysis will assist supervisors in guiding supervisees as they learn to (1) observe and analyze therapy sessions, (2) evaluate clinical performance, (3) maintain clinical and supervisory records, and (4) become progressively involved in the supervisory conference. These same abilities will also allow supervisors to demonstrate basic research strategies in both the clinical and supervisory process. Skillful implementation of a clinical supervision (Cogan, 1973), cognitive coaching (Costa and Garmston, 1994), or the Anderson (1988) continuum of supervision model in conjunction with growth in the interpersonal domain, will enhance supervisors' proficiencies in interacting with clinicians in a helpful manner. This will be particularly true in regard to (1) demonstrating for the supervisee, (2) guiding them as they learn report writing and editing skills, (3) assisting clinicians in refining clinical management and assessment skills, (4) sharing information regarding ethical, legal, regulatory, and reimbursement information, and (5) modeling professional conduct. In summary, each of the thirteen tasks and the underlying competencies may be realized more fully when the supervisor is involved in ongoing professional development.

Summary

This chapter begins with a review of the ASHA adopted tasks of supervision (ASHA, 1985) relevant to the professional development of the supervisor. The related literature from a variety of fields is presented. The status of supervision in practice is described. This is followed by a discussion of potential growth opportunities and examples of career ladders for supervisors. Alternatives for ongoing development of the supervisor are discussed. These include reading, reflecting, data-collecting, modifying, goal-setting, feedback gathering, collaborating, taping, networking, and meeting with others. The topic of formal supervisory training is then considered. It may include continuing education workshops, coursework, or practicums, and may vary widely from one supervisor to another. The final strategy for supervisor growth is involvement in research and other scholarly activities. This chapter highlights the skills relating to the thirteen tasks of supervision that supervisors acquire through training.

REFERENCES

American Speech and Hearing Association, Committee on Supervision in Speech-Language Pathology and Audiology. "Current status of supervision of speech-language pathology and audiology." *American Speech Hearing Association, 20* (1978): 478–486.

American Speech-Language-Hearing Association, Committee on Supervision in Speech-Language Pathology and Audiology. "Clinical supervision in speech-language pathology and audiology. A position statement." *American Speech Hearing Association, 27* (1985): 57–60.

American Speech-Language-Hearing Association, Committee on Supervision in Speech-Language Pathology and Audiology. "Preparation models for the supervisory process in speech-language pathology and audiology." *American Speech Hearing Association, 31* (1989): 97–106.

American Speech-Language-Hearing Association. "Standards for accreditation of graduate education programs in audiology and speech-language pathology." Rockville, Md.: American Speech-Language-Hearing Association, 1999: 1–7.

Anderson, J. "Status of supervision in speech, hearing and language programs in the schools." *Language, Speech and Hearing Services in Schools, 3* (1972): 12–23.

Anderson, J. "Training of supervisors in speech-language pathology." *American Speech Hearing Association, 23* (1981): 79–82.

Anderson, J. *The Supervisory Process in Speech-Language Pathology and Audiology.* Austin, TX: Pro-Ed, 1988.

Barrow, M., and Domingo, R. "The effectiveness of training clinical supervisors in conducting the supervisory conference." *The Clinical Supervisor, 16* (1) (1997): 55–77.

Blair, K., and Peake, T. "Stages of Supervisor Development." *The Clinical Supervisor, 13* (2) (1995): 119–126.

Brasseur, J. "The supervisory process: A continuum perspective." *Language, Speech, and Hearing Services in the Schools, 20* (1989): 274–295.

Brasseur, J., and Anderson, J. "Observed differences between direct, indirect and direct/indirect videotaped supervisory conferences." *Journal of Speech and Hearing Research, 26* (1983): 345–356.

Caracciolo, G., Rigrodsky, S., and Morrison, E. "Perceived interpersonal conditions and professional growth of master's level speech-language pathology students during the supervisory process." *American Speech Hearing Association, 20* (1978): 467–477.

Casey, P. "Casey's supervisory skills self-assessment instrument." In P. Casey, K. Smith, and S. Ulrich, (Eds.), *Self-Supervision: A Career Tool for Audiologists and Speech-Language Pathologists.* Clinical Series No. 10. Rockville Pike, MD: National Student Speech Language Hearing Association, (1988): 95–111.

Cogan, M. *Clinical Supervision.* Boston, MA: Houghton-Mifflin, 1973.

Costa, A. and Garmston, R. *Cognitive Coaching: A Foundation for Renaissance Schools.* Norwood, MA: Christopher Gordon Publishers, 1994.

Crago, M., and Pickering, M. *Supervision in Human Communication Disorders: Perspectives on a Process,* San Diego, CA: Singular Publishing Group, 1987.

Culatta, R., and Seltzer, H. "Content and sequence analyses of the supervisory session." *American Speech Hearing Association, 18* (1976): 8–12.

Curtis, M., and Zins, J. "Effects of training in consultation and instructor feedback on acquisition of consultation skills." *Journal of School Psychology, 26* (1988): 185–190.

Department of Speech and Hearing Sciences, Clinical faculty. Indiana University, Bloomington, Indiana. In-house document, 1989.

DeShon, R., and Alexander, R. "Goal setting effects on implicit and explicit learning of complex tasks." *Organizational Behavior and Human Decision Processes, 65* (1) (1996): 18–36.

Dowling, S. "Supervisory training: Impetus for clinical supervision." *Clinical Supervisor, 4* (4) (1986): 27–34.

Dowling, S. "Research: Past, present, future." In S. Farmer and J. Farmer, (Eds.), *Supervision in Communication Disorders.* Columbus, OH: Merrill Publishing, 1989: 314–340.

Dowling, S. *Implementing the supervisory process: Theory and Practice.* Englewood Cliffs, NJ: Prentice-Hall, 1992.

Dowling, S. "Supervisory training, objective setting and grade contingent performance." *Language, Speech, and Hearing Services in Schools, 24* (1993): 92–99.

Dowling, S. "Supervisory training: Comparison of grade contingent/non-contingent objective setting." In M. Bruce, (Ed.), *Proceedings: International and Interdisciplinary Conference on Clinical Supervision: Toward the 21st Century.* Burlington, VT: University of Vermont, 1994: 180–183.

Dowling, S. "Facilitating clinical training: Issues for supervisees and their supervisors." *Contemporary Issues in Communication Science and Disorders 25,* (1998): 5–11.

Dowling, S. Conference Analysis. Working document. University of Houston, 2000.

Farmer, S., and Farmer, J. *Supervision in Communication Disorders.* Columbus, OH: Merrill Publishing, 1989.

Gavett, E. "Career development: An issue for the master's degree supervisor." In M. Crago and M. Pickering, (Eds.), *Supervision in Human Communication Disorders: Perspectives on a process.* San Diego, CA: Singular Publishing Group, 1987: 55–78.

Glaser, A., and Donnelly, C. "The development of a competency based assessment for supervisors." In M. Bruce, (Ed.), *Proceedings of the 1994 International and Interdisciplinary Conference on Clinical Supervision: Toward the 21st Century.* Burlington, VT: University of Vermont, 1994: 173–179.

Goldberg, B. "The transformation age: The sky's the limit." *American Speech Hearing Association, 37* (1995): 44–50.

Green, T., Knippen, J., and Vincelette, J. "The practice of management: Knowledge versus skills." *Training and Development Journal, 39* (7) (1985): 56–58.

Hagler, P. *Effects of Verbal Directives, Data, and Contingent Social Praise on Amount of Supervisor Talk during Speech-Language Pathology Supervision Conferencing.* Doctoral Dissertation, Indiana University, Bloomington, IN, 1986.

Hagler, P., and McFarlane, L. "A field tested model for supervision of support personnel." Short Course presented at the Annual Convention of the American Speech-Language and Hearing Association, November, 1998.

Harris, H., Ludington, J., Ringwalt, S., Ballard, D., Hooper, C., Buoyer, F., and Price, K. "Involving the student in the supervisory process." *National Student Speech Language Hearing Association Journal, 19* (1991–1992): 109–118.

Heid, L. "Supervisor development across the professional lifespan." *The Clinical Supervisor, 16* (2), (1997): 139–152.

Jensen, J., Parsons, M., and Reid, D. "Supervisory training for teachers: Multiple, long-term effects in an education program for adults with severe disabilities." *Research in Developmental Disabilities, 19* (6) (1998): 449–463.

Kamhi, A. "Research to practice: Defining, developing and maintaining clinical expertise." *Language, Speech and Hearing Services in Schools, 26* (4) (1995): 353–356.

Killion, J., and Harrison, C. "Clinical supervision: Comprehensive training for success." *Journal of Staff Development, 6* (2) (1985): 96–101.

Lafferty, J., and Colletti, L. "Making it in management." *Training and Development Journal, 39* (2) (1985): 86–89.

Manatt, R., and Benway, M. "Teacher and administrator performance evaluation: Benefits of 360-degree feedback." *ERS Spectrum* (1998): 18–23.

Marx, R. "Improving management development through relapse prevention strategies." *Journal of Management Development, 5* (2) (1986): 27–40.

McCrea, E. "Supervision component in undergraduate clinical management class." In K. Smith (Moderator), "Preparation and training models for the supervisory process." Short course presented at the Annual Convention of the American Speech-Language Hearing Association, Washington, DC, 1985.

McCrea, E., Jones-McNamara, S., and Ringwalt, S. "Career ladders for supervisors: The process of promotion and reappointment." Paper presented at the Annual Meeting of the Council of Supervisors in Speech Pathology and Audiology (CSSPA), St.Louis, MO, 1989.

McCrea, E. "Supervision as a master's degree thesis option." In M. Bruce, (Ed.), *Proceedings of the 1994 International and Interdisciplinary Conference on Clinical Supervision: Toward the 21st Century.* Burlington, VT: University of Vermont, 1994: 221–229.

McCready, V. Personal communication, 1999.

Phillips, J. "Training supervisors outside the classroom." *Training and Development Journal, 40*(2) (1986): 46–49.

Rassi, J. *Supervision in Audiology.* Baltimore, MD: University Park Press, 1978.

Rassi, J., and McElroy, M. *The Education of Audiologists and Speech-Language Pathologists.* Timonium, MD: York Press, 1992.

Ringwalt, S. "Reappointment and promotion in a clinical (fixed-term) track: Policies and procedures at one university." *Supervision, 13* (4) (1989–1990): 6–9.

Shapiro, D. "Interactional analysis and self-study: A single-case comparison of four methods of analyzing supervisory conferences." *Language, Speech and Hearing Services in Schools, 25* (2) (1994): 67–75.

Shapiro, D. "Professional preparation and lifelong learning: The making of a clinician." In D. Shapiro, (Ed.), *Stuttering Intervention: A Collaborative Journey to Fluency Freedom.* Austin, Tx: Pro-Ed, 1998.

Shapiro, D., and Moses, N. "Creative problem solving in public school supervision." *Language, Speech, and Hearing Services in the Schools 20,* (1989): 320–332.

Smith, K., and Anderson, J. "Development and validation of an individual supervisory conference rating scale for use in speech-language pathology." *Journal of Speech and Hearing Research, 25* (1982): 243–251.

Stevens, D., Goodyear, R., and Robertson, P. "Supervisor development: An exploratory study in changes in stance and emphasis." *The Clinical Supervisor, 16* (2) (1997): 73–88.

Stoltenberg, C., McNeill, B., Delworth, U. *IDM Supervision: An Integrated Developmental Model for Supervising Counselors and Therapists.* San Francisco: Jossey-Bass, 1998.

Strike-Roussos, C. *Supervisors' Implementation of Trained Information Regarding Broad Questioning and Discussion of Supervision during their Supervisory Conferences in Speech-Language Pathology.* Doctoral Dissertation, Indiana University, Bloomington, IN, 1988.

VanDemark, A., Borton, T., Dowling, S., Nelson, G., Rassi, J., Ulrich, S., and Vallon, J. "Qualifications for supervisors: A proposal for discussion." Annual Convention of the American Speech, Language and Hearing Association, Detroit, MI, 1980.

Watkins, C. "Development of the psychotherapy supervisor." *Psychotherapy, 27* (1990): 202–209.

Watkins, C. "Researching psychotherapy supervisor development: Four key considerations." *The Clinical Supervisor, 13* (2) (1995): 111–118.

APPENDIX 9-A

Promotion Criteria for Supervisors and Clinical Staff

I. **Introduction**

A. Mission of the Department

The instructional mission of the Department of Speech and Hearing Sciences is the provision of comprehensive educational programs leading to the A.B. degree in speech and hearing sciences, and M.A. and Ph.D. degrees in the clinical fields of speech-language pathology and audiology. Training clinical professionals requires a setting combining a broad range of academic coursework with the opportunities to apply academic training to clinical processes. Thus, this Department must provide two types of training, academic and clinical. The mission of the department is carried out by tenure-track academic faculty who are primarily responsible for academic instruction, and clinical faculty, who provide supervised clinical training and teach clinical methods courses.

B. Definition of Clinical Faculty

1. Responsibilities

Clinical faculty have the dual responsibility of ensuring appropriate service to clients and providing the crucial link between students' academic learning and the clinical application of that learning. They must be excellent clinicians themselves and also be able to facilitate the development of clinical skills in students. Clinical teaching includes demonstration or modeling of clinical procedures, on-going observation of clinical work, conferencing and consultation with students, evaluation of students' clinical performance, and assignment of grades. Throughout this process, clinical faculty provide whatever guidance and instruction necessary to assist student clinicians in applying academic training to the delivery of clinical services.

2. Expectations

Clinical training requires that clinical faculty: a) supervise all phases of clinical services provided by student clinicians; b) integrate current research related to valid and reliable techniques of assessment and treatment into the services provided in the teaching clinic; c) participate in classroom teaching where appropriate; and d) participate in research projects (optional), especially those requiring a clinical component.

II. **Clinical Faculty Ranks [Note: The criteria for each rank include those listed for lower ranks.]**

A. Clinical Lecturer

1. The rank for clinical faculty with a Master's degree in speech-language pathology or audiology who:

a. Hold a Certificate of Clinical Competence from the American Speech-Language Hearing Association.

Department of Speech and Hearing Sciences, Clinical faculty. Indiana University, Bloomington, Indiana. In-house document, (1989). Reprinted with permission.

        b. Are eligible for licensure as a speech pathologist or audiologist.

        c. Have at least three years of experience in the provision of clinical services.

        d. Have at least one year of supervisory experience.

B. Clinical Assistant Professor

    1. The rank for clinical faculty with at least four years of clinical experience and who:

        a. Have at least one year of supervisory experience in a teaching clinic.

        b. Have superior skill and knowledge in the area of their clinical specialty (i.e. disorder area, special population), as determined through reviews conducted by an evaluation committee appointed by the chair of the department, as discussed in the final section of this document.

C. Clinical Associate Professor

    1. The rank for clinical faculty who have excelled in the performance of their clinical specialty as indicated in periodic evaluations (final section) and who:

        a. Participate in classroom teaching by serving as the instructor of record for clinical courses or teaching clinical-procedures sections of academic courses.

        b. Participate in applied research (optional) in collaboration with academic or clinical faculty members

        c. Serve on departmental committees, represent the Department to governmental agencies, work with philanthropic support groups and other extra-University organizations.

        d. Contribute to the vigor of the Department and the profession by conducting clinical training workshops at regional and national meetings and through other continuing education activities.

D. Clinical Professor

    1. The rank for clinical faculty whose performance as clinical teachers and clinicians has been superior, as indicated in periodic evaluations (final section), whose professional development, research or creative activity (optional), or service has resulted in a significant contribution to the assessment or treatment of communication disorders or to clinical education at the national, state, or regional level, and who:

        a. Demonstrate leadership in service: chair committees, obtain extramural funding, conduct public relations activities, work with state and local organizations in a leadership role.

        b. Author peer-reviewed publications; conduct presentations, workshops, and continuing education activities.

        c. Provide model service to clients through demonstration of innovative clinical service or supervisory practice.

        d. Conduct clinical research (optional), develop clinical procedures, create areas of study, and generally advance the state of their area of specialization.

    2. Clinical Professors provide administrative service, plan course curricula, plan policy, develop extramural funding and participate in the peer review of their professional colleagues.

III. Evaluation

A. Components

Annual evaluations will be conducted by the department chairperson, with the assistance of the clinic directors and directors of relevant specialty areas within the department. Components of the evaluation will include teaching, clinical practice, service, and, where appropriate, clinical research (optional), and will reflect the candidate's primary responsibility as an academic and clinical teacher. The candidate must normally excel in one of the above categories and be satisfactory in the others.

B. Procedure

Departmental Evaluations for promotions will follow the same basic procedures as those for academic faculty, and will be conducted by a committee made up of all faculty currently holding ranks above the level of the person being evaluated. (No distinction between clinical and academic faculty is made for this purpose.) Dossiers will be prepared in the normal manner, and will include evidence of contributions in the usual three areas. As in the case of annual evaluations, the weights given teaching, clinical practice, service and research (optional) will reflect the clinical faculty member's primary responsibility for clinical teaching and clinical practice. For promotion to Clinical Associate Professor or Clinical Professor, external evaluations of the candidate's contributions to the field, as a teacher, a clinical instructor, a master clinician, or in clinical research (optional) will be solicited both from peers (senior professionals with similar responsibilities in major teaching clinics) and from former students. A portion of these external evaluations will be solicited from individuals identified by the candidate, the remainder will be from individuals selected by the personnel committee.

C. Guidelines: Contents of sections of dossier.
1. Teaching section shall contain evidence of:
    a. supervisory evaluations for each semester or summer session
    b. innovative supervisory practices
    c. departmental lectures or other presentations; "grand rounds"
    d. continuing education lectures
    e. teaching evaluations
    f. supervisory caseload.
2. Clinical-practice section shall contain evidence of:
    a. demonstration therapy
    b. model sessions
    c. external clinical service delivery
    d. private caseload, especially in conjunction with research activity
    e. development of special diagnostic or treatment procedures.
3. Research/Scholarship section (optional) shall contain evidence of:
    a. presentations-peer reviewed; other
    b. extramural funding
    c. grant applications
    d. publications-peer reviewed; other
    e. books as author, editor, contributor
    f. case review publications
    g. technical reports.
4. Service section shall contain evidence of:
    a. work on departmental committees as chair, or member
    b. work on university committees
    c. advising
    d. work with professional organizations: national, regional, local
    e. outreach.

APPENDIX 9-B

Conference Analysis (Dowling, 2000)

Procedure:

Complete in the Following Order

1. Listen to the conference. Then assess the content by completing a Brasseur (Brasseur and Anderson, 1983) Individual Conference Rating Scale.
2. Rewind and let the tape run for two minutes. Then, code the remaining portion using the Culatta and Seltzer (1976) Content and Sequence Analyses of the Supervisory Session observation system.
3. Rewind the tape and collect talk time data for the supervisor and supervises. A tally should be made for each sentence uttered. Count fillers separately.

Supervisor Utterances   *Supervisee Utterances*

Fillers   *Fillers*

4. Rewind the tape and collect data in regard to questions and responses. Count the number of questions asked by the supervisor/supervisee. For each speaker, separate the questions by open/closed and responses by elaborated/simple.

Supervisor   *Supervisee*
Questions   Questions
   Open   Closed   Open   Closed

Responses   Responses
Simple   Elaborated   Simple   Elaborated

5. Rewind the tape and collect data in regard to problem-solving. Was problem-solving occurring? If so, how much and who was doing it?

Supervisor   *Supervisee*
Count

6. Rewind the tape and collect data in regard to strategy development. Was strategy development occurring? If so, how much and who was doing it?

Supervisor   *Supervisee*
Count

ANSWER the following questions in regard to the conference. Base these on your perceptions as a result of listening to the conference.

1. Had data been collected? If so, was it client or clinician oriented?

2. Was there an agenda for the conference? If so, who had planned it?

3. Was the supervisor an active listener in the conference? If so, give examples of the types of things said that made you perceive active listening.

4. What was the interpersonal climate of the conference?

   a. Was a superior/subordinate relationship evident?

   b. Did the clinician appear to comfortable in the relationship?

   c. Using McCrea's (1980) Adapted Scales for Assessment of Interpersonal Functioning in Speech-Language Pathology Supervision Conferences categories as a guide, how would you rate this conference in the following areas?

   Concreteness   Facilitative Genuineness

   Respect   Empathic Understanding

Based on your analysis of the conference, LIST your perceptions of your conference strengths and the areas in which you perceive a need for growth.

Strengths   *Areas for Growth*

A P P E N D I X   9 - C

Student Evaluation of Practicum Supervisor Communication Disorders

Below are listed 13 competencies defined by ASHA's Committee on Supervision. Under each competency is listed one, two or three behaviors of supervisors that demonstrate the competency. Please rate your supervisor on each of these behaviors using the following rating scale: *1 2 3 4 5 NA*. Five (5) indicates the HIGHEST rating; one (1) indicates the LOWEST rating. If an item is not appropriate, circle *NA* (not applicable.)

Name of Supervisor _____   **Date** _____

1. Establishing and maintaining an effective working relationship with the supervisees.

   a. Defines the role of the supervisor and supervisee in the supervisory process
       LOW   HIGH
       1 2 3 4 5 NA

   b. Relates effectively with the supervisee and establishes a supportive working relationship
       LOW   HIGH
       1 2 3 4 5 NA

2. Assisting the supervisee in developing clinical goals and objectives

   a. Assists the supervisee in planning effective client goals and objectives
       LOW   HIGH
       1 2 3 4 5 NA

   b. Assists the supervisee in assigning priority to clinical goals and objectives
       LOW   HIGH
       1 2 3 4 5 NA

3. Assisting the supervisee in developing and refining assessment skills.

   a. Assists the supervisee in developing a rationale for selection and use of appropriate assessment procedures
       LOW   HIGH
       1 2 3 4 5 NA

   b. Assists the supervisee in developing a rationale for integrating assessment findings to make appropriate recommendations
       LOW   HIGH
       1 2 3 4 5 NA

4. Assisting the supervisee in developing and refining management skills

   a. Assists the supervisee in providing rationale for treatment procedures
       LOW   HIGH
       1 2 3 4 5 NA

   b. Assists the supervisee in identifying, adjusting, and evaluating appropriate sequence for client change
       LOW   HIGH
       1 2 3 4 5 NA

   c. Assists the supervisee in describing and measuring client's change
       LOW   HIGH
       1 2 3 4 5 NA

Glaser, A., and Donnelly, C. "The development of a competency based assessment for supervisors." In M. Bruce, (Ed.), *Proceedings of the 1994 International and Interdisciplinary Conference on Clinical Supervision: Toward the 21st Century.* Burlington, VT: University of Vermont, (1994): 173-179. Reprinted with permission.

5. Demonstrating for and participating with the supervisee in the clinical process

    a. Demonstrates or participates jointly in a variety of clinical techniques

        LOW   HIGH
        1 2 3 4 5 NA

    b. Demonstrates or participates jointly in counseling clients and families

        LOW   HIGH
        1 2 3 4 5 NA

6. Assisting the supervisee in observing and analyzing assessment and treatment sessions

    Assists the supervisee in collecting, analyzing, and interpreting data

        LOW   HIGH
        1 2 3 4 5 NA

7. Assisting the supervisee in development and maintenance of clinical and supervisory records

    Assists the supervisee in effectively documenting client progress

        LOW   HIGH
        1 2 3 4 5 NA

8. Interacting with the supervisee in planning, executing, and analyzing supervisory conferences

    a. Holds frequent conferences with supervisee

        LOW   HIGH
        1 2 3 4 5 NA

    b. Provides frequent oral/written feedback to supervisee regardingclinical performance

        LOW   HIGH
        1 2 3 4 5 NA

    c. Assists the supervisee in description and measurement of his/her clinical performance

        LOW   HIGH
        1 2 3 4 5 NA

9. Assisting the supervisee in evaluation of clinical performance

    a. Assists the supervisee in developing skills of self-evaluation

        LOW   HIGH
        1 2 3 4 5 NA

    b. Motivates the supervisee to make changes in clinical performance

        LOW   HIGH
        1 2 3 4 5 NA

10. Assisting the supervisee in developing skills of verbal reporting, writing and editing

    Assists the supervisee in professional reporting, both oral and written

        LOW   HIGH
        1 2 3 4 5 NA

11. Sharing information regarding ethical, legal, regulatory, and reimbursement aspects of the profession

    Communicates to the supervisee an understanding of rules and regulations pertaining to the profession

        LOW   HIGH
        1 2 3 4 5 NA

12. Modeling and facilitating professional conduct

    a. Supervisor models professional and ethical conduct at all times

        LOW   HIGH
        1 2 3 4 5 NA

    b. Supervisor demonstrates continued professional growth

        LOW   HIGH
        1 2 3 4 5 NA

13. Demonstrating research skills in the clinical or supervisory process

Supervisor demonstrates knowledge of current clinical and supervisor research	LOW HIGH 1 2 3 4 5 NA

PART FIVE

Training Vehicles

10 Teaching Clinic: A Vehicle for Clinical and Supervisory Growth

Clinical Supervision Tasks Relevant to Developing Clinical and Supervisory Skills through the Teaching Clinic Methodology

Task 1: Establishing and maintaining an effective working relationship with the supervisee;

Task 3: Assisting the supervisee in developing and refining assessment skills;

Task 4: Assisting the supervisee in developing and refining management skills;

Task 6: Assisting the supervisee in observing and analyzing assessment and treatment sessions;

Task 7: Assisting the supervisee in the development and maintenance of clinical and supervisory records;

Task 8: Interacting with the supervisee in planning, executing, and analyzing supervisory conferences;

Task 9: Assisting the supervisee in the evaluation of clinical performance;

Task 12: Modeling and facilitating professional conduct;

Task 13: Demonstrating research skills in the clinical or supervisory processes.

Literature

The goal of academic and clinical training in the helping professions is to develop qualified, self-supervising professionals. To achieve this end, accurate observation, analysis, and problem-solving abilities must be developed. These skills begin to evolve in preclinical and academic courses. They then emerge, in a more complete form, as a function of the supervisor/clinician interaction during practicum experiences. Both individual and group forms of supervision may be used to stimulate these skills. This chapter will focus on the group methodologies. A variety of group methods are currently in use. Examples from speech-language pathology, social work, psychology, and education will follow.

Speech-Language Pathology

Supervision in speech-language pathology in the United States is predominantly delivered through a traditional one-to-one supervisor–supervisee relationship. As documented by Seal and Runyan (1988), supervisors spend just 11 percent of their time in group conferences. In contrast, in Australia, group conferencing predominates, with supplemental individual conferences when needed. (McAllister and Lincoln, 1994).

Examples of group supervision are microsupervision (Irwin, 1972), case staffing (Farmer and Farmer, 1989), and peer learning (McAllister and Lincoln, 1994). Microsupervision (Irwin, 1972) is the earliest use of group form of supervision proposed for use in speech-language pathology. Case staffings, according to Farmer and Farmer (1989), are used to develop collegiality in the supervisory process. Supervisees meet as a group for clinic meetings in conjunction with clinical practicum. The presenters—the senior clinician, a clinical assistant, and the supervisor—provide a complete case history of the client, pertinent diagnostic information, semester goals for the patient and the clinician involved, a sample lesson plan, and a videotape or live presentation. Discussion follows. Ninety percent of the participants view this procedure as helpful in developing collegiality in the supervisory process. In addition, those in the role of presenter feel it fosters their professional growth. The third type—peer learning (McAllister and Lincoln, 1994)—is the focus of clinical learning for Australian speech-language pathology students. In that country, the majority of supervision is implemented through a group process. One example is that second- and final year students are paired and meet jointly with their supervisor. The second-year student serves as an apprentice and the final year, the more skilled of the pair, assumes a leadership role. This strategy facilitates peer learning.

Social Work

An array of group supervision methods are in use in social work. An example is the consultation circle. Issues that are thought to be appropriate for this method are "values clarification, case direction/action, roles and responsibilities, and exploring ethical dilemmas" (Kuechler and Barretta-Herman, 1998). Participants serve in three roles: facilitator, requestor, and consultant. The requestor asks for input in regard to a specific issue or problem. Each consultant writes down his or her best suggestion. The advice is presented in writing and verbally to the requestor, who then takes the input, acknowledges it, and uses the information to think about the problem and to decide what to do. The suggestions are not discussed or elaborated. The process requires everyone to participate, even those who are typically reticent. It fosters creative problem-solving by increasing the individual's range of options, teaches people how and when to ask for help, and enhances group interdependence (Kuechler and Barretta-Herman, 1998).

According to Chaiklin and Munson (1983), group supervision in the field of social work increases personal learning. It provides opportunities to monitor the ongoing accuracy of one's perceptions. Further, participant involvement necessitates a willingness to take a risk by letting others see what one does and does not know. It requires a desire to learn as well as trust in oneself and others. In addition, it is thought to foster the recognition of peers' knowledge and abilities. Tebb, Manning, and Klaumann (1996) note the use of peer groups allows members to increase their strengths and acknowledge their limitations. They find marginal students, through comparison of their skills with others and with the support of their peers, self-identify their weaknesses and at times opt to remove themselves from practicum. On a more positive note, Powell (1996) says peer group supervision is particularly valuable for working professionals in private or group practice as a vehicle for ongoing growth.

Tebb and colleagues (1996) note several strengths and limitations in the use of peer supervision. A sample of the strengths are that it (1) provides opportunities to teach creativity, (2) provides an arena for openly exchanging ideas, (3) permits students to consider their work in comparison to that of others and to identify areas of strength and weakness, (4) develops a frame of reference for practice and highlights the multiple approaches available in any given situation, and (5) encourages socialization among peers. A sample of the limitations are that it: (1) allows peers to avoid providing constructive feedback, (2) requires the supervisor to have considerable group leadership and comfort skills, and (3) demands significant supervisor skill in organization and planning.

Psychology

Similarly, group supervision methods are used in psychotherapy with students-in-training, in private practices, and in agencies (Cooper and Gustafson, 1985). The structures they describe are informal in nature. Case presentations or discussions of work-related issues serve as the focal point for the interchanges.

Group supervision in counseling psychology is aided by the use of a genogram strategy. The genogram is a drawing of a family in a manner that represents the client and all of the familial relationships at the same time. The family picture emerges from the clinician's case presentation and then serves as the basis for group discussion. The perceived benefits of this process are the structure for problem-solving and learning that emerges and an increase in the flexibility of counselor thought (Pistole, 1995).

Bernard and Goodyear (1998) present an extensive discussion of group supervision for training mental health professionals. They cite numerous advantages of a group approach:

1. economies of time, money and expertise;
2. minimized supervisee dependence;
3. opportunities for vicarious learning;
4. supervisee exposure to a broader range of clients;

5. feedback for the supervisee (greater quantity and diversity);
6. feedback for the supervisee (greater quality);
7. a more comprehensive picture of the supervisee;
8. facilitated risk-taking;
9. greater opportunity to use action techniques;
10. mirroring the supervisees' intervention.

Limitations of the use of groups are also noted:

1. the group format may not allow individuals to get what they need;
2. confidentiality concerns;
3. the group format is not isomorphic with that of individual counseling;
4. certain group phenomena can impede learning;
5. the group may focus too much time on issues not of particular relevance to or interest for the other group members (Bernard and Goodyear, 1998).

Group processes are recommended while alerting users to both the potential strengths and limitations of these approaches.

According to Crutchfield, Price, McGarity, Pennington, Richardson, and Tsolis (1997), the counseling skills of public school counselors are rarely supervised even though these professionals feel they would benefit from supervision. As part of a research project, five counselors from various schools meet once a week for an hour and a half. They each set three professional goals. At the beginning of each meeting they each share situations they have experienced that week. Then they listen to a ten- to fifteen-minute audiotape of a counseling session provided by one of the participants. Peers then provide feedback with each representing a different perspective depending on the role assigned before listening to the tape. Examples are from the viewpoint of a teacher, parent, or sibling. The participants all feel their counseling improves as a result of the process and they report feeling professionally energized by the group meetings (Crutchfield et al., 1997).

Education

Loiselle, St. Louis, and Dupey-Walker (1998) describe a group supervision process for preservice teachers. The participants, using a computer listserv, discuss their concerns about teaching with peers, cooperating teachers, and the university supervisor. They all contribute and provide feedback via computer and are pleased by the outcomes. Another similar, but nontechnology-based style of group supervision is suggested by Reiman and Thies-Sprinthall (1998) for beginning teachers. They feel it reduces the stress and feelings of isolation new teachers often experience.

Glickman (1985) suggests the use of informal peer groups for classroom teachers. He views the process of teachers turning to each other for professional growth as being highly productive. To increase participation though, he feels the meetings need to take place during the school day. He suggests using planning periods or having individuals relieved for a class period by substitutes or the supervisor. Anderson, Vail, Jones, and Huntington (1994), too, support the idea of peer coaching. They find that it increases the use of new strategies that are retained long-term. This school district, similar to the idea presented by Glickman (1985), fosters this endeavor by hiring paraprofessionals to assume nonteaching responsibilities such as monitoring the lunchroom and bus duty. This frees the teachers to observe each other.

Chrisco (1989) describes another peer group method. Again, the desire for professional growth draws teachers to a peer assistance strategy. The process, in this setting, typically consists of a preobservation meeting, the actual observation, and then a follow-up discussion. Teachers help each other on a one-to-one basis. According to Robbins (1991), as a result of peer coaching, the teachers

1. report a stronger sense of their professional skill and efficacy;
2. are better able to analyze their own teaching behavior;
3. have a better understanding of teaching and how students learn;
4. are better teachers as a result; and
5. feel stronger ties to colleagues (Robbins, 1991).

Further, Buttery and Michalak (1974) indicate teachers and administrators perceive group methods of supervision as valuable staff development tools. In particular, these educators feel it provides an opportunity to observe and learn from others. It also creates a positive milieu for discussing instructional problems. They also learn observational techniques and strategies for phrasing supportive yet objective comments to peers. In addition, group supervision gives them the occasion to experiment with personal goals, to identify and develop strengths, and a chance to obtain feedback. Finally, they value the process as a means to develop self-analysis and self-evaluation skills. Practicing school counselors, in general, find peer group supervision to be helpful (Crutchfield and Borders, 1997). Further, Ludlow, Wienke, Henderson, and Klein (1998) recommend group supervision for persons adding a new teaching endorsement to their credentials as a method for retooling teachers to teach in underserved areas.

Group supervision, as reported, is diverse in nature. Varying uses are seen within a professional field and across disciplines. These approaches are shown to benefit both beginning and experienced professionals.

New Directions

Three supervisors, Miranda Jones, Michael Sanders, and Chris Ramirez are meeting for lunch.

MIRANDA: Today has sure been a whirlwind. I had so many observations to do today, a committee meeting and four conferences with supervisees to squeeze in.

CHRIS: Me too. Whew!

> **MICHAEL:**   We need to come up with some way to make our supervision more efficient. I feel like I say so many of the same things to each of my clinicians. I sometimes feel like I am a tape recorder stuck on replay.
>
> **MIRANDA:**   So many of my clinicians are having trouble figuring out what works and what doesn't. Others are always right on. I've wondered about doing some type of group supervision so they could benefit from each others' viewpoints.
>
> **MICHAEL:**   I heard about a peer group form of supervision, the teaching clinic, at a workshop. That would give a us a structure to implement group supervision. I also liked the way people seemed to learn to problem-solve from participating in the teaching clinic.
>
> **MIRANDA:**   Maybe the teaching clinic would improve the quality of our supervision and take less of our time.
>
> **CHRIS:**   Let's let the students know we are going to implement group supervision next term so they have time to get used to the idea.
>
> **MIRANDA:**   That will give us time to find out more about the teaching clinic, too.
>
> *Michael nods in agreement.*

Teaching Clinic Method

A group supervision approach is a logical alternative to traditional supervision. As noted from the literature, group supervision may vary in form from an open discussion to structured methods such as the teaching clinic, the topic of this chapter. The approach originates from the work of Olsen, Barbour, and Michalak who designed it for use in teacher education (1971). Dowling and Michalak (1976) later adapted it for use in speech pathology.

The teaching clinic (Dowling, 1979, 1992) is a peer-group form of supervision in which one of the participants brings a videotape of his/her therapy to the meeting for discussion. The teaching clinic members assume the following roles: clinic leader, demonstration clinician, peer, and group monitor. The clinic leader is usually assumed by the supervisor but is adopted by others as they grow in comfort and skill. The clinic leader monitors and encourages the teaching clinic ground rules and guides participants to fulfill their designated responsibilities. This same person also stimulates discussion and interaction among the peers as the role is primarily one of facilitation. The demonstration clinician volunteers to bring a videotape of therapy to the teaching clinic for group observation and discussion. The peers are the demonstration clinician's colleagues. Everyone observes the therapy session presented, collects data during the observation, and discusses this information with the demonstration clinician. The participants also assist in the generation of strategies for future clinical intervention and suggest alternative approaches to reach a specified goal. The group monitor observes the group process, notes whether team members meet the responsibilities defined by their roles, and determines if the clinic ground rules are observed.

The teaching clinic itself consists of six sequential phases: (1) review of the previous teaching clinic, (2) planning, (3) observation, (4) data analysis and critique preparation, (5) problem-solving and strategy development, and (6) clinic review. Each will be discussed in greater detail in the material that follows.

Phases

Review of the Previous Teaching Clinic.   This phase maintains the continuity of supervision from one teaching clinic to the next. During this stage, the demonstration clinician from the previous clinic shares the outcomes of strategies implemented as a result of the last meeting. Following this brief discussion, the group monitor restates the clinic ground rules. If weaknesses in the group process were noted during the previous clinic, the difficulties are outlined and procedural modifications made to prevent their recurrence.

Planning Session.   The second phase of the teaching clinic is the planning session. The demonstration clinician presents the therapy objectives and plan to the team members. This presentation is intended to be informative. It is therefore *not* appropriate for team members to critique either the objectives or plan. The demonstration clinician may then request that specific types of information be collected during the observation of the therapy segment. For example, this person may request data about the implementation of the reinforcement schedule, use of closure, or the appropriateness of objectives.

After the demonstration clinician presents the therapy plan and objectives and requests feedback, the clinic leader outlines the type of information to be collected and may also suggest procedures for doing so. The leader then assigns data collection tasks. It is the responsibility of each peer to collect at least one type of data. This may take the form of response counting, use of a formal observation system, or informal data strategies. Data-gathering, in some form, is critical to the success of the teaching clinic.

Observation.   The observation session is the third phase of the teaching clinic. The team members, including the demonstration clinician, observe the videotaped session. The observation may be live but it then excludes the demonstration clinician from viewing the therapy segment. In addition, it increases the complexity of scheduling the group process.

The therapy segment to be observed should be approximately ten minutes in length. Such a portion focuses discussion as it limits the number and type of behaviors that occur and yet provides a representative view of therapy (Schubert and Laird, 1975). Observation in excess of fifteen minutes lengthens the teaching clinic unnecessarily while adding limited amounts of new information.

Data Analysis and Critique Preparation.   At the beginning of the data analysis and critique preparation session, the demonstration clinician leaves the group to analyze the observed therapy independently. Meanwhile, the peers tabulate and analyze the data collected during the observation session. Then the group problem-solves and determines a strategy for providing feedback to the demonstration clinician in the most supportive manner. The clinic leader guides this discussion to insure the material being prepared for the clinician is balanced, a combination of both positive and negative, and is pertinent to the supervisee's stated needs.

Problem-Solving and Strategy Development.   The fifth phase of the clinic is the problem-solving and strategy development session. The demonstration clinician returns and shares aspects of the completed self-analysis. Following this input and/or at appropriate points, peers interject their observations and suggestions. The purpose of this phase is to problem-solve and generate strategies for future clinical use. Thus, a variety of alternatives for reaching a specific goal may be considered. Throughout this segment, the clinic leader guides and facilitates interaction but does not monopolize it. Therefore, interaction among all group members is expected. Figure 10.1 illustrates how the interaction evolves.

Clinic Review.   The sixth and final phase of the teaching clinic is the clinic review. Accordingly, the group monitor assesses the effectiveness of the group's interaction. This is done by noting if all members have participated and if the ground rules were observed.

The focus of the teaching clinic is clinical behavior. It is based on observation, analysis, and problem-solving. The strategies or techniques proposed by peers and/or the clinic leader are advisory only. The teaching clinic is not intended to be coercive. Therefore, the person in the role of demonstrator may choose to implement or disregard suggestions.

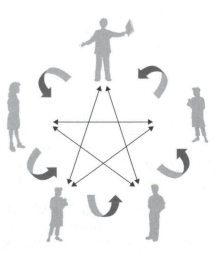

FIGURE 10.1   Communication during the Problem-Solving and Strategy Development Phase.

Ground Rules

For the teaching clinic to be optimally effective, four procedural ground rules are to be observed. The first is predominantly a housekeeping rule. It states that an agenda must be prepared by the demonstration clinician and given to each participant at least one day in advance of the teaching clinic. The agenda includes the data and starting time for the meeting, the location, the type of disorder exhibited by the client, and the objectives for the therapy that is to be viewed. The second rule states the analysis and discussion throughout the teaching clinic are directed to the clinical behavior of the demonstration clinician, not to that individual as a person. Rule three stipulates all observer comments must be supported by recorded data. The fourth is that all comments made during the teaching clinic remain in the room in which they were made.

Ground rules two, three, and four are critical and are intended to protect the demonstration clinician and the integrity of the process. The purpose of the teaching clinic is to analyze and improve clinical behavior. Discussions of a clinician's personality or idiosyncracies are not pertinent or appropriate unless these behaviors directly impact clinical performance. Further, only comments based on collected data may be made. Therefore, if the observer wants to state a technique is either effective or ineffective, this person must be able to demonstrate that the statement is true based on gathered information. In addition, confidentiality of the contents of teaching clinics lays the foundation for honest analysis, willingness to open one's clinical self to the scrutiny of others, and the building of trust among the group members. It also underlies group cohesiveness. These last three rules safeguard the process because personality directed and/or gut reactions and/or violations of privacy can be destructive to individuals and the group.

Training

Participants must be trained prior to use of the teaching clinic if it is to be used effectively. The trainer begins this process by presenting the philosophy and content of the method. The phases are discussed as are the events that occur within each. (The training material in Appendix A can be used as a tool and reference during both training and later teaching clinic implementation.)

The final component of this process is a teaching clinic simulation. The trainer provides an agenda and a videotape of therapy to be analyzed. Note that the first phase, the review of the previous clinic, does not occur during training. The trainer states that normally the clinic begins with feedback from the prior clinic but, because one has not occurred, a summary of what typically transpires will be substituted.

During the second phase, the planning session, the events that should occur are summarized. Then, in the persona of the demonstration clinician, the trainer presents the therapy plan and requests that certain types of information be collected. The trainer then guides the clinic leader as data collection tasks are assigned to peers.

The videotaped therapy is then shown in phase three, the observation. Immediately following, the trainer identifies the next stage, four, as the data analysis and critique preparation phase and outlines the content. At this time, it may also be helpful to reiterate the ground rules and note that the demonstration clinician typically leaves to complete a self-analysis at that time. The trainer then fades into the background leaving the clinic leader to guide the discussion. If the ground rules are being violated or if members fail to assume appropriate responsibilities, the trainer may interject and request compliance by calling this to the clinic leader's attention.

At the beginning of phase five, problem-solving and strategy development, the trainer restates the intended content of this segment. The trainer then assumes the role of the demonstration clinician viewed on the videotape. This is done so that the analysis, discussion, and generation of potential strategies can occur. If feedback is lopsided during this phase, the demonstration clinician may interject a comment to guide participants into a more balanced discussion.

The final component, phase six, of the simulated teaching clinic is the clinic review. The trainer assists the group monitor in assessing the effectiveness of the group process. The last step is to select a demonstration clinician for the first real teaching clinic. When this is completed, formal training ends.

To insure effective implementation, it is best if the trainer observes the group's first actual teaching clinic. The purpose is to answer questions that arise and to insure the members understand and use the method optimally. Following this, the trainer may continue, as needed, as a resource person for groups implementing the procedure.

Rationale for Training Components

As individuals are trained to participate in the teaching clinic process, it is suggested that the trainer role-play the demonstration clinician. The reason is that the teaching clinic is designed to build clinical self-development and/or supervisory skills through observation, analysis, and problem-solving. It is best to teach the technique in an emotionally neutral environment. The therapy or supervision viewed and analyzed in the training session is then not colored by anxiety or emotion because it is not the product of any of the participants. Therefore, they can focus on learning the process without psychological interference.

The trainer assuming the persona of the demonstration person also makes a valuable contribution during the problem-solving and strategy development phase. Participants often perceive feedback as telling someone what is wrong. They tend to focus on the negative, overlooking the positive. If this is occurring, the trainer, as demonstration person, can specifically request positive feedback. Similarly, some groups will whitewash performance, ignoring areas needing modification. Constructive feedback should be data-based and have positive as well as negative components. The trainer needs to be sure that this occurs during the training session. Having the instructor assume the demonstration role makes this easy to accomplish.

Facilitation

The optimum number of participants (Olsen, Barbour, Michalak 1971) for a teaching clinic is seven. It is thought effectiveness is impaired when three or fewer individuals participate or when the number involved exceeds seven. When there are less than four peer observers, a group monitor, demonstration clinician, and clinic leader, the diversity of viewpoints within the group tends to be reduced. This may lead to limited problem-solving and strategy development. In contrast, a large group can become unwieldy due to the number of individuals gathering data and sharing ideas. Of interest, Buttery and Weller (1988) routinely use groups consisting of five members, four peers and a clinic leader. Shapiro (1990) reports effective usage with a group of four peers and a supervisor as well. Mawdsley (1990) uses the teaching with as few as three persons. Williams (1995) includes from three to ten peers plus a supervisor when implementing a modified teaching clinic. Thus, there appears to be some room for variability in the number of members participating in a particular clinic.

A teaching clinic consisting of all six phases should last 60 to 75 minutes. The data analysis and critique preparation segment must be monitored and curtailed if the clinic is lasting longer than this. During this phase, the demonstration person leaves the room for the purpose of self-analysis. The discussion, in the group that remains, can become theoretical, tangential, or overly specific. It is important that these members remain on-task because it is unnerving for the demonstration person to be left to self-analyze for an extended period of time.

During training or at the outset of the first actual clinic, it is helpful to alert the clinic leader to a strategy for increasing participant interchange. Often the designation of a person as clinic leader causes members to direct comments to this individual rather than to other members. Recall the intent during the data analysis and critique preparation and the problem-solving and strategy development phases is to have an exchange similar to that reflected in Figure 10.1. If the clinic leader perceives comments are being inappropriately aimed at her/him, this may be discouraged by actively avoiding eye contact with the speaker. Typically, this will redirect the comments to other group members.

Participation in the teaching clinic and in the role of demonstration person is best when it is voluntary. When individuals volunteer, it shows a willingness to share their professional selves and their clinical performance with group members. Until individuals are psychologically ready to reveal this aspect of themselves, they should not be coerced to do so. Nonetheless, a decision to become involved in the process also indicates a readiness, at some point, to serve in the demonstration role.

Value

The teaching clinic requires participants to observe therapy, collect and analyze data, and generate clinical strategies. It provides the tools and then trains participants to critically examine clinical behavior. Cause and effect become a prime consideration. The use of videotaped therapy is also an advantageous component of the process. The participants view the therapy sample and then direct their discussion to the observed behavior. Because they share a common frame of reference, there is little need to describe events that have occurred in therapy. As a result, the focus of the discussions shifts appropriately from the recounting of events to the analysis of behavior.

The participants benefit from the role of peer as well as that of demonstration person. They learn to analyze their own work through the consideration of others' behaviors. It also provides the opportunity for peers to increase their knowledge beyond the scope of their own direct involvement.

Applicability

The teaching clinic potentially has a wide range of applicability, ranging from the beginning clinician to those who are employed. On one end of the continuum, it may by used with students in the pre-clinical phase of their training. Teaching clinics with an array of client types exposes them to a variety of disorders and gives them the opportunity to devise and contemplate clinical strategies. In addition, if these preclinical students know the value of data collection, problem-solving, and openly discussing clinical behavior, they can function with more flexibility and innovativeness at a later point in their career.

The teaching clinic may also be used with students during their clinical training. At this level, it may be used to guide students as they develop the observation, analytic, and problem-solving skills that form the foundation for professional growth. During training, the participants in the teaching clinics may be selected on the basis of client disorders, academic level, or willingness to participate. Homogeneous or heterogeneous groups may be used effectively. In addition, the focus of the exchange may be either diagnosis or treatment.

For student teachers, interns, and employed professionals, the teaching clinic is an ideal vehicle for ongoing growth. A factor often cited by these individuals is their isolation and subsequent lack of opportunities for professional development. By meeting in a central location and using the teaching clinic format, these persons may share and evolve strategies for challenging clients. This also allows them to continue to build their own clinical skills through data collection, problem-solving, and generation of potential strategies.

New Directions Revisited

Near the end of the next term, the three supervisors, Miranda, Chris, and Michael, are talking while they eat lunch.

> **MICHAEL:**   You know, I'm really glad we decided to implement group supervision using the teaching clinic. The clinicians have really grown professionally.
>
> **MIRANDA:**   Yeah. Their ability to sort out what works and seeing them come up with a plan for next time has been fun to watch.

CHRIS: They all tell me they have learned so much from each other. They said they had no idea how much help their peers could be.

MICHAEL: The exposure to a variety of clients has helped them, too. I think they learn as much from being a peer as being the demonstration clinician.

MIRANDA: I am concerned about one of my clinicians, Sandra. She has had trouble both as a peer and as demonstration clinician. She seems overwhelmed by the process. My sense is she needs to have individual conferences with me instead of participating in the group.

MICHAEL: Yeah. I have one clinician, too, who is not doing well in the group. He is really struggling in therapy. He probably isn't ready for group supervision.

CHRIS: You know, we required everyone to participate in group supervision this term. Maybe we ought to give them the choice. We could invite them to participate but let them pick the type of supervision they want.

MIRANDA: That's an idea. I think I'd like to use the teaching clinic next term but have at least a few individual conferences with each clinician as well. I really like the growth I see in their problem-solving when they are in the group. But I think some of my clinicians would like more time with me.

MICHAEL: Yeah. We still have to work the bugs out of this process and get the right balance. I'm going to ask my clinicians what they would pick—teaching clinic, individual, or a combination of both. You know, I've grown as a supervisor too from really analyzing and discussing therapy.

CHRIS: It has been stimulating. I am glad we implemented it. Good show guys!

Miranda, Michael, and Chris's discussion highlights successes when using the teaching clinic. They perceive that both they and the clinicians grew professionally from active participation. They also note issues that emerge from a group supervision process. Two key matters are the appropriate balance of group and individual supervision and participants' abilities to function successfully in a group. These and other topics will be discussed in the material that follows.

Teaching Clinic Adaptations

When the teaching clinic is first described in speech-language pathology (Dowling, 1976), it is being implemented with two matched groups of graduate students with clients exhibiting a similar disorder. It is reported to work well in this circumstance. But it is unknown, at that time, whether it will be equally effective with heterogeneous supervisees and/or clients. Subsequently, it is used in a variety of ways. Examples follow. Videotaped segments of both treatment and diagnosis are the focus of the clinic. Mixed peer groups, consisting of both undergraduates and graduates, implement teaching clinics. At other times, participants are exclusively graduate or undergraduate. The patients assigned to the group members are diverse, as compared to homogeneous, in the disorders they exhibit. It is even used with preclinical supervisees. Thus, the initial questions about the potential breadth of teaching clinic applicability are answered with its continued use.

The teaching clinic method is currently in use in the United State, Canada, and Australia. Alternate uses as well as modifications are being and have been made to meet individual needs (Dowling, Fey, Glaser, Shapiro, and Mawdsley, 1990; McCrea, 1994; Williams, 1995). Several examples follow.

Fey (1990) reports requiring supervisees in a training environment to bring two short segments of videotape to the clinic. One is reflective of something with which they were pleased, relating either to client or clinician behavior. The second piece is a portion of the session that did not go well or as planned. Fey indicates this guides supervisees in gaining a "balanced picture" of their skills and helps them identify both strengths and weaknesses. This idea parallels the one Crago (1987) suggests for individuals preparing for a traditional one-to-one supervisory conference.

In addition, Fey says, during summer terms, when enrollments are small, all students are involved in the teaching clinic. Thus, the number varies. In addition, two or three supervisors participate. She feels the concurrent immersion of the supervisors increases supervisory consistency. It also provides these persons with an opportunity to update their skills in areas in which they typically do not supervise.

Finally, Fey omits the data analysis and critique preparation session and the clinic review. In regard to the former, she states the data collection and analysis process regarding the observation focuses supervisees sufficiently to eliminate the need for the demonstration clinician to leave the group. In relation to the clinic review, she ceases to use it after a time because compliance with the ground rules consistently occurs. Glaser (1990) also deletes a phase, but she eliminates the review of the previous clinic when using the method.

Shapiro (1990) states one of his groups opted to have the demonstration clinician remain during the data analysis and critique preparation phase. He indicates the individuals involved felt comfortable giving and receiving feedback. As a result, he reports there is not a need to have the supervisee leave to ease the discussion.

In a situation such as this, the data analysis and critique preparation phase and the one that follows, problem-solving and strategy development, merge. For groups selecting this alternative, the time necessary to complete a clinic is reduced. But in all cases, having the supervisee remain should emerge at the group's wish. Under no circumstance should it be forced on them.

Shapiro (1990), due to scheduling conflicts, reports having five participants rather than the usual seven. He also reports another innovative use of the process. After several teaching clinics, the group engages in one "live" for approximately fifty observers including faculty, graduate, and undergraduate students. Shapiro states the participants and observers react positively to the experience. The observers feel the teaching clinic offers a nonthreatening vehicle to collaborative learning. Further, the facility contemplates requiring all graduate students to serve as demonstration clinician at least once with all faculty and students present.

Of interest, Sbaschnig (1989) reports trying various modifications to the teaching clinic method over the years. She discovers not explicitly following the ground rules reduces the effectiveness of the process. But she finds she always comes back to the original structure as it consistently meets supervisor/supervisee needs.

Williams describes using an adapted form of the teaching clinic called the modified teaching clinic (MTC) (1995). The structure of the process is reduced and the phases are renamed: (1) introduction, (2) focus, (3) observation, (4) problem-solving, (5) resolution, and (6) integration. A number of other aspects differ as well. For example, the ground rules are generated by the group rather than being preset. The supervisor remains as the clinic leader throughout the process rather than rotating this role among participants, although the supervisor does encourage increasing collaboration from the participants over time. The presenting clinician remains in the room throughout the process as Williams feels this increases levels of trust among group members. During the observation phase, the videotape may be stopped at any point to ask questions or discuss a particular occurrence. Also, comments, feelings, and viewpoints may be stated without supporting data. At the end of the modified teaching clinic, the participants discuss what they have learned from the process rather than reviewing the group process. This modified teaching clinic retains certain aspects of the teaching clinic and alters others. In doing so, Williams presents an interesting variation of the teaching clinic.

Professional Growth

Three speech-language pathologists, Estelle, Jerome, and Tram, are meeting for lunch.

ESTELLE: I'm glad we could get together for lunch. I feel so isolated at times.

JEROME: Me, too. Sometimes I really get stuck with a client and would like to talk to someone else to get some ideas.

TRAM: I know. I keep feeling like I'm continually reinventing the wheel at my school!

ESTELLE: Would you be interested in getting together once a month to discuss job issues?

JEROME: I'd like that. I'm really frustrated with a client's lack of improvement. If I brought a tape, could we look at it and talk about ways I could make changes?

TRAM: I also have a client who has me really puzzled. I'd like input.

JEROME: I read about the teaching clinic. Maybe we could implement one every other month and talk about other concerns in the months in between.

ESTELLE: I've read something about that, too. I have two other friends working in long-term care homes that might be interested.

TRAM: My friend, Jo, who's at an acute care hospital, and her colleague might be interested, too.

> **JEROME:**   Yeah, that way we would have enough people to make the group process work.
>
> **ESTELLE:**   This sounds great. I sometimes feel like I am in a rut. I'd like the chance to learn some new things.
>
> **TRAM:**   Let's pick a date for our first meeting and see if we can get everybody together. Do you want this first meeting to be one where we just talk or do we want the first to be a teaching clinic?
>
> **ESTELLE:**   Let's get everybody together and get acquainted the first time and see what everyone is most interested in. We can also get ready for our first teaching clinic for the following month.
>
> **JEROME:**   How about the first Friday of every month?
>
> **TRAM, ESTELLE:**   That will work. See you then.

These working professionals are actively seeking ways to grow and to reduce their sense of isolation. The teaching clinic is a tool that works equally well with pre-service or working professionals. In the material that follows a variety of uses of the teaching clinic are described.

Alternate Uses

The traditional focus of the teaching clinic is hands-on treatment or diagnostic clinical skill development. But innovative alternative applications are also in use. Weiseth (1990) indicates the speech pathologists in the Washington state Northshore School District are using the teaching clinic for the purpose of peer-based professional development. They hold these clinically focused meetings after school hours. She says they wrote a grant so that members are compensated for participating in this form of in-service education. Fey (1990) feels the teaching clinic approach is a viable mechanism for supervision in-services. The taped segment serves as a focal point for discussion of supervision skills. Supervisors initiate exchanges in areas in which they perceive a need for input. She feels this is particularly helpful in remote areas of the country where contact among supervisors is minimal.

This model is also used by Mawdsley (1990), Godden (1989), Crago (1987), and Scholten (1990) to teach supervisory skills. Thus, the conference rather than treatment is the focus of data collection, analysis, and problem-solving. Mawdsley indicates supervisors learn how to ask for data and feedback. She also feels it facilitates their skills in providing information to others.

McCrea (1994) also uses the teaching clinic to assist master's level graduate students apply supervisory skills learned in a supervision course. The participants bring a segment of videotape in which they are in the role of supervisor. Each of the steps of the teaching clinic is implemented with the demonstration supervisor having the option to leave or remain during the critique and strategy development session. McCrea indicates this process provides a controlled laboratory experience for trainees. They also become more self-aware, are able to self-analyze, and develop skill in modifying their supervisory behaviors.

Glaser (1990) describes using the teaching clinic as a global forum for teaching specific clinical skills. For example, it might be used to define the characteristics of good therapy. Similarly, Williams and Boggs (1990) use the structure to consider a variety of topics such as a review of current therapy approaches or clinic procedures. They even incorporate guest speakers or "experts" as needed. In this modified teaching clinic, the presenting clinician introduces a case and raises questions for consideration. Immediately following, the tape of this client is viewed and the group discusses the issues stated by the clinician at the outset. The findings are then summarized and participants share ideas they have learned as a result of the exchange. The Williams and Boggs usage appears to parallel the case-staffing strategy implemented by Farmer and Farmer (1989).

Benefits

A number of advantages are attributed to the teaching clinic process. According to Dowling (1983b), the approach fosters the development of self-supervision skills. The focus on data collection, analysis, problem-solving, and strategy development teaches the skills supervisees need to learn in order to observe and then modify their own behavior. Further, the phases of the teaching clinic methodology parallel the components of the clinical supervision model (Cogan, 1973). Both incorporate planning, data collection, analysis, problem-solving, collaborative interactions, and an ongoing supervisory process. Thus, many aspects of clinical supervision are built into this peer group method.

As stated above, Fey (1990) indicates the process assists the supervisee in developing a balanced view of his or her professional self. Fey also feels it saves time as the same information is imparted to several persons at a time. In addition, Glaser (1990) reports it is an effective technique to teach specific clinical skills. She states the parameters of an effective therapy session, appropriate planning, articulation cues, language prompts, response rate, and reinforcement have been explored using this process. In addition, she thinks it teaches problem-solving skills and that the supervisee's exposure to a variety of clients is beneficial. Shapiro (1990) says it is perceived as a nonthreatening vehicle for collaborative learning. In addition, Sweda (1989) feels it fosters nondefensive discussions.

Sbaschnig (1989) states use of the teaching clinic leads to self-supervision because supervisees develop skills to modify their own behavior. In addition, she feels participants develop observation and analytic skills from participation. Sweda (1989) further reports that it fosters objectivity in observation and evaluation. In this same vein, Bountress (1989) senses supervisees brainstorm and solve more problems when they are in groups than they do on an individual basis. She also feels it provides students opportunities to demonstrate leadership skills, and decreases supervisee dependence on the supervisor. Similarly, Godden (1989) indicates the process helps supervisees take risks and to learn there are no "right or wrong" answers.

Liabilities

This process also has potential pitfalls as well. When the teaching clinic is used as the primary or only supervisory strategy, supervisees are not receiving the benefits of a one-to-one supervisor–supervisee relationship. In addition, certain persons do not work well in groups. Finally, in general, group methods are not efficient for basic goal-setting, providing valuative information, or dealing with crisis situations. Other specific concerns expressed in regard to the process follow.

Glaser (1990) reports the major disadvantage of the process is the initial uneasiness felt by persons in the role of demonstration clinician. Scholten (1990) also expresses this concern, although she finds that the ground rules quickly establish that sharing ia a positive experience for all concerned. In addition, Scholten says finding the time to schedule a clinic is sometimes a problem. Also, if the process is seen as an extra responsibility rather than an integral part of supervision, supervisee resentment emerges (Sweda, 1989). In a markedly different realm, Bountress (1989) feels that, at times, inappropriate alternatives are generated by the peers. She states this is difficult to redirect without appearing critical of the suggestion.

In sum, both advantages and disadvantages exist when a group supervision methodology is employed. Overall, the positives appear to outweigh the negatives. In addition, the liabilities may be minimized through conscious awareness and efforts by those who implement the strategy.

Research Summary

Research on the teaching clinic process is limited. Several observations may be made from that which is reported. It appears to be at minimum, equivalent in types of talk behaviors generated and in perceived effectiveness to traditional one-to-one meetings (Dowling and Shank, 1981; Dowling, 1983a). In regard to participant anxiety, supervisory relationship perceptions, clinical self-concept, and clinical effectiveness, the two methods are similar (Johnson and Fey, 1983). All participants are actively involved in the exchange. Thus, the supervisor does a lot of talking but so do the supervisees (Dowling, 1983b). Superiors continue to set the tone for the exchange as participants parallel the talk modeled by the supervisor in both category type and quantity (Dowling, 1987a). Also, serving as the demonstration clinician is less stressful than previously thought (Dowling, 1987a; Sleight, Power, Cluver, and Calloway, 1987). Clinicians and supervisors reflect satisfaction and even a preference for group supervision (Dowling, 1983b; Sleight, Power, Cluver, and Calloway, 1987; Williams, 1995). On a continuum of satisfaction, the teaching clinic is closer to their perceptions of an ideal conference than it is to one-to-one conferencing (Dowling, 1987b). In addition, supervisees do engage in behaviors characteristic of self-supervision by discussing methods/objectives, giving opinions/suggestions, and actively participating (Dowling, 1983b). They also learn to collect and analyze data and translate this information into clinical problem-solving. Finally, they report an increase in their ability to observe, evaluate and modify their own behavior (Dowling, 1983b).

Teaching Clinic Summary

Some closing thoughts are relevant to the discussion of the teaching clinic. First, the teaching clinic format is flexible and may be modified depending on the needs of the facility and or participants. A viable example is the modified teaching clinic described by Williams (1995). The modification most often made is having the demonstration clinician remain in the room during critique preparation, which combines that phase with the next. This strategy is appropriate as long as the decision to do so emerges from the participants. In practice, it is more likely to emerge from a cohesive group than from one that is not.

To be effective, participants must be trained to use the procedure and the ground rules observed when it is implemented. In particular, three of the rules are critical to the success of the clinic: Comments must be based on collected data, the focus is on clinical rather than personal behavior, and the contents of discussions do not leave the room in which they occur. These rules protect both the participants and the integrity of the teaching clinic process. Failure to observe them may be damaging to the individuals involved and make the process destructive. The exception to the third rule is a situation such as that described by Shapiro (1990) in which the teaching clinic is planned to be viewed by others. Participant consent to share the contents legitimizes that procedure, but even one dissent should prevent the process from being used in this manner.

One of the appealing aspects of the teaching clinic is the potential time it can save for supervisors. In practice, one conference takes the place of many. In this regard, the author views the teaching clinic as a supplement to traditional supervision rather than a substitute. As mentioned earlier, this approach is not particularly effective with goal-setting, grade assignment, or for dealing with crisis situations. Recall also that not all persons function well in a group. In taking these factors into account, it may be best to start out with individual conferences. Then a move to group conferences might be made while, at the same time, providing supervisees the opportunity to schedule individual conferences as needed. Another general alternative is to have supervisees meet periodically with individual supervisors and use the teaching clinic strategy for weekly group clinic meetings. The key point, as in all supervision, is that the supervisees' needs are being met.

The teaching clinic approach may also be used to build supervisory skills. It is currently being used on a limited basis (Crago, 1987; Fey, 1990; Mawdsley,

1990; McCrea, 1994). The focus of the teaching clinics is a videotape of a supervisory conference. Data collection, analysis, and problem-solving occur just as they do in regard to the clinical process with an eye toward the implementation of clinical supervision (Cogan, 1973), the appropriate stage of the Anderson (1988) continuum of supervision, or cognitive coaching (Costa and Garmston, 1994). Specific supervisory skills such as verbal/nonverbal mirroring of the supervisee's behavior, using of open-ended questions, reducing supervisor talk time, fostering clinician problem-solving and strategy development may be targeted. Again, the supervisor serving in the demonstration role will share the objectives for the conference and request specific feedback from the peer observers. Using the teaching clinic process for supervisor growth is filled with promise.

The teaching clinic may also serve as a vehicle for professional growth in other disciplines as well. It would be applicable in nursing, psychological counseling, social work, occupational and physical therapy, medicine, and education. Again, the focus of the process may be the clinical and/or supervisory process, depending on the area being developed at a given time.

Relationship of the Teaching Clinic Approach to the Specified Supervision Tasks

The teaching clinic may be used to facilitate both clinical and supervisory skills. Nine of the thirteen tasks of supervision can be addressed, in part, with this methodology. In regard to establishing and maintaining an effective working relationship with the supervisee, the process minimizes the superior–subordinate relationship as the supervisor is likely to serve in a peer role. In addition, the demonstration person's colleagues are likely to act as "supervisor" by collecting information and providing feedback. Also, the data-based, analytic focus minimizes the valuative tone of interactions. In this regard, Farmer and Farmer (1989) say this mechanism fosters colleagiality and Shapiro (1990) states it is a nonthreatening vehicle for collaborative learning. In addition, the supervisor as peer or demonstration clinician provides multiple opportunities for this individual to model professional conduct. Four related tasks are also readily addressed in the teaching clinic: Task 6, assisting the supervisee in observing and analyzing assessment and treatment sessions; Task 9, assisting the supervisee in the evaluation of clinical performance; Task 3, assisting the supervisee in developing and refining assessment skills; and Task 4, assisting the supervisee in developing and refining management skills. The heart of teaching clinics is data-based analysis and problem-solving. Participants are required to collect and interpret data and then use it to solve problems and generate suggestions for future implementation. As a result of involvement in this process, supervisees do learn to observe and then analyze behavior. Therefore, they also have the tools to arrive at valuative conclusions. Because either treatment or assessment sessions may be presented by the demonstration clinician, supervisees have the opportunity to develop and refine either assessment or treatment skills depending on the focus of the particular clinic. In terms of planning and executing the supervisory conference, the demonstration clinician prepares the agenda for the meeting and requests specific feedback from the observers. As a result, this method mandates active supervisee involvement in the planning and executing of the conference. The remaining two tasks are less directly taught through teaching clinics. The maintenance of clinical and supervisory records only tangentially emerges as clinicians become increasingly skilled in data collection during observations. Similarly, research skills are alluded to indirectly. Asking clinical and supervisory questions and then gathering data to measure outcomes is basic to quality research (Kamhi, 1995). In sum, the teaching clinic may be considered as a tool for cultivating nine of the thirteen tasks of supervision.

Summary

This chapter begins with a consideration of the ASHA (1985) tasks of clinical supervision relevant to the use of the teaching clinic for clinical and supervisory training. Then the literature relevant to group supervision methodologies and vignettes about a search for supervisory alternatives are presented. Immediately thereafter the teaching clinic method is described. This begins with an iteration of the phases and ground rules. Training procedures and the underlying rationale are noted. These sections are followed by strategies that facilitate teaching clinic implementation. The advantages and applicability of the process are then discussed. Modifications of the approach currently in use are reported. Applications other than that outlined in the original format are given as are the perceived benefits and liabilities noted by current users. A summary of teaching clinic research is presented. Summary thoughts about the teaching clinic process are discussed. The last segment relates the teaching clinic to the acquisition of nine of the thirteen tasks of supervision. (Training materials to use when initiating the teaching clinics will be found in Appendix A.)

REFERENCES

American Speech-Language-Hearing Association. Committee on Supervision in Speech-Language Pathology and Audiology. "Clinical supervision in speech-language pathology and audiology: A position statement." *ASHA*, 27 (1985): 57–60.

Anderson, D., Vail, C., Jones, K., and Huntington, D. "Professional collaboration: Empowering school personnel through peer coaching." Paper presented at the Annual Convention of the Council of Exceptional Children, Denver, CO, April, 1994.

Anderson, J. *The Supervisory Process in Speech-Language Pathology and Audiology.* Austin, TX: Pro-Ed, 1988.

Bernard, J., and Goodyear, R. *Fundamentals of Clinical Supervision* (2nd ed.). Boston, MA: Allyn and Bacon, 1998.

Bountress, M. Old Dominion University. Personal communication, 1989.

Buttery, T., and Michalak, D. "Competency based teacher preparation and humanistic education: A supervisory approach." *The Teacher Educator, 9* (3) (1974): 34–40.

Buttery, T., and Weller, D. "Group clinical supervision: A paradigm for preservice instructional enhancement." *Action in Teacher Education, 10* (1) (1988): 61–73.

Chaiklin, H., and Munson, C. "Peer consultation in social work." *The Clinical Supervisor, 1* (2) (1983): 21–34.

Chrisco, I. "Peer assistance works." *Educational Leadership, 46* (8) (1989): 31–32.

Cogan, M. *Clinical Supervision.* Boston: Houghton Mifflin, 1973.

Cooper, L., and Gustafson, J. "Supervision in a group: An application of group theory." *The Clinical Supervisor, 3* (2) (1985): 7–25.

Costa, A., and Garmston, R. *Cognitive Coaching: A Foundation for Renaissance Schools.* Norwood, MA: Christopher Gordon Publishers, 1994.

Crago, M. "Supervision and self-exploration." In M. Crago and M. Pickering, (Eds.), *Supervision in Human Communication Disorders.* San Diego, CA: Singular Publishing Group, 1987: 137–167.

Crutchfield, L., and Borders, D. "Impact of two clinical peer supervision models on practicing school counselors." *Journal of Counseling and Development, 75* (3) (1997): 219–230.

Crutchfield, L., Price, C., McGarity, D., Pennington, D., Richardson, J., and Tsolis, A. "Challenge and support: Group supervision for school counselors." *Professional School Counseling, 1* (1) (1997): 43–46.

Dowling, S. *A Comparison to Determine the Effects of Two Supervisory Styles, Conventional and Teaching Clinics, in the Training of Speech Pathologists.* (Doctoral dissertation, Indiana University, 1976). *Dissertation Abstracts International, 37,* 889B. (University Microfilms No. 77-01, 883).

Dowling, S. "The teaching clinic: a supervisory alternative." *American Speech Hearing Association, 21* (9) (1979): 646–649.

Dowling, S., and Shank, K. "A comparison of the effects of two supervisory styles, conventional and teaching clinic, in the training of speech-language pathologists." *Journal of Communication Disorders, 14* (1981): 51–58.

Dowling, S. "An analysis of conventional and teaching clinic supervision." *The Clinical Supervisor, 1* (4) (1983a): 15–29.

Dowling, S. "Teaching clinic conference participant interaction." *Journal of Communication Disorders, 16* (1983b): 385–397.

Dowling, S. "Teaching clinic conferences: Perceptions of supervisor and peer behavior." *Journal of Communication Disorders, 20* (1987a): 119–128.

Dowling, S. "Teaching clinic participation: Impact on conference perceptions." In S. Farmer, (Ed.), *Clinical Supervision: A Coming of Age,* A National Conference on Supervision. Las Cruces, NM: New Mexico State University, (1987b):72–77.

Dowling, S. *Implementing the Supervisory Process: Theory and Practice.* Englewood Cliffs, New Jersey: Prentice-Hall, Inc. 1992.

Dowling, S., Fey, S., Glaser, A., Shapiro, D., and Mawdsley, B. "Teaching clinic application and adaptations." Miniseminar presented at the Annual Convention of the American Speech-Language and Hearing Association, Seattle, WA, 1990.

Dowling, S., and Michalak, D. "The teaching clinic: A supervisory alternative." Paper presented at the Annual Convention of the American Speech-Language Hearing Association, Houston, TX, 1976.

Farmer, S., and Farmer, J. *Supervision in Communication Disorders.* Columbus, OH: Merrill Publishing, 1989.

Fey, S. The University of Western Ontario. Personal communication, 1990.

Glaser, Johnson, A. Miami University. Personal communication, 1990.

Glickman, C. *Supervision of Instruction: A Developmental Approach.* Boston, MA: Allyn and Bacon, 1985: 263–269.

Godden, A. University of Western Ontario. Personal communication, 1989.

Irwin, R. "Microsupervision: A study of the behaviors of supervisors of speech clinicians." Paper presented at the Annual Convention of the American Speech-Language Hearing Association, San Francisco, CA, 1972.

Johnson, D., and Fey, S. "Comparative effects of teaching clinic versus traditional supervision methods." *Supervision, 7* (1) (1983): 2–4.

Kamhi, A., "Research to practice: Defining, developing and maintaining clinical expertise." *Language, Speech and Hearing Services in Schools, 26* (4) (1995): 353–356.

Kuechler, C., and Barretta-Herman, A. "The consultation circle: A technique for facilitating peer consultation." *The Clinical Supervisor, 17* (1) (1998): 83–93.

Loiselle, J., St. Louis, M., and Dupuy-Walker, L. "Giving professional help to pre-service teachers through computer-mediated communication." Paper presented at the Annual Meeting of the Association of Teacher Educators, Dallas, TX, Feb. 1998.

Ludlow, B., Wienke, W., Henderson, J., and Klein, H. "A collaborative program to prepare mainstream teachers: Using peer supervision by general and special educators." In *Coming together: Preparing for Rural Special Education in the 21st Century. Conference Proceedings of the American Council on Rural Special Education*, Charleston, SC, March, 1998.

Mawdsley, B. Wichita State University. Personal communication, 1990.

McAllister, L., and Lincoln, M. "Facilitating peer learning in clinical education." In M. Bruce, (Ed.), *Proceedings of the 1994 International and Interdisciplinary Conference on Clinical Supervision,* Burlington, VT: University of Vermont (1994): 184–189.

McCrea, E. "Supervision as a master's degree option." In M. Bruce, (Ed.), *Proceedings of the 1994 International and Interdisciplinary Conference on Clinical Supervision,* Burlington, VT: University of Vermont (1994): 221–229.

Olsen, H., Barbour, C., and Michalak, D. "The teaching clinic: A team approach to improved teaching." *Association of Teacher Educators Bulletin 30, (1971):* 1–33.

Pistole, M. "The genogram in group supervision of novice counselors: Draw them a picture." *The Clinical Supervisor, 13* (1) (1995): 133–143.

Powell, D. "A peer consultation model for clinical supervision. *The Clinical Supervisor, 14* (2) (1996): 163-169.

Reiman, A., and Thies-Sprinthall, L. *Mentoring and Supervision for Teacher Development.* New York: Longman, 1998.

Robbins, P. *How to Plan and Implement a Peer Coaching Program.* Alexandria, VA: Association for Supervision and Curriculum Development, 1991.

Sbaschnig, K. Wayne State University. Personal communication, 1989.

Scholten, I. South Australian College of Advanced Education. Personal communication, 1990.

Schubert, G., and Laird, B. "The length of time mecessary to obtain a representative sample of clinician-client interaction." *Journal of National Student Speech and Hearing Association 3* (1975): 26–32.

Seal, B., and Runyan, E. "Time management in clinical supervision: A descriptive study of time allocation." *American Speech Hearing Association, 30* (1988): 59–61.

Shapiro, D. Western Carolina University. Personal communication, 1990.

Sleight, C., Power Cluver, E., and Calloway, M. "Student reactions to group supervision." *Human Communication Canada, 11* (1) (1987): 5–10.

Sweda, J. Cleveland State University. Personal communication, 1989.

Tebb, S., Manning, D., and Klaumann, T. "A renaissance of group supervision in practicum." *The Clinical Supervisor, 14* (2) (1996): 39–51.

Weiseth, C. Northshore School District, Bothell, WA. Personal communication, 1990.

Williams, L. "Modified teaching clinic: Peer group supervision in clinical training and professional development." *American Journal of Speech-Language Pathology, 4* (3) (1995): 29–38.

Williams, L., and Boggs, T. "Peer group supervision: Modified teaching clinic." Paper presented at the Annual Convention of the American Speech-Language and Hearing Association, Seattle, WA, 1990.

APPENDIX 10-A

Teaching Clinic Training Material

The Teaching Clinic

The Teaching Clinic, a peer-group form of supervision, consists of the following six sequential steps:

1. Review of the previous Teaching Clinic;
2. Planning Session;
3. Observation Session;
4. Data Analysis and Critique Preparation Session;
5. Problem Solving and Strategy Development Session;
6. Clinic Review.

THE TEACHING CLINIC

CLINIC LEADER
Individual who guides the discussion
and stimulates interaction among peers

DEMONSTRATION CLINICIAN
Clinician being observed

PEERS
Observers assisting in collecting and
analyzing data and problem solving
with the demonstration clinician

GROUP MONITOR
Individual who monitors the group
process

Teaching clinic procedure is based on Dowling (1979, 1992). Reprinted with permission from Dowling, S., *Implementing the Supervisory Process: Theory and Practice.* Englewood Cliffs, NJ: Prentice-Hall, 1992.

PHASE 1   REVIEW OF PREVIOUS CLINIC

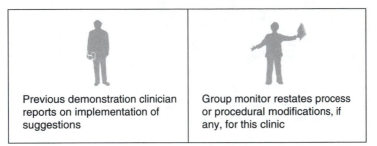

Previous demonstration clinician reports on implementation of suggestions

Group monitor restates process or procedural modifications, if any, for this clinic

PHASE 2   PLANNING SESSION

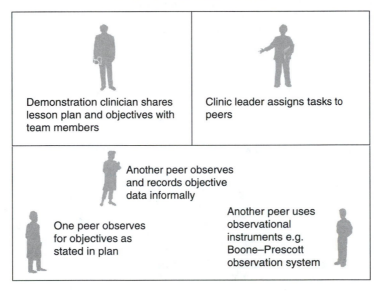

Demonstration clinician shares lesson plan and objectives with team members

Clinic leader assigns tasks to peers

Another peer observes and records objective data informally

One peer observes for objectives as stated in plan

Another peer uses observational instruments e.g. Boone–Prescott observation system

PHASE 3   OBSERVATION SESSION

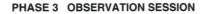

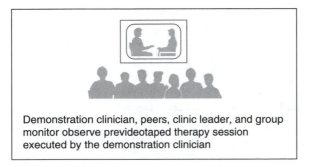

Demonstration clinician, peers, clinic leader, and group monitor observe prevideotaped therapy session executed by the demonstration clinician

PHASE 4   DATA ANALYSIS AND CRITIQUE PREPARATION

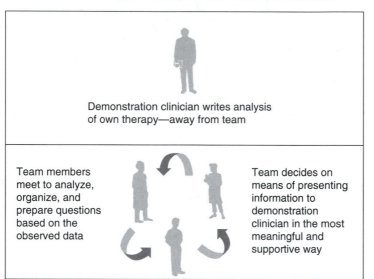

Demonstration clinician writes analysis
of own therapy—away from team

Team members
meet to analyze,
organize, and
prepare questions
based on the
observed data

Team decides on
means of presenting
information to
demonstration
clinician in the most
meaningful and
supportive way

PHASE 5   PROBLEM SOLVING AND STRATEGY DEVELOPMENT

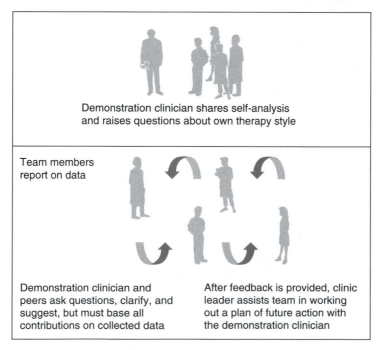

Demonstration clinician shares self-analysis
and raises questions about own therapy style

Team members
report on data

Demonstration clinician and
peers ask questions, clarify, and
suggest, but must base all
contributions on collected data

After feedback is provided, clinic
leader assists team in working
out a plan of future action with
the demonstration clinician

PHASE 6 TEACHING CLINIC REVIEW AND FUTURE PLANNING SESSION

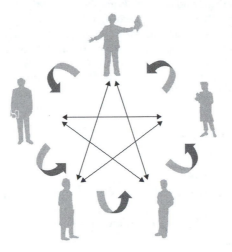

Group monitor reviews and assesses the group process and suggest modifications, as needed

A new demonstration clinician is selected and the time and place of the next teaching clinic is decided

Ground Rules*

1. An agenda must be prepared and given to each participant in advance of the teaching clinic. The agenda includes:
   a. Date of the teaching clinic and starting time;
   b. Location of the meeting;
   c. Objectives for the segment to be viewed/observed.
2. Analysis and discussion throughout the teaching clinic are directed to the teaching behavior of the demonstration clinician, not to that individual as a person.
3. All observer comments must be supported by recorded data.
4. For the purpose of confidentiality, all comments made during teaching clinics remain in the room in which they occurred.

Roles of Teaching Clinic Participants

I. Clinic leader

   A. Encourage all group members to participate.
   B. Guide group members so that they fulfill their roles and observe the Teaching Clinic ground rules.
   C. Assign observation tasks to group members during the Planning Session.

---

*Adapted in part from the ground rules in H. Olsen, C. Barbour, and D. Michalak. *Teaching Clinic: A Team Approach to Improved Teaching.* Washington, D.C.: National Education Association, 1971.

    D. Encourage group members to generate alternative therapy approaches during the Data Analysis and Critique Preparation and the Problem Solving and Strategy Development Phases of the Teaching Clinic.

    E. At the end of the Data Analysis and Critique Preparation session, summarize the peer observations and guide the observers as they determine their approaches to provide feedback to the demonstration clinician.

    F. Guide the discussion during the Data Analysis and the Critique Preparation and the Problem Solving and Strategy Development sessions so that positive as well as the negative aspects of the therapy are considered.

    G. Direct peer feedback so that the demonstration clinician is not overwhelmed by the amount or type (positive and/or negative) of feedback that he or she is receiving.

II. Demonstration Clinician

    A. Prepares an agenda and distributes it to the group members.

    B. Presents her therapy objectives to the group.

    C. Requests specific information about his or her therapy.

III. Peer Observers

    A. Collects observable data.

    B. Provides feedback to the demonstration clinician.

IV. Group Monitor

Answer these questions as a guide to review the group process in the Teaching Clinic.

    A. Were the ground rules observed?

        1. Was agenda prepared and distributed?

        2. Was the analysis and discussion throughout the Teaching Clinic directed to the teaching behavior of the demonstration clinician?

           a. Was it oriented to him or her as a person?

        3. Were observer comments supported by recorded data?

    B. Did group members fulfill their roles?

        1. Demonstration clinician presented objectives and asked for information about specific aspects of her therapy.

        2. Clinic leader assigned tasks for the Observation session.

        3. Clinic leader encouraged group participation and interaction.

        4. Peer observers collected observable data.

    C. Did all group members participate?

11 Teaching Supervisory Skills through Role-Playing and Simulation

Clinical Supervision Tasks Relevant to Teaching Supervisory Skills through Role-Playing and Simulation

Task 1: Establishing and maintaining an effective working relationship with the supervisee;

Task 2: Assisting the supervisee in developing clinical goals and objectives;

Task 3: Assisting the supervisee in developing and refining assessment skills;

Task 4: Assisting the supervisee in developing and refining clinical management skills;

Task 5: Demonstrating for and participating with the supervisee in the clinical process;

Task 6: Assisting the supervisee in observing and analyzing assessment and treatment sessions:

Task 7: Assisting the supervisee in the development and maintenance of clinical and supervisory records;

Task 8: Interacting with the supervisee in planning, executing, and analyzing supervisory conferences;

Task 9: Assisting the supervisee in evaluation of clinical performance;

Task 10: Assisting the supervisee in developing skills of verbal reporting, writing, and editing;

Task 11: Sharing information regarding ethical, legal, regulatory, and reimbursement aspects of professional practice;

Task 12: Modeling and facilitating professional conduct.

Beginning Thoughts

Tom is a professor in a university training program. Shannon is a supervisor in a public school system, and Sonia is the supervisor in a large healthcare organization. They have worked together on a number of projects in their professional community. Tom is offering a course at the masters level in Clinical Supervision this fall and Shannon is gearing up to train certified speech-language pathologists in her district to supervise the new speech-language pathology assistants being added to the district's staff. Sonia would like to involve more staff members in some aspects of supervision. They are discussing strategies that might work with each of these groups. Snippets of their conversation follow:

TOM: I agree that we need to begin with a model of supervision to give people a foundation for their supervision. But, I don't think just telling people about it is enough. Sometimes, I think the students are saying, "oh yeah, right" to themselves and setting aside the information once they take the test because they haven't had a chance to apply it.

SHANNON: I think that is true of the people on my staff as well.

TOM: Several students told me last term they learn best when they have the opportunity to experience a situation.

SHANNON: I did two supervision workshops last year and their were a number of comments on the evaluation forms saying they really enjoyed the workshop but didn't know if they would be able to apply some of the ideas we discussed.

SONIA: I've been thinking about roleplay. We have talked about collaboration in our staff meetings but when I observe my staff supervising interns, they are doing a lot of telling and almost no collaboration. Maybe roleplaying conferences would be a way to help them develop their supervision. I've read a couple of articles that said it works.

SHANNON: That's an interesting idea.

TOM: I have also been thinking about having them assume the role of a supervisor in a simulation where they would have to deal with issues that might arise.

SONIA: That would be particularly good if they had a chance to be a supervisor in varied work settings because working in a rehabilitation facility is sure different than an acute care hospital or the schools.

SHANNON: I am going to try roleplay and see how it works. Maybe we could each come up with some and share them.

TOM: Yeah, That's a good idea. I'm also going to think about a simulation for my class. As I put it together, maybe we could talk about it some more. You know, I bet you could use it too, Shannon. When you do longer workshops, "in and out basket" situations would work well for audience participation.

SONIA: Wow. Look at the time. I've got to go. Let's all write some roleplays and try a couple before we get together next month. I'll be interested to see how your simulations are coming Tom.

TOM: Good plan, I'll see you both next time.

Role-Playing and Simulation

Tom, Shannon, and Sonia touch on the issue of how to assist people in incorporating new information into their professional repertoires, and they think role-playing and simulation may be helpful. This chapter will explore these topics as tools to teach supervisory skills.

Role-playing and simulation share certain features, but are unique as well. In role-playing, a given dilemma provides the context. Individuals assume roles and interact with each other in regard to a particular circumstance. Dyads are often used but it can also involve a group, for example, a family interaction. The purpose of this process may be to practice a specific skill, such as active listening, or to learn ways to manage a given situation.

In simulation, persons assume a role and then deal with a variety of events from the perspective that they adopt. For example, one may deal with phone calls, memos, and anticipated meetings. In some games, persons actually receive simulated phone calls or, if it is a computerized simulation, the scene might develop in reaction to the participant's responses. The factor that differentiates role-playing from simulation is that the latter tends to be an integrated ongoing event rather than isolated episodes. The two strategies may also be used in conjunction with each other. For example, a decision may be made to role-play a particularly thorny circumstance occurring in the simulation. An example of intertwining role-playing and simulation is an educational unit designed to increase participants' understanding of global climate change (Williams and Mowry, 1997). These participants are involved in a five-day simulation in which they role-play key events.

Role-playing will be addressed first and then simulation. Relevant aspects of the literature will be presented regarding each. Key considerations in using these approaches will be addressed. Implementation of these methods and their relevance to twelve of the thirteen tasks of supervision will be discussed. Example role plays and a simulation game will also be provided for the reader's use.

Role-Playing Literature

The Use of Role-Playing

Varied Applications. Role-playing approaches are implemented for a variety of purposes. In cooperative vocational education classes, role-playing is viewed as a mechanism to bridge the gap between education and the workplace (Grubb and Badway, 1998). It is used in law enforcement to teach peer debriefing skills (Seigel and Driscoll, 1995). It is also effective in teaching conflict management skills to adolescents and their parents (Wood and Davidson, 1993). In addition, child psychiatrists employ both group discussions and role-playing to assist speech pathologists in applying a family systems approach to increase their effectiveness in working with disorganized families and their children (Marks, 1983).

Educational Process.   Maier (1989) states role-playing can be used for three distinct reasons in the educational process: to teach skill acquisition, to enhance knowledge, and to cause a change in affect. Joyce, Weil, and Showers (1992) feel its primary purpose is to create empathy for others in a given situation. According to Rieke and Curtis (1981) behaviors demonstrated during role-playing transfer to real-life situations.

McCarthy, Linnan, and Muryn (1996) suggest role-playing as a teaching strategy for skills needed as part of a clinical education. They also recommend using it as a means to adapt teaching to individual learning styles. Crago (1987) endorses it as an option a supervisee might choose for use during the supervisory conference to practice and evaluate alternate treatment strategies.

A unique type of role-playing is used to train physicians, involving a person who plays a patient with a given diagnosis. In one example, the physician trainees are being taught how to present bad news. They role-play the situation with the patient who then provides feedback to the trainees. In a follow-up role play with a second patient, the physician trainees perform significantly better, demonstrating the effectiveness of role-playing (Viadya, Greenberg, Patel, Strauss, Pollack, 1999). Simulated patient role plays are also found to be effective in the training of paramedics (Johnson, Macias, Dunlap, Hauswald, and Doezema (1999) and physicians during residency (Madan, Caruso, Lopes, and Gracely (1998).

Rabinowitz (1997) describes the use of a semester-long role play that shares many similarities with a simulation. In a counselor education course, as the instructor, he role-plays a client for whom he has developed a case history and a psychological profile. For ten weeks, the professor assumes the persona of the client and the students alternately counsel this character as the remainder observe. Each of the role-play class periods begins with a discussion of the client, hypotheses about his behavior, and predictions of his presenting demeanor that day. This is followed by a forty-five-minute role play in which the instructor assumes the client persona. The class period closes with a debriefing. This approach allows the students to see the progression of therapy, experience issues that might arise in therapy, and explore a variety of counseling strategies. In general, the students find the process helpful and they are surprised at how invested they become in the counseling situation. They do voice some criticisms about the process as well. In particular, they would like the instructor to break from character and provide feedback at specific points. The instructor feels this would undermine the cohesiveness of the process. He suggests the use of a teaching assistant to allow him to stay in character while providing more immediate feedback to participants.

In regard to the planning process, Munson (1983) indicates the concept to be taught must be developed by the leader prior to the role play. He further suggests participants be selected based on their ability to perform a given role and that a warm-up period precede the actual roleplay. If an audience is viewing the exchange, observation guidelines are to be shared prior to the activity.

Regarding the technique of monitoring during implementation, Munson indicates the instructor might be an observer or serve as one of the participants to insure the role play is kept on-task. If subjects have significant difficulty assuming the role, he suggests abandoning the attempt after several brief assists. He also states the characters played by particular persons may need to be shifted if the individuals are unable to perform as assigned.

At the completion of the role play, Munson feels, as part of the evaluation process, it is critical to review and highlight the concepts that are learned. He states the views of all involved, instructor, participants, and observers should be shared as each is likely to have a unique contribution. He indicates both the "observed" and "felt" realms need to be explored. During the final component, the debriefing, he stresses the importance of saying that the "as if" experiences might not occur in real situations.

Further, Bredemeier and Greenblat (1981) report that debriefing may be the key to maximum learning as generalizations can be identified from the participants' concrete experiences. Maier (1989) indicates a review of the process is particularly important when the intent of the episode is to change the way participants feel about a situation. Brannon (1985) and West (1984) also cite the importance of this summation process.

The Impact of Role-Playing

Hunt (1982) indicates role-play materials may be blended effectively into course content. He cites the work of Elgood (1976) in stating that such a strategy results in "enjoyment, releasing knowledge already possessed, presenting new knowledge, encouraging the practice of skills, provoking behavior and stimulating thought." Bernard and Goodyear (1998) cite the work of Borders (1989) who feels role-playing can be used to create heightened interest when peer group processes stagnate. Hunt also feels gaming type procedures assist in bridging the gap between theoretical and practical learning. Even though participants are not truly on the job in a role-play, they are given the opportunity to apply information as it is learned. In particular, in regard to supervisory training, Loganbill and Hardy (1983) point out role-playing facilitates the supervisee's assumption of a supervisor "mindset" and overall attitude. A prime example of this type of application is the strategy implemented by Rassi (1978) in training supervisors of audiology. Trainees supervise the course instructor as she role-plays a beginning audiology clinician assessing the hearing of patients whose roles are enacted by other staff members.

Regarding the value of role-playing, Delamater, Conners, and Wells (1984), in a twenty-one-week study, find that role-playing is more effective than either an in-service or direct feedback in modifying the behavior of nurses and aides in an inpatient psychiatric unit. Isaacs, Embry, and Baer (1982) determine that both family therapists and the involved families benefit from training that contains a simulated component. Similarly, Jackson (1984) finds a rapid increase in a group's skills when these strategies are used. But research indicates that the impact of participation may vary within subjects (Bredemeier and Greenblat, 1981). These authors cite both personality variables and cognitive styles as impacting willingness to become involved and subsequent perceptions of gains from the activity. Brown and Bourne (1996) suggest the nearer the role play is to the real thing, the more productive it is likely to be.

The author feels role-playing is extremely valuable in training those involved in the clinical and supervisory process. Through simulated situations, participants can glimpse and begin to experience a role prior to actual involvement. In particular, it allows them to apply new concepts to a specific situation or event. For the trainee, employee, or supervisor desiring further growth, this procedure can be used to develop specific conferencing skills. For the supervisee, role-playing an aspect of therapy with the supervisor during the conference provides an opportunity to practice alternate strategies in an environment in which feedback is readily available and experimentation is encouraged. In addition, the person in the role of supervisee may provide specific reactions to the supervisor's efforts and/or style. In particular, the "felt" aspects may be explored. This method, then, is potentially beneficial for both the supervisor and supervisee.

Implementing Role-Playing

Advance Preparation

In designing role plays for use in a conference, a workshop, classroom, or work setting, thought must be given to the nature and appropriateness of the situation to be enacted. Once this is determined, a strategy for keeping the interaction on track must then be planned. Finally, guidelines for evaluating the exchange and a format for debriefing need to be developed.

Munson (1983) expresses concern that confidential emotions might be revealed in a role play. He states that inadequate planning by the trainer or failure to note the release of emotion may leave the person feeling vulnerable and embarrassed. In the author's use of role play, a similar situation has surfaced only once. A simulated conference in which a failing clinician was being encouraged to seek an alternate career was enacted. One participant, who by chance was playing the supervisee, had been told several years earlier that she was failing and would benefit from career counseling. The emotions previously experienced resurfaced. This precipitated the need and the opportunity to discuss the supervisee's current feelings as well as the sense of rage and disappointment she had felt at the time of the initial event. This was an unanticipated event that necessitated sensitivity and debriefing for the participants and observers.

Application Strategies

A variety of situations may be role-played. They may range from the supervisee who wants to enact a situation in therapy, the clinician or supervisor interacting with families to the implementing of aspects of supervisory conferences. In the training of supervisors, it is the author's opinion that experience needs to be provided in role-playing conferences with supervisees who are performing successfully, those who are having difficulty clinically, and at least one who is failing and has a accompanying need for career counseling or, in the work setting, has to be laid off. This later circumstance is painful for both members but it is a reality of supervision. This is particularly true if one works in a training program or health-care setting where downsizing may necessitate layoffs and terminations. One's personal ability to work with a failing supervisee or fire/lay off an employee may be a factor in an individual's ultimate decision to seek a supervisory position.

Before beginning a role play, the ideas to be learned should be thought out. For example, a specific conference style, such as indirect or collaborative (Anderson, 1988), might be targeted for implementation. The goal might be to increase supervisee problem-solving. The supervisor and supervisee may choose to engage in behaviors reflective of active listening such as clarifying, restating, or summarizing. Increasing the facilitative nature of interpersonal conference climate through verbal and nonverbal pacing may be the intent. In other instances, the goal may be learning to manage a particularly difficult situation. In considering alternatives to address, the reader may wish to review the chapters on conferencing and feedback for additional ideas.

Following each role play, several issues may be considered during the debriefing process. For example, did the supervisor deal with the affective aspects of the exchange? Did the supervisor convey positive regard? Was the conference direct/indirect /collaborative in style? Was problem-solving occurring and, if so, by whom? Did the supervisor meet the supervisee's needs? What was the supervisor's agenda? What was the supervisee's agenda? How were the participants likely to feel as a result of the conference? Was the discussion successful? Was the method used perceived as effective? Were there alternative strategies that might have been employed?

These questions may be answered at the discretion of the group leader and the participants. This decision may depend on the circumstance and the purpose of the role play. The role-play leader, in most cases, will play a significant role by integrating the experience and highlighting salient points. This person also needs to be alert and attentive to personal emotions that may have been triggered by the experience.

There are a limited number of variations for role playing. Munson (1983) suggests using a stage and theatrical lighting. Actors may also be used. One alternative is to identify three or four dyads for the remaining participants to observe. The author typically has all members, in groups of two, implement the role play concurrently. This simultaneous involvement seems to allow persons to move quickly into the roles as concerns about others observing are diminished.

Some participants are initially more adept than others in implementing role play. Those more proficient rapidly assume the assigned identity and role. Others have more difficulty doing so. The latter may be revealed by off-task behavior or an apparent inability to interact with appropriate dialogue. Generally, a restatement of the purpose of the interaction or modeling by a more effective pair resolves this problem. It is important to recall that personality style or an individual's general tendency to participate in novel situations may impact that person's inclination to assume an alternate persona (Bredemeier and Greenblat, 1981) and thus may be a marked factor during the initial stages of this procedure.

The author continually encourages participants to pick a new partner as role plays are incorporated in various class periods or at different points during a workshop. Although there is no literature to support this procedure, it makes sense on an intuitive level. Initially, participants tend to pick a friend or someone they already know. If the pairings remain static, learning may not be optimal as a set pattern of interaction may emerge. Also, if a particular pair proves to be less than functional, changing the makeup of the duo the next time minimizes the impact of that circumstance. A side benefit of requiring varied twosomes is that class or workshop members all get to know each other and a sense of camaraderie and group cohesiveness typically emerges.

Similarly, each time the author incorporates role play in a workshop or the classroom, at least two situations are enacted. If one person is the supervisor in one exchange, the other assumes this role in the second. This provides both participants an opportunity to practice specific skills and to experience the impact of the situation from the supervisee's viewpoint. This is particularly valuable when the trainee is trying to implement specific supervisory strategies. Because both participants are aware of the goal, the supervisee is able to provide very specific feedback to her or his partner.

Relationship of Roleplaying in Teaching Supervisory Skills to the Specified Supervision Tasks

Nine of the tasks listed at the outset of the chapter are those that may be impacted through role-play activities. Some may be addressed more directly than others. For example, conferences may be simulated to focus on the development of those skills necessary for establishing and maintaining an effective working relationship with supervisees, and discussing assessment and treatment in ways which facilitate supervisee problem-solving and growth. Regarding the interaction with clinicians to plan, execute, and analyze the supervisory process, the supervisor and supervisees might role-play a conference in which the supervisor implements different strategies during various segments. Then the supervisees may select the style they feel would benefit them most in future conferences. Two of the remaining tasks are clinically oriented within the context of supervision. They relate to issues such as supervisor demonstration and participation in the clinical process and the evaluation of clinical performance. In this regard, the supervisor and supervisee may role-play an aspect of treatment to provide the clinician with the opportunity to see or try alternative strategies and then assess the outcomes. Verbal reporting and aspects of professional and ethical conduct may be handled in a similar fashion. Thus, role-playing may be used as a tool to develop aspects of nine of the thirteen tasks of supervision.

Examples of Role-Playing

The role plays that follow relate to the ASHA supervision tasks (1985) cited above. They are not intended to be exhaustive but rather to serve as a stimulus for readers to develop others on their own. Additional role-play ideas may be gathered from the material in the section of the text devoted to simulation. The reader may choose to add, delete, or edit the examples provided. Further, additional concrete planning will need to occur prior to actual use. For example, decisions must be made about the goal for each role play, the make-up of the dyads, the implementation procedures, and the debriefing method. It will be important to encourage participants to assume the persona of the persons described in the role play and to respond as those individuals might. A judgment will also need to be made regarding the number of situations to be incorporated in an ongoing class or workshop. The role-play examples that follow will be clustered in regard to the specific supervisory task addressed.

Tasks 1, 3, 4, 5, 9

Task 1: Establishing and maintaining an effective working relationship with the supervisee;

Task 3: Assisting the supervisee in developing and refining assessment skills;

Task 4: Assisting the supervisee in developing and refining clinical management skills;

Task 5: Demonstrating for and participating with the supervisee in the clinical process;

Task 9: Assisting the supervisee in evaluation of clinical performance.

Role Play 1, Tasks 1 and 4. The supervisor, M. Green, is meeting for the second conference with S. Goodman, a clinician who has previously accrued one hundred clock hours of supervised practice. The supervisee wants specific suggestions on how to proceed with her/his ten-year-old language-delayed client. This clashes with the supervisor's preferred indirect supervisory style. When M. Green encourages him to generate the alternatives for the next therapy session, he becomes demanding and hostile.

Role Play 2, Tasks 1 and 9.   A first semester clinician, D. Armand, is doing excellent clinical work with her/his preschool hearing-impaired client. But, during conferences, s/he is overly critical of her/his own performance. In fact, s/he verbalizes that a "good" clinician should be judgmental about her/his own work. The supervisor, R. Smith, senses that the supervisee must become more realistic and confident in assessing her/his abilities.

Role Play 3, Task 1.   A clinician, L. Middleton, arrives late for a conference. The tone of her/his voice as well as her/her mannerisms convey the message that s/he would rather not be there at all. When treatment is broached, s/he becomes defensive, bordering on belligerent. Her/his client is an adult with aphasia.

Role Play 4, Tasks 1, 4, and 5.   A beginning clinician, R. Todd, has been seeing a client for four weeks. The child is consistently off-task. The clinician is upset and wants to change clients because of the lack of progress. S/he is feeling angry at the child because of his misbehavior. The supervisor, S. Williams, feels role-playing specific behavior management strategies might be helpful.

Role Play 5, Tasks 1, 3, and 5.   The supervisee, M. Jackson, has requested the supervisor, L. Andersen, demonstrate during her/his therapy session this week. The client is a head-injured adolescent exhibiting cognitive/reasoning deficits. The specific skills the supervisee would like demonstrated and procedures for assessing the outcomes of each of the approaches are the topic of discussion in the conference.

Role Play 6, Tasks 1, 3, and 5.   J. Sanders, the supervisor, is conferencing with J. Neff, whose work is average but disorganized. Although the clinician says s/he understands what has been discussed, it is clear s/he is not accurately processing the information. In particular, s/he is confused about test administration protocol and the scoring of the assessment data.

Role Play 7, Tasks 1 and 9.   You, G. Gomez, are supervising a clinician, P. Waters, who you feel is incompetent. P., in contrast, perceives her/himself as an outstanding clinician. The client involved is a severely language-impaired child with Down syndrome.

Role Play 8, Tasks 1, 4, and 9.   A clinician, S. Krousou, has worked at this facility for fifteen years. She continues to do therapy in the same manner as she was originally trained. The supervisor, T. Pisoni, feels that some of the techniques are questionable and, in particular, are outdated. Suggestions to try alternatives have been ignored. Some of S. Krousou's caseload, particularly those with closed-head injuries, are of serious concern to T. Pisoni.

Role Play 9, Task 1.   You, J. Levine, assumed a new supervisory position six months ago. You have just observed and are conferencing with F. Martinez, a staff clinician. F. is indicating to you that you couldn't possibly have anything to offer him/her. This is particularly true because F. has worked in this facility for twelve and a half years and has worked with this specific population for ten of those years.

Role Play 10, Tasks 1 and 9.   A clinician, S. Samuels, has been doing poor clinical work throughout the semester. Her/his performance has markedly deteriorated since midterm. Grades have been tabulated and s/he has failed practicum. S/he will not be receiving credit or clock hours for her/his work. The conference in which this information is to be discussed is ready to begin.

Role Play 11, Tasks 1, 3 and 9.   John, a third semester graduate student majoring in audiology, appears to arrive at decisions prematurely. For example, in threshold testing, he feels the first patient response is representative. Thus, he does not present stimuli again to check for consistency. He prides himself on completing diagnostic evaluations quickly. When these issues have been noted and he has been required to more thorough, he has become defensive and hostile. The conference to discuss these concerns is about to begin.

Task 10

Task 10: Assisting the supervisee in developing skills of verbal reporting, writing, and editing.

Role Play 12, Task 10.   A clinician, J. Smith, held an initial meeting with a patient's (Mr. Green) family to discuss the impact of his stroke on his ability to communicate. The family left the meeting confused. Some of the information presented by J. was too technical. Other data was highly appropriate but was given in a disorganized fashion. As a result, the family was unable to gather a clear picture of Mr. Green's problem and prognosis. You are meeting with J. to assess the content and outcome of the family conference and to discuss strategies to improve the clarity of J.'s information transmission.

Tasks 11 and 12

Task 11: Sharing information regarding ethical, legal, regulatory, and reimbursement aspects of professional practice;

Task 12: Modeling and facilitating professional conduct.

Role Play 13, Task 11.   B. C. Nelson has just come into your office. S/he is a beginning graduate student. S/he has been approached by a neighbor who has a language-delayed preschooler. S/he would like some ideas for treating this child in the parent's home.

Role Play 14, Task 11.   Material is being taken from the clinic and the clinician work area. One of the clinicians is suspected of stealing or borrowing the material without checking it out. During an observation, the supervisor, L. Nicodemus, sees one of her/his supervisees, G. Heinz, use items that have been missing for several weeks. G. Heinz is just arriving for her/his weekly conference.

Role Play 15, Tasks 11 and 12.   You are an ASHA certified speech-language pathologist contracting with a school district and provide service in several buildings. In talking with the speech-language pathology assistant at two different sites, you realize they are not getting the supervision specified by state licensure. Both assistants are seeing some students with no supervision at all. You are in a quandary about what to do ethically. You run into the primary speech-language pathology supervisor of the district as you are leaving for the day.

Role Play 16, Task 12.   A clinician, J. Cooper, is having a personality conflict with a current supervisor. S/he feels s/he may be failing clinic. S/he approaches R. Applegate, a previous supervisor, to solicit help in resolving the problem.

Role Play 17, Task 12.   M. Grant is seeing a patient who she suspects has a psychological disorder. Without asking her client, M. Grant has contacted her client's boss/employer. She did this to find out if there is a record of substance abuse, a referral for psychological counseling, or a clinical diagnosis in the client's personnel file. You are meeting with M. Grant to discuss the inappropriate contact she has made with her client's employer.

Role Play 18, Tasks 11 and 12.   Mrs. Ware, a parent, has arrived at your office. Her child is being seen in a hospital outpatient facility/local elementary school by B. Chambers. The parent is extremely unhappy with the services provided by B. Chambers. She wants you to assign a different speech-language pathologist to her child. Mrs. Ware has arrived unannounced, without an appointment.

Role Play 19, Task 12.   You are in your office waiting for the arrival of J. Smit. His/her work has continued to deteriorate. You have documented the problems and the implementation of the due-process intervention plan. His/her performance has not improved but has actually become worse. You are going to fire him/her. J. Smit has just arrived.

Task 8

Task 8: Interacting with the supervisee in planning, executing, and analyzing supervisory conferences.

Role Play 20, Task 8.   Supervisor S. Morgan and supervisee L. Grant have briefly discussed their last supervisory conference. The supervisee has asked the supervisor to increase the frequency of active listening in the conference. Unclear as to specifics, the supervisor has asked the supervisee to switch roles so that L. Grant may demonstrate the types of behaviors s/he feels will be more beneficial to her/him in future conferences. The discussion revolves around L.'s client, an adult who stutters.

Role Play 21, Task 8. MaryJane is an audiologist completing her clinical fellowship year. She has not had previous exposure to some of the test procedures in use at the hospital where she is employed. She requested a meeting with her supervisor, L. West, to discuss ways for her to gain the skills she needs to be successful. She also wants to talk to her supervisor about the way L. West gives feedback. Mary-Jane prefers a delay in the provision of valuative information, while L. West tends to give it on the spot. The conference is ready to begin.

Role-Playing Summary

It is hoped that the reader has enjoyed the material on role-playing. The situations presented are issues that arise in supervision and are ones likely to stimulate lively interaction. You are encouraged to use these role plays in your setting. The section that follows moves beyond the individual events used in role-playing to provide a cohesive, longer term, integrated tool for training supervisory skills. This segment begins with some introductory thoughts and information from the literature about simulation. It ends with a simulation game.

Simulation

Simulation is a strategy the author has used extensively to teach supervisory skills in a graduate clinical supervision course. It may also be implemented as a tool for fostering clinical development. For example, Diedrich and Driscoll (1987) state it may be utilized to develop cognitive, performative, and interpersonal skills prior to actual clinical involvement. Godden and Fey (1990) report using simulation to teach both clinical and supervisory skills. This tool may also be used in employment settings to develop either clinical or supervisory skills. Readers may wish to utilize this material in a supervision workshop or course.

Simulation: Literature

Teacher Education

Simulation is used in a variety of ways in teacher education. For example, it is suggested as a strategy to assist preservice teachers in developing realistic ideas about the teaching profession (Jesus and Paixao, 1996). It is implemented as a method to increase educators' awareness of their own cultural attitudes, thereby increasing their effectiveness with culturally diverse children in the classroom (Hinchcliff-Pelias and Elkins, 1995). Overbaugh (1995) reports designing an interactive video computer-aided simulation game to teach preservice teachers classroom management skills. Simulation is also being used as a tool to foster teaching skills in college teaching assistants (Goodlad, 1997).

A teacher training game and its effects are reported by Strang (1997). He summarizes research on the effects of the Curry Teaching Simulation. The computer-based simulation allows preservice teachers to interact with a classroom of children. The simulated children respond differently depending on the action of the teacher. The students' behaviors are designed to reinforce or punish targeted teacher behaviors. The method is found to be effective in building fundamental teaching behaviors such as giving feedback, managing behavior, and in facilitating accurate teacher self-evaluation. Regarding the latter, an important part of the simulation is the opportunity teachers have to compare their perceptions of their performance to an objective measure. Many are surprised that they have overestimated their skills. Of significance is the finding that gains made during the simulation are maintained when measured at a later time.

A multimedia simulation is in use in education for training educator observation skills (Fitzgerald, Nichols, and Semrau, 1998). This "Classroom Behavior Record Observation Training Program" is presented by videodisc containing both audio and video segments of children in the classroom and play groups. Participants using the system can control the speed of delivery of the segments and are provided feedback about their performance. Data indicate the simulated training is efficient and effective. Fitzgerald and colleagues feel that instructional design, authenticity of materials, and ability to provide learner-controlled instruction are critical components contributing to the effectiveness of the program.

McQuillen and Ivy (1986) discuss the use of simulation in the educational process. They feel experience with "real life" situations provides students an opportunity to use and assess new behaviors and skills. These occasions also bridge the gap between cognitive understanding and application. Because constituents report enjoying this process, it is also thought to increase motivation. Finally, a key advantage of gaming for individuals is the vicarious learning that occurs from observing the experiences of the other participants.

Health Care Education

Isaacs, Embry, and Baer (1982) implement a training program with a simulation aspect to teach family therapists to guide parents in carrying out compliance management with their preschool children. In nursing, a self-paced simulated laboratory is used to update clinical skills (Wood, 1994). In nursing, simulation is shown to enhance students' abilities to collect data and make clinical judgments. It also makes them aware of their biases in decision making (Weber, 1994).

Barak (1990) examines the acquisition of empathic understanding in nine beginning graduate students in counseling psychology. These subjects participate in a simulation called the Empathy Game. In groups of three, they read a statement from a "client." Their task is to understand the feelings, thoughts, and needs of the writer of the statement. One person from each subgroup then reads the "client's" comments while portraying appropriate nonverbal behavior for the "client" to the members of the other two groups. The viewers' task is to ask questions of the reader to further increase their understanding of that individual. The final step for the viewers is to complete a multiple-choice instrument describing their impressions of the "client." Barak (1990) finds that participants significantly increase their levels of empathic understanding, and use these skills in written, simulated client–counselor verbal interactions. In sum, he feels simulation is an appropriate methodology for teaching specific clinical skills to trainees.

Mosher-Ashley (1995) suggests caution when considering the impact of geriatric training simulations in altering persons' views of the elderly. She reports that participants find the simulation process enjoyable but questions whether persons learn more than they do from didactic instruction. Her work reviews the literature in gerontological education. Her primary point is that the research that has been done has not been adequately controlled or designed to legitimately answer the question.

Rieke and Curtis (1981) examine the effects of simulation training in an academic setting on later job performance. They find that, for school psychologists, behavior exhibited during a simulation is highly predictive of later work implementation. Thus, skills learned through gaming can be expected to emerge in real work situations.

Business Applications

Jacobs and Baum (1987) review the literature concerning simulations in corporate training and development environments. They state these games are experiential in nature and are an appropriate application of adult learning theory. In addition, they report that these strategies are performance oriented because individuals have the opportunity to observe others, to practice a skill, and to receive immediate feedback. They indicate both experimentation and creativity are encouraged in a flexible, low-risk environment. Tarnopolsky (1998) suggests that instead of using a preset simulation, business students benefit from being allowed to shape the content and processes used in the simulation while addressing specific course topics. He reports the dynamic nature of the task is highly motivating to participants.

Consistent with these views, Thornton and Cleveland (1990) discuss the varied use of simulation in developing managerial skills. They describe three primary uses of managerial gaming: (1) research, (2) assessment and diagnosis, and (3) training. Observing managers in a simulated activity/setting allows for an analysis of the process and a determination of individual adeptness. Performances below optimum are directly targeted for improvement through simulations designed to teach specific skills.

The Synthetic Economy for Analysis and Simulation (SEAS) project is a sophisticated game allowing participants to participate in large-scale economic experiments (Chaturvedi and Mehta, 1999). Dealing with stock, bonds, labor, and money markets are the tasks of the participants. The game changes depending on the actions of the players. As a result, they gain an understanding of the economic process and the impact of their behavior. It also allows them opportunities to explore the effects of taking certain actions. Debriefing is an important part of this process because their insights grow by reviewing their performances and analyzing different aspects of their decision making and the related effectiveness.

In summary, simulation games are identified as a strategy to teach behavior, provide immediate feedback, and modify attitudes. It is found to provide a realistic teacher-training environment and a format for instructing health-care professionals. In business, it is used to train managers. Simulations give participants an opportunity to expand their viewpoints by experiencing a new job or event. The participants broaden their perspectives and learn as a result of their and others' experiences. Skills gained during gaming are found to be retained and later transferred to real-life work situations. The complexity of simulations varies. With advances in technology, computerized simulations with branching capabilities are emerging along with those that are multimedia and interactive.

Relationship of the Use of Simulation to the Specified Supervision Tasks

At the outset of the chapter, eleven of the thirteen tasks of supervision were identified as relevant to the use of simulation in supervisory training. Specific foils may be designed to teach each of the tasks, even the two that are excluded, numbers five and thirteen. Four of the remaining tasks may be fostered with simulation, although other methods are likely to be more efficient for these particular items: (1) assisting the supervisee in the development and maintenance of clinical and supervisory records, (2) interacting with the supervisee in planning, executing, and analyzing supervisory conferences, (3) assisting the supervisee in developing skills of verbal reporting, writing, and editing, and (4) sharing information regarding ethical, legal, regulatory, and reimbursement aspects of professional practice.

For those tasks remaining, simulation may be readily used to directly teach components of each. In particular, issues relating to the establishment and maintenance of an effective working relationship often emerge in regard to the supervisee who is openly hostile or is interacting less than optimally in the conference. Similarly, the refinement of clinical objectives, rather than the initial development, is often a topic of discussion with a supervisee who is struggling or is having difficulty controlling task difficulty in therapy. The development and refinement of assessment skills may emerge relative to issues regarding patient dismissal or in regard to the establishment of goals grounded in accurate, complete data. The development and refinement of treatment skills as well as the ability to collect and analyze data are at the heart of supervisory conferences and thus, are likely to occur frequently in simulated exchanges. In addition, numerous opportunities occur, particularly in regard to data collection and analysis, to assist the supervisee in analyzing professional performance. The modeling and facilitating of professional conduct is likely to be directly considered in a supervision simulation game as the need to deal with events or actions reflecting inappropriate professional conduct arise. In sum, eleven of the thirteen tasks of supervision may be appropriately addressed with simulation activities.

Simulation Game

The remainder of this chapter is a supervisory training simulation game. This exercise is designed to provide "on the job" experience for participants. The issues and circumstances presented parallel the real-world work environment. It is this writer's feeling that the assumption of the supervisory role causes individuals to think about the process and to develop the attitudes and a portion of the skills necessary to function proficiently. Individuals often approach situations in the game with the strategy they personally would take. These persons see the array of options available in a given circumstance through discussion of the situations and the likely outcomes with others. The intent of this game is to increase the participants' repertoire of responses. It is further hoped that when these persons become supervisors, they will, as a result of this experience, be able to avoid obvious pitfalls, define their role, and actively negotiate responsibilities.

This material is intended for use with a class or as a supplement to a series of workshops. After the participants read the orientation and review the simulation example, they are to select, as a unit, two work environments as the focus for the game. Once this has been completed, each individual is expected to respond to the events for the first section independently. Each person's task is to generate the responses that will be described more completely in the orientation section. A specific due date for each segment of the simulation will also need to be assigned. On the day the material is to be submitted, the group will meet to discuss the range of issues and options for each of the presented cases. During this exchange, the group leader may opt to identify the array of acceptable outcomes or guide the participants to arrive at a decision. As this activity is intended to increase critical thinking and to broaden the participants' viewpoints and ranges of experience, the goal is not necessarily consensus. It is important for participants to understand there isn't a right or wrong answer. The underlying issues and varying perspectives are intended to be brought to light. The leader's task is to actively encourage each person's contribution to the discussion and to invite diversity of thought.

At the completion of the discussion, the written materials independently prepared in response to the simulation may be submitted for review. This is true if it is to constitute a portion of a course grade or serve as a required component of a workshop. Procedurally, participants should be limited to the simulation segment being addressed at the time and should be discouraged from perusing the events that occur in a later segment such as Winter and/or Spring. The basic procedure of completing the work independently, then meeting as a group to discuss the events, and, when appropriate, submitting the written material for evaluation is the same for each of the three simulation segments.

Simulation Orientation

To: Chris (Christine/Christopher) Green

You have accepted a highly competitive and unusual supervisory position. It is in the metropolitan Matador area. It is a joint appointment with the participant selecting two of three work environments: the Matador Public Schools, Matador University, or the Matador Trauma and Rehabilitation Hospital/Matador House. You are the supervisor of Speech Pathology and Audiology Services if you select the Matador Public Schools or the Matador Trauma and Rehabilitation Hospital/Matador House. In both of these settings, you will discover that you are the first person to be given this title in this setting. At Matador University, you are a part-time supervisor reporting to the Coordinator of Clinical Services. Your position at each of the two selected facilities is half-time. Thus, your schedule is negotiated as needed.

You hold dual certification (CCC-SLP and CCC-A) from the American Speech-Language and Hearing Association in the areas of Speech-Language Pathology and Audiology. Although you are dually certified, your focus has been predominantly Speech-Language Pathology. You have outstanding clinical skills and have completed an academic course and a practicum in supervision. You are somewhat nervous about the positions you have accepted but are confident that you will do well.

The year has started smoothly. You are spending all day Monday and Friday as well as Wednesday mornings at one facility and the remaining time at the other. If you select the Matador Public schools, your staff members have completed all preliminary testing and are about to initiate treatment. At Matador University, the clinical program is just about to begin and at the Matador Trauma and Rehabilitation Hospital/Matador House, the ongoing program is at the beginning of the fiscal year. The time period covered in the simulation exercise is nine to twelve months: Set A focuses on issues likely to occur initially, and then the issues in sets B and C emerge as the year progresses.

The sections that follow will be a series of situations that you, as Chris Green, must handle. The circumstance may or may not suggest or require a response. You should determine whether you feel action is appropriate, and if so, what type. You may choose to respond by writing a letter, memo, or by making a note to yourself that could be used in a discussion or phone conversation. You may also choose to analyze the letters, memos, and phone calls for their communicative effectiveness. If you decide to do so, determine if the form, style, and tone are appropriate given the situation. You might also outline the alterations needed to focus and increase the impact of these messages.

For each situation, identify the issues involved and generate as many alternatives as possible for each problem. Some of the issues are obvious while others may be hidden agendas. For each issue identified, be sure to have at least one option for action. Then, identify the one(s) you feel is optimal given the circumstance. Thoroughness in considering the range of alternatives is critical to success with this material. A broad array of options is more important than the conclusion reached.

Each situation has a code in the upper right hand corner, for example, (Fall, S1, Sch). This translates to outset, event 1, public schools. "Univ" equals university and "Hosp," hospital. In responding to each, your response should contain: (1) the coded identifier, (2) a list of the possible issues, (3) the array of potential options for dealing with the issues, (4) an identification of the optimal choice and your logic for making this decision. Also include the nature of the action taken, such as a memo or phone call and the persons involved. An example of a solution follows for the first school simulation. See page 352.

Example of Response

Fall, S1, Sch.

Issues:

1. Did you tell Ms. Candry not to take playground duty?

2. Should the speech pathologist assume playground duties and attend staff meetings at each school on his/her caseload?

3. What is the procedure to establish district policy?

4. Is Chris Green really out-of-line?

5. Can Stan Smith override Green's decisions?

6. How much autonomy does Chris Green have in terms of job description and responsibilities?

7. What is the chain of command re: building principals, the supervisor of speech-language services, and the director of special education?

Options:

1. Tell Ms. Williamson to assume playground duties and attend staff meetings at all buildings.

2. Stand firm on the issue and take the steps necessary to establish district wide policy on the duties of speech pathologists.
   a. Do extensive public relations with the building principals and staff members;
   b. Clarify the tasks of the speech pathologist, indicating children are not being served as extensively as possible due to caseload size;
   c. Share information about the types of reports and paperwork needed in order to do a good job as a speech pathologist;

   d. Point out that playground time prevents children from being diagnosed and treated;

   e. Each speech pathologist also needs to actively promote his/her program in the building;

   f. The speech pathologist also must let others know she serves other buildings during the times she is absent from a given school;

   g. The speech pathologist should not be seen wasting time or taking frequent breaks in the teachers' lounge.

   3. For public relations purpose, the speech pathologist should attend faculty meetings and assume limited outside responsibilities at the home school.

   4. Call Ms. Williamson and tell her she should have contacted Chris directly and state one of the above positions.

   5. Call or drop by to see Stan Smith.

   a. Collect information about his perceptions of the situation and go along with whatever he says;

   b. Present your point of view for discussion and request his support in this decision and express that you expect him to trust your judgment in the future;

   c. Set up a time when you can discuss your role, responsibilities, and authority.

   6. Have Stan Smith return the call to Ms. Williamson to resolve the problem based on the outcome of the above meeting between Stan Smith and Chris Green.

   7. If Chris Green did not tell Ms. Candry to refuse playground duty, call or see Ms. Candry to point out the problem this has caused and to make it clear that it should not recur.

Solution(s):

The participant would select the option(s) s/he thinks would be most effective. A brief statement of the logic behind the decision(s) would also be included.

Cast of Characters

The following is a partial list of professionals at the Matador Independent School District, Matador University, and the Matador Trauma and Rehabilitation Hospital/Matador House. The latter is a long-term care facility affiliated with the hospital. Other professionals are involved at each facility, but only those having direct contact with Chris Green during the simulations will be included.

Matador Independent School District

   Stanley Smith—Director of Special Education

   Chris Green—Supervisor of Speech-Language Pathology Services

   Diedra Williamson—Principal of Dupree Elementary School

Russell Smith—Principal at Westside Elementary and High School

Jim Waters—Principal of North Oaks Elementary School

Melissa Santee—Speech-Language Pathologist at North Oaks and White Oaks Elementary School

Vanessa Candry—Speech-Language Pathologist at Dupree Elementary and Whitehall Elementary School

Tom Litton—Speech-Language Pathologist at Eastside Elementary School

Marge Lopez—Speech-Language Pathologist at Waterloo Elementary and Granville Elementary School

Linda Verlinde—Speech-Language Pathologist at Westside Elementary and High School

Arnold Ramirez—Speech-Language Pathology Assistant

Matador University

Sandra Renault—Coordinator of Clinical Services

Chris Green—Half-time Supervisor of Speech and Language Services

Martha Writley—Supervisor of Speech and Language Services

Student Trainee Speech-Language Pathologists

   Margarite Bradley—Graduate Student

   Randy Linwood—Graduate Student

   Ron Sanders—Graduate Student

   Mary Ann Rossi—Undergraduate Student

   Renee Williams—Undergraduate Student

Matador Trauma and Rehabilitation Hospital/Matador House

Herbert Gilke—Chairman of the Board

Robert Marganti—Director of Rehabilitation Services

Dr. Carmen White—Neurologist

Chris Green—Supervisor of Speech Pathology and Audiology Services

Ramona Galvez—Supervisor of Nursing

Bettye Snider—Speech-Language Pathologist

Reginald Smith—Audiologist

Frank Miller—Speech-Language Pathologist

Jo McKay—Speech-Language Pathologist

Prabha Patel—Speech-Language Pathologist

Melinda Wright-Speech-Language Pathologist (CFY)

Vo Tran—Speech-Language Pathology Assistant

Simulation: Fall

MATADOR INDEPENDENT SCHOOL DISTRICT

MEMORANDUM

From: Stanley Smith, Director of Special Education

To: Chris Green

I had planned to call you today but realized you would be out of the office until Friday. It's important so I wanted to get this to you as soon as possible.

Diedra Williamson, building principal at Dupree Elementary School, called me. One of your staff members, Vanessa Candry, provides speech pathology services at that school. Ms. Candry is refusing to take noon playground duty, supposedly as you directed. This is creating quite a flap among the other teachers. They already feel Ms. Candry receives special treatment in that she is only there for three hours twice a week, sees only 30 children, and then in such small groups. She doesn't attend building staff meetings, etc.

Ms. Williamson feels you have no business interfering in her building. I told Ms. Williamson I would get back to her. I feel you may have been out-of-line here. This needs to be resolved. Contact me immediately.

MATADOR INDEPENDENT SCHOOL DISTRICT

MEMORANDUM

From: Stanley Smith, Director of Special Education

To: Chris Green

I just returned from a conference for Special Education Directors. Speech-language pathology assistants are being employed at several school districts. Is having an assistant viable here? I heard that it really saves money and it makes it possible to provide service to a lot more children. You know the budgetary pressure we are under. Maybe this would be a solution. Let's talk about it when we meet on Monday.

MATADOR INDEPENDENT SCHOOL DISTRICT

Dear Chris,

I have some information or maybe a problem to share with you. I'm so glad to finally have someone to whom to direct these irritants. As you know, I provide speech and language services on the westside. I'm having continual petty problems at Westside Elementary and High School. They are little things but are starting to get me down.

Mr. Russell Smith is the principal at both of these schools. I've spoken with him about the problems below but have gotten nowhere. I'd appreciate your assistance in resolving these issues.

The amount of available supplies such as paper, paper clips, stationary, dittos, and construction paper is extremely limited. I'm finding a need to supplement these materials at my own expense, which I don't feel is appropriate. The proportion of supplies I receive seems to be much less than those of the other teachers.

Mr. Smith feels it is inappropriate for me to contact parents more than the minimal amount spelled out in the rules and regulations for children receiving special services. In addition, I am required to get a signed approval from him before calling parents or making home visits. This seems to be unreasonably restrictive. I feel it is hurting the quality of the services I provide.

The other problem is at Westside High School. The pass system is driving me crazy. Time I spend writing hall passes for students to return to class could be devoted to much better use. Mr. Smith just won't bend on this issue.

I'd appreciate your assistance as soon as possible.

Yours truly,
Linda Verlinde

MATADOR INDEPENDENT SCHOOL DISTRICT

MEMORANDUM

From: Stanley Smith, Director of Special Education

To: Chris Green

Tom Litton, the speech pathologist on the eastside dropped by today. He indicated you were out and observed him during therapy on three different occasions last week. He said he didn't mind your coming by to observe but was somewhat surprised and apparently irritated when you suggested ways he might change therapy.

This brings up something I have been meaning to discuss with you. When you were hired and during your interview, we both knew that this supervisory position had just been created and as a result was ambiguous. The need for a supervisor evolved from a need to coordinate forms and procedures. I do recall that during the interview, you indicated a desire to provide guidance for the staff that seemed, at the time, like a good idea. Now that you are settled in, we need to talk more specifically about your job and the associated responsibilities. Jot down some ideas and let's plan to talk sometime Monday.

♦   ♦   ♦   ♦

MATADOR UNIVERSITY

MEMORANDUM

From: Sandra Renault, Coordinator of Clinical Services

To: Chris Green

Welcome aboard Chris! There is a schedule for your clinical supervision this semester in your mailbox. Tentatively, you are scheduled with fifteen clinician–client pairs. Most of the clinicians have more than one client so you will actually be supervising about eight students. As I told you before, I am particularly excited that you have had some supervisory training.

In a nutshell, the department's philosophy toward our supervisory staff is a very good one. Our supervisors are highly competent and, as such, have a substantial amount of freedom as to supervisory methodology, approaches to therapy, etc. We do ask that you observe students a minimum of one out of every four therapy sessions and have a standing conference time with each of them on a weekly basis.

If there is any way I may help you, please let me know.

MATADOR UNIVERSITY

MEMORANDUM

From: Chris Green

To: Chris Green

Ron Sanders, a graduate clinician in his third term of therapy, just left following our first conference. He will be working with Tim Way, an eight-year-old who stutters. After reading Tim's file, Ron is convinced that Tim wouldn't stutter if it weren't for his parents. He cites marital problems, an older brother with an IQ of 150, and the parents' desire for upward mobility as causative and maintaining factors in the stuttering behavior.

Ron is thoroughly convinced and not as open-minded as I would like. He wants to have a parent conference after the first week. Ron and I agreed on two points: to discuss the advisability and content of a parent consultation during our conference next week, and to finalize initial treatment procedures.

MATADOR UNIVERSITY

MEMORANDUM

From: Chris Green

To: Chris Green

Renee Williams, a beginning clinician, just left my office. She has been assigned an articulation client and an adult who stutters who is at the carryover stage. She has had coursework in both areas but doesn't feel she knows where to begin therapy. The clients will all be in on Monday. After some probing, I felt she had the basic knowledge to decide where to initiate treatment.

When I refused to outline a plan for her, she became angry and demanded that I, as the supervisor, tell her what to do. I suggested a couple of articles for her to read. At that point, she stomped out of my office. She will be back for her regular conference tomorrow. What strategy should I take?

MATADOR UNIVERSITY

MEMORANDUM

From: Sandra Renault, Coordinator of Clinical Services

To: Faculty and Staff Members

We have had a wave of referrals for two-, three-, and four-year-old children who were "crack" babies. This population is underserved in the Matador metropolitan area. Is it an area that we want to move into? It will be an agenda item for the staff meeting on Monday. Consider the following in preparation for that discussion:

1. Can we serve this group effectively?
2. What additional training will students need?
3. What types of staff in-services would be appropriate?
4. Are there unique support services, equipment, and/or materials required if this population is targeted by our facility?
5. Will these children be good "training" cases for our students?

♦   ♦   ♦   ♦

MATADOR TRAUMA AND REHABILITATION HOSPITAL/MATADOR HOUSE

MEMORANDUM

From: Bob Marganti, Director of Rehabilitation Services

To: Chris Green

When you interviewed for the supervisor position we indirectly talked about the assets and liabilities of the department you are heading up. Now that you are in place, we need to talk further. Let's meet sometime early this week. I'd like you to be thinking about the following:

1. A strategy to smooth out and increase the efficiency of treatment scheduling for patients.
2. A way to increase the visibility of your department and possibly to develop a greater range of services.
3. The apparent friction among three staff members: Bettye Snider (Speech Pathologist), Reginald Smith (Audiologist), and Ramona Galvez (Nursing supervisor).
4. How you will deal with Reginald Smith because he feels he should have been named supervisor instead of having you brought in from the outside.
5. How to respond to the budgetary crunch we are experiencing.

MATADOR TRAUMA AND REHABILITATION HOSPITAL/MATADOR HOUSE

Subject: Phone Call

From: Jo McKay

To: Chris Green

Jo just called and won't be in due to a family emergency. She has a stroke patient intake evaluation scheduled at 8:30 and 7 other patients to see. She said her case file notes for patient Jones, the subject of today's rounds, are on her desk. She indicated the data may need to be supplemented since she was under the weather on Friday and wasn't thinking clearly at the time. She was sure she would have had time to complete the evaluation and round out the notes this morning. She apologized for not being able to come in.

MATADOR TRAUMA AND REHABILITATION HOSPITAL/MATADOR HOUSE

MEMORANDUM

From: Chris Green

To: Chris Green

After reviewing personnel, caseloads, past scheduling, and service delivery, the following impressions emerge:

1. Staffing levels are adequate.
2. Each person schedules his/her own patients and caseloads stay relatively constant. The exception is Frank Miller, who appears overloaded. Jo McKay's patient contact looks like it has been down for the last two months. Reason?
3. All staff members hold the certificate of clinical competence, except Melinda Wright, who is completing her CFY. The majority of the staff members have been on staff for 2 to 3 years.
4. Three speech-language pathologists serve Matador House, a long-term care facility.
5. A speech-language pathology assistant is a new staff member.
6. The patient load is primarily post-stroke and head-injured patients. A few patients have had laryngectomies and a limited number of children are seen through the pediatric division.
7. The hospital is a nonprofit agency but extreme pressure is put on individual departments to be self-supporting and to offset the total hospital deficit. A financial crisis surfaced during the year due to a drop in patient load, changes in insurance reimbursement, and medicare variability. Layoffs may be looming.

Fall, H4, Hosp.

MATADOR TRAUMA AND REHABILITATION HOSPITAL/MATADOR HOUSE

Subject: Phone call

From: Ms. Reba Smith, parent of Joshua Smith

To: Chris Green

Ms. Smith just called and said she needed to speak to her speech-language pathologist, Vo Tran. She has been thinking about Ms. Tran's recommendation to have Joshua seen by an acupuncturist to help him control his temper outbursts. She still has a few questions that she needs answered and she would like a recommendation for a person who does acupuncture.

Fall, H5, Hosp.

MATADOR TRAUMA AND REHABILITATION HOSPITAL/MATADOR HOUSE

MEMORANDUM

From: Chris Green

To: Chris Green

Vo Tran is a speech-language pathology assistant. Vo has not discussed the idea of using acupuncture or her rationale for doing so with you. Acupuncture is not in the patient's treatment plan.

Fall, H6, Hosp.

MATADOR TRAUMA AND REHABILITATION HOSPITAL/MATADOR HOUSE

MEMORANDUM

From: Ramona Galvez, Nursing Supervisor

To: Chris Green

Chris, see me as soon as possible. Bettye Snider has created havoc in my department again. John Cooper, an adult with aphasia, was scheduled for physical therapy at two today. Bettye insisted on seeing him, so he missed physical therapy. When one of my nurses tried to work out the problem, Bettye tore into her. She also told the same nurse to leave when she came in to deliver medication and to change his soiled bedding. There is a limit. We are short three nurses on this shift and are having trouble covering as it is without continuous interference from Bettye. She also expects us to do tongue and swallowing exercises with Mr. Cooper before meals. Give me a break!

Simulation: Winter

MATADOR INDEPENDENT SCHOOL DISTRICT

MEMORANDUM

From: Stan Smith

To: Chris Green

Chris, I wanted to tell you what a fine job you are doing. From the feedback I'm getting, your in-service workshop for the building principals was a success. They are telling me that for the first time they are beginning to really see the ways in which speech pathologists can facilitate their programs. I thought you would like to know that Diedra Williamson called me. She is sorry about the run-in you two had in the fall. She feels that you are an asset to the school system. Well done, Chris.

MATADOR INDEPENDENT SCHOOL DISTRICT

MEMORANDUM

From: Chris Green

To: Chris Green

Vanessa Candry, the speech pathologist at Whitehall Elementary School, has contacted me in relation to a problem that has come up. Sandy Osborn, a severely mentally retarded child, has been on Vanessa's caseload for over three years. The child has not made any gains in approximately six months. Vanessa feels that Sandy has achieved her potential. She has decided to dismiss Sandy from treatment and feels strongly about it. Sandy's parents are angry and want speech pathology services continued. They have indicated that they will sue the school system if services are not provided.

MATADOR INDEPENDENT SCHOOL DISTRICT

MEMORANDUM

From: Chris Green

To: Chris Green

A problem has repeatedly arisen during your bimonthly staff meetings. There are two highly vocal clinicians on your staff. Independent of the issue, they tend to end up on opposing sides during discussions. As a result, meetings have essentially been nonproductive because it is difficult to remain on-task or to get any type of agreement. The remaining clinicians are getting annoyed and are beginning to feel staff meetings are a waste of time.

MATADOR INDEPENDENT SCHOOL DISTRICT

MEMORANDUM

Subject: Phone Calls

From: Martha Mitchell's Mother
Tom Widner's Mother

To: Chris Green

Both parents have called to tell you how pleased they are with the speech and language services being provided to their children by Linda Verlinde at Westside Elementary School.

Winter, S5, Sch.

MATADOR INDEPENDENT SCHOOL DISTRICT

MEMORANDUM

Subject: Phone call

From: Marge Lopez

To: Chris Green

Marge Lopez, the speech pathologist at Waterloo and Granville Elementary Schools, has just called. She indicated that she has reached the limits of her patience. The only place available to her at Waterloo Elementary School is the hall outside the lunch room. The school is large and lunch periods are staggered over a two-hour period, so there is not only traffic in and out of the lunchroom, but also a constant barrage of noise. She is beginning to feel that her therapy is a waste of time.

Winter, S6, Sch.

MATADOR INDEPENDENT SCHOOL DISTRICT

MEMORANDUM

From: Arnold Ramirez
          Speech-language pathology assistant
          Westside Elementary School

To: Chris Green

When I was hired, it was agreed that both you and Linda Verlinde would be my supervisors. In general, that is working out ok, but I am frustrated and need to talk to you. Russell Smith, the building principal, has come to me three times this week and told me to fill in for classroom teachers who need to be away from their rooms for an hour or so. Last week, they couldn't find a substitute for a first-grade teacher so I was told to take the class for the day. Linda was always busy when this happened and was of no help. Also Linda was out sick two days last week and was angry that I met with a parent who insisted on seeing the speech-language pathologist. This position isn't working out like I thought it would. When can we meet?

◆ ◆ ◆ ◆

MATADOR UNIVERSITY

MEMORANDUM

From: Chris Green

To: Chris Green

Randy Linwood is a first-term graduate student working with a voice client. He also sees a child with an articulation disorder. He is demonstrating the potential to become an excellent clinician. He tends to plan thoroughly and appears to give treatment a great deal of thought. Because he thinks through his approaches, he tends to feel that he consistently arrives at the right decision. At times, he does not. I specifically told him to change his voice production technique. When I observed the last two sessions, he had not. In conferences, he doesn't argue with me but his nonverbal reactions tell me that he is rejecting my suggestions on the spot. His weekly conference is today at three.

MATADOR UNIVERSITY

MEMORANDUM

From: Chris Green

To: Chris Green

Ron Sanders, a graduate clinician in his third term of therapy, has been working with Tim Way, an eight-year-old stutterer, for about five weeks. Ron feels that Tim's stuttering is largely related to Tim's family, Although Ron has not conferenced with Mr. and Mrs. Way, he has, in less than subtle ways, communicated his feelings to Tim's parents.

Mr. and Mrs. Way have just arrived at my office. They initiated the conference by saying that if Ron Sanders continues to see Tim, they are going to seek services elsewhere. They feel that Ron has no right or training to probe into their personal lives. They sincerely want to help Tim and are willing, within reasonable limits, to do anything to help him. They are angry and are seeking your advice.

MATADOR UNIVERSITY

MEMORANDUM

From: Chris Green

To: Chris Green

Mary Ann Rossi is near completion of her bachelor's degree. This is the fifth week of the term. Mary Ann is working with a client with a moderate articulation disorder and a language client who, at times, is a behavior problem. There is no logic to her treatment program. Although we jointly outlined client objectives and possible procedures, there is no continuity to her work. From observing her therapy, I cannot discern her objectives or the purpose of her activities. She does have excellent client behavior management skills.

MATADOR UNIVERSITY

MEMORANDUM

From: Chris Green

To: Chris Green

Chris, you are in your office at Matador when a student who is doing therapy during the time you usually observe, but is not your supervisee, comes to your door. Margarite Bradley, a graduate student, is telling you that she is having a problem with her supervisor. Her supervisor is Martha Writley, a full-time supervisor at Matador. Margarite feels that she is being graded unfairly and that the supervisor is suggesting and insisting on treatment techniques that are inappropriate.

◆   ◆   ◆   ◆

Winter, H1, Hosp.

MATADOR TRAUMA AND REHABILITATION HOSPITAL/MATADOR HOUSE

MEMORANDUM

From: Chris Green

To: Chris Green

I observed Jo McKay twice this week. On Monday, her therapy was well organized and her control of task difficulty appeared to be excellent. Mr. Jones worked hard and appeared to be making progress. Today, everything fell apart. Jo went through the motions but it was obvious she hadn't given it much thought. She was disorganized and at one point snapped at Mr. Jones when he couldn't figure out what she wanted him to do.

Winter, H2, Hosp.

MATADOR TRAUMA AND REHABILITATION HOSPITAL/MATADOR HOUSE

MEMORANDUM

From: Bob Marganti, Director of Rehabilitation Services

To: Chris Green

I have just reviewed your staff evaluations and recommendations for salary increments. With the exception of McKay, you make them all sound like they can walk on water. Chris, I know you have a good group of people but you are going to need to come up with a way to distinguish among them. The kinds of dollars you are requesting just aren't there. Even if they were, I would be reluctant to approve such glowing across-the-board evaluations. You realize your credibility is at stake here. Unfortunately, it is looking more and more like a major layoff is coming. Think about which of your staff members is expendable if revenues continue to drop. If you have a choice between no raise, pay cuts, or layoffs, where will you stand?

Winter, H3, Hosp.

MATADOR TRAUMA AND REHABILITATION HOSPITAL/MATADOR HOUSE

Subject: Phone Call

From: Bob Marganti, Director of Rehabilitation Services

To: Chris Green

Mrs. Peterson died last month in the Rehabilitation unit. She was six months post-stroke. She had dysphagia and a swallowing workup was done. Subsequently, when she was positioned incorrectly, the bolus of food or liquid by-passed the trachea and entered the esophagus. She died from pneumonia. The family is suing because it appears she aspirated fluids and apparently some solids as well. They claim negligence and wrongful death.

In talking to Ramona Galvez, the Nursing supervisor, Melinda Wright told the duty nurses that Mrs. Peterson was better so the nurses didn't need to continue adjusting her body position before feeding. Was that a mistake? Apparently, the lung fluid buildup was rapid and fatal. The nurses weren't aware she was having a problem until an hour before she expired.

We need to discuss this as soon as possible. Tell your staff members to keep a lid on it.

Winter, H4, Hosp.

MATADOR TRAUMA AND REHABILITATION HOSPITAL/MATADOR HOUSE

MEMORANDUM

From: Herbert Gilke, Chairman of the Board

To: Chris Green

Congratulations! The Westmoreland family has donated $10,000 to be used for equipment, materials, and staff development in the speech pathology and audiology department. Their son has fully recovered from the head injury that resulted from his motorcycle accident. They felt Frank Miller was instrumental in his language recovery.

MATADOR TRAUMA AND REHABILITATION HOSPITAL/MATADOR HOUSE

MEMORANDUM

From: Robert Marganti, Director of Rehabilitation Services

To: Chris Green

The decision to add the speech-language pathology assistant was a good one. Several people tell me Vo Tran is a real asset to the department. I'd like to see her have more responsibility without it taking up more of your time. With all of the funding issues limiting services, is there any way we can use Tran to further maximize services? I was thinking it may be possible to lay off one of the full-time staff and have Ms. Tran pick up the slack. Let's talk later this week.

MATADOR TRAUMA AND REHABILITATION HOSPITAL/MATADOR HOUSE

MEMORANDUM

From: Chris Green

To: Chris Green

The biweekly meeting of my staff members was yesterday afternoon. Reginald Smith, the audiologist, made numerous comments to Melinda Wright, Frank Miller, and Jo McKay who were sitting near him. From their embarrassed reaction, I'm sure he was sniping at me. I am getting concerned that the team isn't pulling together as well as I thought it would. They all, with the exception of Melinda Wright, react when I come in to observe. Frank Miller actually bristled last week when I shared the data I had collected while observing his session.

Simulation: Spring

MATADOR INDEPENDENT SCHOOL DISTRICT

MEMORANDUM

From: Stan Smith

To: Chris Green

I just received a packet of information from Jim Waters, principal of North Oaks Elementary School. A note is attached stating that he will call on Friday. Melissa Santee is the speech pathologist in that school. She is itinerant but is in that building three days a week.

The packet of information is related to Ms. Santee's performance. According to Jim Waters, Ms. Santee has been absent twenty days, with the absences always occurring on Monday or Friday. On five of those occasions, she did not call to indicate that she would not be in the office that day. She sporadically cancels one or two hours of treatment by sending a note to teachers saying she will not be seeing specific children that day. There is no evidence that she does anything constructive during these times.

In addition, petty cash kept in the special education area has disappeared. Mr. Waters feels she may be responsible. Mr. Waters wants her contract terminated.

MATADOR INDEPENDENT SCHOOL DISTRICT

MEMORANDUM

From: Chris Green

To: Chris Green

Melissa Santee is completing her second year in the school system. Her personnel records contain excellent references although they are training experience recommendations. As this is her first job, there are none from previous employers. My contact with Melissa Santee has been limited to general staff meetings and one brief observation. She is enthusiastic and appears competent.

MATADOR INDEPENDENT SCHOOL DISTRICT

Dear Chris,

After the last staff meeting, several of us got together to talk about services for the hearing-impaired children who will be transferred to our buildings next year. We are all uneasy because of the limited experience we have had with this population. I'm the only one who has had any course work in this area and it was a long time ago. Can you be of assistance? We will probably need new equipment and materials once we identify a basic strategy for dealing with these children. Help!

Yours truly,
Vanessa Candry

MATADOR INDEPENDENT SCHOOL DISTRICT

Subject: Phone Call

From: Stan Smith

To: Chris Green

Stan has just received a memo from Russell Smith, principal of Westside Elementary and High School. As a result of your meeting with the principals, Mr. Smith feels he better understands your job responsibilities. He recalls that you said you would be evaluating the speech pathologists in all buildings. He has thought about it and has decided it isn't a good idea, at least in his building. He indicates that he has attended conferences on special education and feels competent in evaluating *all* of his staff members.

MATADOR INDEPENDENT SCHOOL DISTRICT

MEMORANDUM

From: Stan Smith

To: Chris Green

I just received a call from the Kiwanis. They would like to have one of the special education staff members speak at their meeting on May 19. Are you interested?

MATADOR INDEPENDENT SCHOOL DISTRICT

MEMORANDUM

From: Arnold Ramirez
Speech-language pathology assistant
Westside Elementary School

To: Chris Green

Linda Verlinde was away at a conference three days last week. She expected me to twiddle my thumbs on all but the day you were here. I didn't appreciate it. I have done a really good job of implementing Linda's therapy plans. I've written one Individual Education Plan and have given a couple of diagnostic tests. I felt really competent in what I did. I have seen all of Linda's caseload this week because she has been buried in the end of the year testing and paperwork. In general, I'd like more responsibility and independence because I've proven I can do the work. When can we talk about this?

♦   ♦   ♦   ♦

MATADOR UNIVERSITY

MEMORANDUM

From: Sandra Renault

To: Chris Green

I just received a call from Mrs. Way, Tim's mother. She terminated Tim's therapy at Matador. There are only four weeks left in the term but she is unwilling to reconsider. Apparently Ron Sanders told Mrs. Way yesterday, in no uncertain terms, that if she would get off Tim's back about school, home responsibilities, and his speech, he wouldn't be stuttering. She told Ron she didn't feel confident in the treatment Tim was receiving. Ron then told her he couldn't understand why the Ways had children if they couldn't be better parents. Apparently, it was a very angry exchange.

Chris, we need to talk about how this is to be handled. See me as soon as possible.

MATADOR UNIVERSITY

MEMORANDUM

From: Chris Green

To: Chris Green

Mary Ann Rossi will be coming in at 3:00 today. I talked to her briefly after therapy yesterday. She was so upset that we both felt it was best to wait and talk today. Her sessions aren't going well. We've planned together repeatedly and I've done demonstration therapy with each of her clients. Yesterday she knew things were going awry but she couldn't turn them around. Jimmy, her language client, was so frustrated that he hit her. I saw her right after therapy and she was on the verge of tears. Unfortunately, the quality of her treatment is consistently poor.

MATADOR UNIVERSITY

MEMORANDUM

Subject: Phone Call

From: Mrs. Widner

To: Chris Green

Mrs. Widner called to say how pleased she has been with Renee Williams. Renee works with her son Ricky. Ricky is speaking so much clearer that even his grandparents and babysitter can consistently understand him. She is particularly happy with Renee's professional manner.

MATADOR UNIVERSITY

MEMORANDUM

From: Chris Green

To: Chris Green

Chris, you are in your office when a graduate student, Margarite Bradley, drops in to see you. You are not her supervisor but she feel comfortable talking to you. She is very upset. She is ready to graduate and has begun job-hunting. There are only two jobs open in the entire Matador area and they aren't the kind of positions she was hoping she would find. There are least 5 other people competing for those two positions. She says she really needs to talk to you about how to move forward and what her options are.

MATADOR UNIVERSITY

MEMORANDUM

From: Sandra Renault

To: Chris Green

Randy Linwood has just been in to see me. Randy is angry because he feels he has not been graded fairly. He wants me to raise his grade at least one letter. He says he is highly competent and, as a result, the grade you recommended is totally inappropriate.

◆   ◆   ◆   ◆

MATADOR TRAUMA AND REHABILITATION HOSPITAL/MATADOR HOUSE

MEMORANDUM

From: Chris Green

To: Chris Green

Jo McKay has called in sick four times in the last two weeks. Her sick time was used up a month ago. Her therapy continues to be erratic. Sometimes it is excellent and other times extremely poor. She tore up the evaluation form the last time I observed. Emotionally, she seems to have up and down days. Unfortunately, the hospital due-process procedures in situations like this are vague.

MATADOR TRAUMA AND REHABILITATION HOSPITAL/MATADOR HOUSE

MEMORANDUM

From: Chris Green

To: Chris Green

Reginald Smith just left. Apparently he just had a blowup with Bettye Snider. He says he can't just drop everything when Bettye says she needs to have a hearing test for one of her patients. Bettye was in earlier. She was still angry about her exchange with Reginald. She said rehabilitation patients are worked into the audiology schedule at Reginald's pleasure. Since some of the patients are not covered by insurance for audiological assessment once they leave the hospital, she feels he needs to be more cooperative. His apparent cavalier attitude upset her even further. Ramona Galvez, the nursing supervisor, stormed in as Bettye left saying she can't and won't continue to have these shouting matches between Bettye and Reginald in the middle of her floor.

MATADOR TRAUMA AND REHABILITATION HOSPITAL/MATADOR HOUSE

MEMORANDUM

From: Frank Miller

To: Chris Green

I just received the summary of my job evaluation and the related salary for the next fiscal year. I thought your evaluation was reasonably fair although it was much lower than last year's rating by Bob Marganti, Director of Rehabilitation Services. My real concern lies in the related change in my salary. Can you honestly think I will happy with what you are suggesting? I feel that my performance deserves more. I have attached documentation concerning the hours I work, the number of cases seen, the number of evaluations completed, and the progress my patients have made. I have also attached salary comparables for speech-pathologists with my number of years of service. After you have had time to review this information, we need to talk.

Spring, H4, Hosp.

MATADOR TRAUMA AND REHABILITATION HOSPITAL/MATADOR HOUSE

Subject: Phone call.

From: Melinda Wright

To: Chris Green

Melinda Wright just came from Grand Rounds. Although she felt somewhat awkward, she thought I needed to know about comments made at the meeting. In reviewing two different cases, the neurologist, Dr. Carmen White, indicated audiology had missed the boat by failing to assess patients thoroughly. In one case, indications of a tumor on the eighth cranial nerve were overlooked and, in another, a hearing aid was fitted without a complete evaluation. Dr. White also stated Frank Miller overstepped his limits when he told a family that he thought their child was misdiagnosed.

Spring, H5, Hosp.

MATADOR TRAUMA AND REHABILITATION HOSPITAL/MATADOR HOUSE

Subject: Phone call.

From: Bob Marganti

To: Chris Green

Bob Marganti just came from a Board meeting. The hospital's financial deficit climbed during the last month. Effective next Monday, a 20% reduction in total staff hours worked and a 25% decrease in total funds expended needs to be implemented. Further cuts are pending. The cuts are likely to be much deeper in the rehabilitation unit due to the uncertainty of funding for extended care. According to Bob, the methods to reduce spending are at my discretion. I need to think about how I can decrease staff/hours worked while maintaining patient care.

MATADOR TRAUMA AND REHABILITATION HOSPITAL/MATADOR HOUSE

MEMORANDUM

From: Chris Green

To: Chris Green

Prabha Patel is the speech-language pathologist serving Matador House, an extended care facility affiliated with the Matador Trauma and Rehabilitation Hospital. Two other speech-language pathologists also served that facility but have been layed-off. Funding cuts have severely limited rehabilitation services. Ms. Patel no longer has a full caseload. Robert Marganti, Director of Rehabilitation Services, is suggesting that I need to give Prabha the opportunity to move to a contract position with no benefits or lay her off. Even worse, I am going to have to tell her that on days when her caseload dips, she will need to go home early without pay. Do I have any options here? I don't want to lose Prabha.

REFERENCES

American Speech-Language Hearing Association, Committee on Supervision in Speech-Language Pathology and Audiology. "Clinical supervision in speech-language pathology and audiology: A position statement." *American Speech Hearing Association, 27* (1985): 57–60.

Anderson, J. *The Supervisory Process in Speech-Language Pathology and Audiology.* Boston, MA: College Hill, 1988.

Barak, A. "Counselor training in empathy by a game procedure." *Counselor Education and Supervision, 29* (1990): 170–178.

Bernard, J., and Goodyear, R. *Fundamentals of Clinical Supervision.* (2nd ed.). Boston, MA: Allyn and Bacon, 1998.

Borders, L. "Structured peer supervision." Paper presented at the Annual Convention of the American Association for Counseling and Development, Boston, MA, 1989.

Brannon, D. "Adult learning principles and methods for enhancing the training role of supervisors." *The Clinical Supervisor, 3* (2) (1985): 27–41.

Bredemeier, M., and Greenblat, C. "The educational effectiveness of simulation games." *Simulation & Games, 12* (3) (1981): 307–332.

Brown, A., and Bourne, I. *The Social Work Supervisor.* Philadelphia, PA: Open University Press, 1996.

Chaturvedi, A., and Mehta, S. "Simulations in economics and management. *Communications of the Association for Computing Machinery, 42* (3) (1999): 60–61.

Crago, M. "Supervision and self-exploration." In M. Crago and M. Pickering, (Eds.), *Supervision in Human Communication Disorders: Perspectives on a Process.* San Diego, CA: Singular Publishing Group, 1987.

Delamater, A., Conners, C., and Wells, K. "A comparison of staff training procedures: Behavioral applications in the child psychiatric inpatient setting." *Behavior Modification, 8* (1) (1984): 39–58.

Diedrich, W., and Driscoll, M. "Clinical simulation in speech-language pathology." Paper presented at the Annual Convention of the American Speech-Language and Hearing Association, New Orleans, LA, 1987.

Elgood, C. *Handbook of Management Games.* London: Gower Press, 1976.

Fitzgerald, G., Nichols, P., and Semrau, L. "Training in observation skills for health care professionals: Interactive multimedia." Paper presented at the National Convention of the Association for Educational Communications and Technology, St. Louis, MO, February, 1998.

Godden, A., and Fey, S. "Simulation: A tool for teaching clinical and supervisory skills." Paper presented at the Annual Convention of the American Speech-Language and Hearing Association, Seattle, WA, 1990.

Goodlad, S. "Responding to the perceived training needs of graduate teaching assistants." *Studies-in-Higher-Education, 22* (1) (1997): 83–92.

Grubb, W., and Badway, N. "Linking school-based and work-based learning: The implications of LaGuardia's Co-op seminars for school-to-work programs." Berkeley, CA: National Center for Research in Vocational Education, 1998.

Hinchcliff-Pelias, M., and Elkins, M. "The Intercultural Informant: An experiential learning resource for teacher training." Paper presented at the Annual Meeting of the Speech Communication Association, San Antonio, TX, Nov., 1995.

Hunt, I. "Developing a design philosophy for business games." *Simulation/Games for Learning, 12* (3) (1982): 95–112.

Isaacs, C., Embry, L., and Baer, D. "Training family therapists: An experimental analysis." *Journal of Applied Behavior Analysis, 15* (4) (1982): 505–520.

Jackson, R. "Gate summer academy: A leadership curriculum." *Roeper Review, 7* (2) (1984): 109–111.

Jacobs, R., and Baum, M. "Simulation and games in training and development: Status and concerns about their use." *Simulation & Games, 18* (3) (1987): 385–394.

Jesus, S., and Paixao, M. "The 'Reality Shock' of the beginning teacher." Paper presented at the International Conference of Fedora, Coimbra, Portugal, Sept., 1996.

Johnson, D., Macias, D., Dunlap, A., Hauswald, M., and Doezema, D. "A new approach to teaching prehospital trauma care to paramedic students." *Annals of Emergency Medicine, 33* (1)(1999): 51–55.

Joyce, B., Weil, M., and Showers, G. *Models of teaching.* (4th ed). Boston, MA: Allyn and Bacon, 1992.

Loganbill, C., and Hardy, E. "Developing training programs for clinical supervisors." *The Clinical Supervisor, 1* (3) (1983): 15–21.

Madan, A., Caruso, B., Lopes, J., and Gracely, E. "Comparison of simulated patient and didactic methods of teaching HIV risk assessment to medical residents." *American Journal of Preventive Medicine, 15* (2) (1998): 114–119.

Maier, H. "Roleplaying: Structures and educational objectives." *Journal of Child and Youth Care, 4* (3) (1989): 41–47.

Marks, F. "Description and evaluation of a brief workshop run by child psychiatrists for a group of speech therapists to help them in their work with disorganized families from a deprived city area." *Child Care, Health and Development, 9* (5) (1983): 293–299.

McCarthy, M., Linnan, K., and Muryn, M. "Clinical education: Alternative teaching strategies." In B. Wagner, (Ed.), *Proceedings of the 1996 Conference on Clinical Supervision: Partnerships in Supervision: Innovative and Effective Practices.* Grand Forks, ND: University of North Dakota, 1996: 100–105.

McQuillen, J., and Ivy, D. "Simulations: Addressing competence and performance." *Education, 107* (1) (1986): 71–75.

Mosher-Ashley, P. "Use of simulations in gerontological and geriatric training: A review." *Gerontology and Geriatrics Education, 16* (2) (1995): 53–70.

Munson, C. *An Introduction to Clinical Social Work Supervision.* New York: The Haworth Press, 1983: 228–235.

Overbaugh, R. "The efficacy of interactive video for teaching basic classroom management skills to pre-service teachers." *Computers-in-Human-Behavior, 11* (3–4) (1995): 511–527.

Rabinowitz, F. "Teaching counseling through a semester-long role play." *Counselor Education and Supervision, (36)* (1997): 216–223.

Rassi, J. *Supervision in Audiology.* Baltimore: University Park Press, 1978.

Rieke, S., and Curtis, M. "The consistency between consultant performance during simulated and real-life consultations." In S. Rieke and J. Zins, (Eds.), *The Theory and Practice of School Consultation.* Springfield, IL: Charles C. Thomas, 1981.

Seigel, J., and Driscoll, S. "Law enforcement critical incident teams: Using psychodynamic methods for debriefing training." *Journal of Group Psychotherapy-Psychodrama-and-Sociometry, 48* (2) (1995): 51–60.

Strang, H. "The use of curry teaching simulations in professional training." *Computers in the Schools, 13* (3–4) (1997): 4135–4144.

Tarnopolsky, O. "Business English teaching: Imaginative continuous simulation and critical analysis tasks." Paper presented at the Annual Meeting of the International Association of Teachers of English as a Foreign Language, Manchester, England, April, 1998.

Thornton, G., and Cleveland, J. "Developing managerial talent through simulation." *American Psychologist, 45* (2) (1990): 190–199.

Viadya, V., Greenberg, L., Patel, K., Strauss, L., and Pollack, M. "Teaching physicians how to break bad news: A 1-day workshop using standardized patients." *Archives of Pediatric Adolescent Medicine, 153* (4) (1999): 419–422.

Weber, J. "Using a gaming-simulation to teach students how to collect data and make clinical judgments." *Nurse Educator, 19* (1) (1994): 5–6.

West, J. "Utilizing simulated families and live supervision to stimulate skill development of family therapists." *Counselor Education and Supervision, 24* (1) (1984): 17–27.

Williams, M., and Mowry, G. "Global responses to potential climate change: A simulation." Santa Fe, NM: Project Crossroads, 1997.

Wood, C., and Davidson, J. "Conflict resolution in the family: a PET evaluation study." *Australian Psychologist, 28* (2) (1993): 100–104.

Wood, R. "Use of the nursing simulation laboratory in reentry" programs: An innovative setting for updating clinical skills. *Journal of Continuing Education Nursing, 25* (1) (1994): 28–31.

INDEX

Abbott, A., 74, 76, 90

Accountability, 223

Acculturation
of beginning clinicians, 158–160
of externs, 179
organizational, 195

Acheson, K., 33, 78, 165, 170, 174, 201, 224

Achievement, need for, 7

Active listening, 138–139

Agan, J., 228–229

Agenda
for supervisory conferences, 126–128, 225
for teaching clinics, 311

Alderfer, C., 7, 20

Alexander, R., 8, 156, 221, 283

American Speech-Language and Hearing
Association (ASHA), 16
Certificate of Clinical Competence, 279
code of ethics, 260
Committee on Supervision, xiii–xiv, 249–250,
272, 274–275, 285–286, 287, 288–289
"Guidelines for the Training, Credentialing,
Use, and Supervision for Speech-Language
Pathology Assistants," 189–193, 201
"Preparation Models for the Supervisory
Process in Speech-Language Pathology and
Audiology," 249–250
Standards for Accreditation of Graduate
Education Programs in Audiology and
Speech-Language Pathology, 279
Subcommittee on Supervision of the Council
on Professional Standards in Speech-
Language Pathology and Audiology, xiv
Tasks of Supervision. See Tasks of Supervision
(ASHA)

Amundson, N., 41–42, 49, 90, 221

Andersen, C., 82, 83, 153, 158

Anderson, D., 307

Anderson, J., xiii, xv–xvi, 13, 20–21, 31–32, 34,
35, 43–44, 48, 52–54, 73, 86, 89–91, 119,
122–126, 128–129, 131, 139–140, 141,
153, 154–156, 163, 165, 169, 170, 176,
192, 196, 216, 219–221, 224–226, 248,
251–253, 272–273, 274, 282, 285,
287–288, 289, 322, 337

Anderson, J. B., 264

Anderson, N., 78, 79

Anderson Continuum of Supervision, 13, 54–55

Arygle, M., 138

Ashelman, P., 229

Assistants. See Supervising speech-language
pathology assistants

Audiotapes
journaling with, 89
in professional development process, 263, 284
as supervisory tool, 88, 200

Autonomy, 176, 237

Average clinicians, supervision of, 167–172, 177

Babad, E., 136–137, 138

Badway, N., 333

Baer, D., 335, 344

Bailey, D., 14

Baker, R., 236

Ballard, D., 161, 249, 252, 272

Balloun, L., 83

Bandura, A., 74

Barak, A., 344–345

Barbour, C., 308, 313, 329

Baretta-Herman, A., 219, 304

Barlow, J., 15, 229–230, 238

Barrett-Lennard Relationship Inventory, 135–136

Barrow, J., 10, 19

Barrow, M., 154, 273–274, 278

Bartlett, C., 120

Baseline, 32

Baum, M., 345

Baxley, B., 93

Bazerman, M., 239

Beginning clinician, supervision of, 158–160

Bengala, D., 75, 136

Benway, M., 283–284

Bernard, J., 121, 305–306, 335

Bernstein, B., 74

Best practice protocols, 258–259

Bias, supervisor, 157–158, 227–228

Bice-Stephens, N., 219

Billings, B., 92

Birdwhistle, R., 138

Birnbach, L., 9

Bittel, L., 6, 237

Blair, K., 275

Blake, R., 12, 21, 125–126
Blakeney, R., 7
Blanchard, K., 12–13, 152–153
Bleuer, J., 32
Bliss, L., 80, 156
Block, F., 75, 120, 230
Blodgett, E., 157–158
Bloom, A., 47–48
Blumberg, A., 35
Bobko, P., 48
Boggs, T., 319
Boone, D., 35, 55, 88, 263–264
Borders, D., 307
Borders, L., 176, 335
Borgen, W., 41–42, 49, 90, 221
Borton, T., xiii, 274
Bountress, M., 319, 320
Bourne, I., 336
Bowers, L., 93
Bowman, J., 14
Brannon, D., 335
Brasseur, J., 140, 154, 254, 272–274, 278, 287
Bredemeier, M., 335–336, 338
Brenway, M., 228
Brewer, N., 74
Brooks, M., 133–134, 225
Brookshire, R., 35
Brown, A., 336
Brown, E., 75, 120, 230
Bruce, M., 16, 23, 175–176, 234, 260, 265
"Bug-in-the-ear" feedback strategy, 87–88, 154
Buhler, C., 239
Buoyer, F., 161, 249, 252, 272
Burnout, 235
Business
    simulation in, 345–346
    in supervisor professional growth, 276–278
Buttery, T., 307, 313

Calloway, M., 320
Caracciolo, G., 135–136, 137, 171, 226, 253, 278
Career development, 238
Career ladders, 236, 279–280
Carkuff, R., 135
Carlsmith, J., 138
Caruso, B., 334
Case file, 255
Case staffing, 304
Casey, P., 33, 35, 78, 122, 248, 263, 283
Cashwell, C., 128
Category systems, 33, 34

Caven, C., 120
Centralization, 234
Cervone, D., 74
Chaiklin, H., 305
Chamberlain, M., 157
Chambers, R., 153
Champness, B., 138
Chang, L., 13
Charting, 257–258
Chaturvedi, A., 345
Chrisco, I., 307
Cimorell-Strong, J., 75, 153
Classroom Systems Observation Scale, 34
Clem, R., 153
Cleveland, J., 217, 345
Client assessment, 255–256
Client objectives, 256–257
Clinical practicum guide forms, 103–106
Clinical Supervision (Cogan), xv
Cluver, E., 320
Cogan, M., xv–xvi, 13, 20–21, 31–32, 73, 90, 119,
        132, 139, 140, 152, 153, 174, 215, 226,
        229, 248, 251, 273, 289, 319, 322
Cognitive coaching, 126, 226, 252
Cognitive Coaching (Costa and Garmston), xv
Cohen, S., 13, 14
Cole-Holliday, P., 237
Collaborative style, 125–126, 224–225, 251–252,
        284
Colletti, L., 277, 278
Communication
    effective, 225–226
    nonverbal, 138
    verbal, 133–135
Competency-based assessment, 85–86, 87
Competency-based objectives form, 107–117
Conferences, supervisory, 118–148
    for average clinicians, 171–172, 177
    for beginning clinicians, 161
    conference initiation, 132–133
    conference reflections, 120
    content of, 139–142
    effective communication and, 225–226
    for externships, 180–181
    facilitative behaviors, 133–139
    issues in, 225
    literature review, 119–120
    for marginal clinicians, 165–166
    preconference planning, 123–132, 225
    relationship to supervision tasks, 142–143
    for speech-language pathology assistants, 202

strategies for, 224–225
student evaluation form, 298–300
supervisee expectations, 120–122
in supervisee preparation, 254
tasks relevant to, 118–119, 142–143
typical conferences, 122–123
Conflict management, 137
Conners, C., 335
Conover, H., 35
Content and Sequence Analysis of Speech and
      Hearing Therapy, 88
Continuous process improvement, 16, 22, 175,
      234–235
Continuum of supervision
   in clinical training, 154–156, 161, 169, 171, 173
   in supervisee preparation, 251–254
   in supervising in the workplace, 224
   in supervisor professional growth, 273, 281,
      282, 284
Continuum of Supervision (Anderson), xv
Control
   autonomy and, 176, 237
   job satisfaction and, 239
   self-directed growth and, 262–267
Cooper, L., 305
Cory, M., 153
Costa, A., xv, 73, 90, 122, 126, 132, 133, 134–135,
      139, 202, 226, 252, 261, 289, 322
Counseling, in supervisor professional growth,
      275–276
Cousins, J. B., 76, 227, 228, 239
Crago, M., 76, 86, 88, 90, 91, 131–132, 147, 200,
      282, 316, 318, 321, 334
Creating value for services, 216, 222, 223
Crespi, T. D., 128, 219
Critical thinking, 16–17, 23, 175–176
Cron, W., 238–239
Cross-training, 277
Crutchfield, L., 306, 307
Culatta, R., 35, 122–123, 140, 153, 248, 251, 253
Curry Teaching Simulation, 344
Curtis, M., 277–278, 334, 345

Daley, D., 48
Data collection, 29–47
   application to supervisory process, 52–62
   continuum, 34–35
   and goal-setting options, 61–62
   implementation, 54–61
   individually designed systems, 33, 34, 35–40,
      55–58

in professional development process, 263–264,
      282–283
relationship to supervision tasks, 62
sequential strategies, 40–43
strategies, 33–45, 54
supervisee introduction to, 45–47
in supervisee preparation, 257–258
in supervising speech-language pathology
      assistants, 199
in supervisory conferences, 131
as supervisory tool, 29–31, 222–223
tasks relevant to, 29, 62
terminology, 32–33
tools, 33
Davidson, J., 333
Davis, H., 9
Davis-LaMastro, V., 233
Deal, T., 254
Decentralization, 234
Delamater, A., 335
Delworth, G., 275
Deming, W., 16, 234
Demonstration therapy, 164, 199
Densmore, A., 94
DeShon, R., 8, 156, 221, 283
Developing people, 235–236
Developmental levels of thought, 176
Diedrich, W., 343
Dissatisfiers, 6–7, 237
DiVenere, N., 260
Dixon, G., 48
Doezema, D., 334
Domingo, R., 154, 273–274, 278
Donnelly, C., 87, 161, 264, 283, 298
Dorsey-Gaines, C., 229
Dowling, S., xiii, 8, 16, 23, 32, 34, 36–37,
      40–41, 45, 47, 48, 52, 75, 77–78, 80,
      86, 88, 91, 121, 122, 126, 140, 153,
      154, 156, 157, 160, 162–163, 164,
      167–168, 172–173, 175–176, 181,
      192, 199, 200, 219, 220, 225, 226,
      234, 248, 253, 263, 265, 274, 278,
      282, 283, 284, 288, 296, 308, 315,
      316, 319, 320, 321, 326
Driscoll, M., 343
Driscoll, S., 333
Drucker, P., 3, 4, 9, 14, 16, 21–22, 234
Dunlap, A., 334
Dunning, D., 47, 49, 74, 85, 163, 165–166
Dupuy-Walker, L., 306
Dussault, G., 136

Earley, C., 8
Earley, P., 238
Education
    group supervision in, 306–307
    role-playing in, 334–335
    simulation in, 343–345
    in supervisor professional growth, 275
Eisenberger, R., 233
Eldridge, C., 138
Elgood, C., 335
Elkins, M., 343
Ellis, M., 136, 237
Ellsworth, P., 138
Embry, L., 335, 344
Empathy, 138
Empathy Game, 344–345
Ensley, K., 75, 153
Entrepreneurship, 232
Ersoz, C., 16, 175
Ethington, C., 176
Evans, M., 8, 9–10, 48, 75, 120–121, 123,
        125–126, 136
Evans, R., 239
Evidence-based practice, 123, 203, 223, 258
Exline, R., 138
Externship experience, supervision of, 178–181
Eye contact, 138

Fahey, R., 82, 83
Family interaction, 260–261
Farmer, J., xv, 52, 92–93, 122, 123, 136, 192, 282,
        304, 319, 322
Farmer, S., xv, 34, 52, 122, 123, 128, 132–135,
        136, 137, 139, 153, 192, 224, 225, 261,
        282, 301, 304, 319, 322
Fasolo, P., 233
Feedback, 73–117
    and direct observation, 77–87
    effective feedback criteria, 75–76
    grades and salary increment determination,
        94–95
    literature review, 73–77
    nature and effects of, 74–75
    relationship to supervision tasks, 95–96
    strategies, 87–91
    supervisee experiences, 76–77
    about supervision experiences, 180, 181–183
    in supervisor professional growth, 283–284
    tasks relevant to, 73, 95–96
    timing, 91–92
    on written material, 92–94

Felicetti, T., 80
Fey, S., 316, 318, 319, 320, 321, 343
Fidler, H., 229
Filley, F., 13, 81, 156
Fish, M., 34
Fisher, C., 74, 156
Fisher, K., 15, 231
Fitch, J., 223
Fitzgerald, G., 344
Flahive, L., 81
Flanders, N., 31
Flat organizations, 234
Fleuridas, C., 48
Flynn, P., 79
Fong, M., 176
Foti, R., 237
Frase, L., 237–238
Frederick, E., 48
Freedman, S., 236
Freeman, E., 76, 78, 83, 84, 86, 91
Freiberg, H. J., 264
Freiberg, J., 32, 48, 86
French, E., 236
French, N., 192, 194
Friedlander, M., 136, 237
Furniture, for supervisory conferences, 129–131

Gall, M., 33, 78, 165, 170, 174, 201, 224
Gallagher, T., 157
Gardner, W., 157
Garett, K., 219
Garmston, R., xv, 73, 90, 122, 126, 132, 133,
        134–135, 139, 202, 226, 252, 261, 289, 322
Gavett, E., 238, 279
Genograms, 305–306
Georgia State Department of Education, 236
Gergeron, C., 260
Glaser, A., 87, 107, 161, 283, 298, 316, 319, 320
Glickman, C., 239, 306–307
Glover-Dorsey, G., 229
Goal-setting
    for average clinicians, 168–169
    for beginning clinicians, 160
    criteria for student clinician form, 100–102
    in job satisfaction, 239–240
    for marginal clinicians, 163
    as motivational strategy, 8
    options for, 61–62
    for outstanding clinicians, 173
    in professional development process, 267
    supervisee, 220–221

in supervising speech-language pathology assistants, 196–198
in supervisor professional growth, 283
Godden, A., 318, 320, 343
Goldberg, B., 160, 219, 261, 262, 280
Goodlad, S., 343
Goodyear, R., 121, 128, 276, 305–306, 335
Gracely, E., 334
Grades, 94–95
Green, T., 276, 287
Greenberg, L., 334
Greenberger, D., 239
Greenblat, C., 335–336, 338
Greenfield, C., 10
Group discussion, in supervisor professional growth, 284
Group supervision. *See also* Teaching clinic method
in psychology, 305–306
in speech-language pathology, 304
Grover, R., 74
Grubb, W., 333
Guinty, C., 153
Gully, S., 8, 221
Gustafson, J., 305

Hagan, E., 221, 222, 236, 237
Hagler, P., 78, 82, 83, 87, 94, 154, 156, 159–160, 189, 193, 194, 195, 196, 197, 205, 210
Hagler, R., 274
Halfond, M., xiii
Hall, D., 238
Hanson, L., 238
Hardy, F., 335
Harkins, S., 221, 230
Harris, H., 75, 136, 161, 249, 252, 272
Harris, M., 80
Harrison, C., 275
Hatfield, M., 120
Hauswald, M., 334
Hayes, D., 13, 81, 156
Health care education, simulation in, 344–345
Heflich, D., 217
Heid, L., 280
Henderson, J., 307
Herbert, T., 9
Hersey, P., 12–13, 152–153
Herzberg, F., 6, 18, 236–237
Hess, C., 121, 136
Hewlett, Bill, 15
Hewlett-Packard, 15
Hinchcliff-Pelias, M., 343

HongBo, W., 198
Hooper, C., 161, 249, 252, 272
Horney, M., 86, 87, 159, 160, 255, 264
Housley, W., 128
Huber, V., 74
Human Synergistics, Inc., 277
Hunt, I., 335
Huntington, D., 307
Hygienic factors, 6–7

Ilgen, D., 74, 156
Implementation
of data collection, 54–61
of role-playing, 336–338
of supervision, 219–227
in teaching clinic method, 312
of simulation, 347–374
Individually designed data collection systems, 33, 34, 35–40, 55–58
Individual Supervisory Conference Rating Scale, 274
Ingrisano, D., 153
Integrative Task-Maturity Model of Supervision (ITMMS), 13, 20–21
Interaction analysis systems, 33
Interpersonal behaviors, 135–138
Irwin, R., 304
Isaacs, C., 335, 344
Ivy, D., 344

Jackson, R., 335
Jacobs, R., 345
Jacobson, L., 156
Jans, L., 78, 90
Jensen, J., 32, 48, 275
Jesus, S., 343
Jimenez, B., 140
Job initiation, 218–219
Job rotation, 277
Job satisfaction, 197–198, 236–240, 280
Job-sharing, 239
Johnson, A., 217
Johnson, D., 320, 334
Joint planning, 199
Jones, J., 75, 90–91
Jones, K., 307
Jones-McNamara, S., 279–280
Joshi, S., 153
Journals, 89
Joyce, B., 48, 218, 334
Juhnke, G., 90, 124, 126, 262

Kacmar, M., 254–255
Kamhi, A. G., 62, 87, 160, 177, 219, 220, 261–263, 265, 280, 323
Kampfe, C., 156
Kanfer, R., 8
Kansas Inventory of Self-Supervision, 33, 164
Kennedy, K., 75
Killion, J., 275
Kinesics, 138
Kingsley, G., 75, 136
Kinicki, A., 6, 7, 47–48
Kjelgaard, M., 221, 230
Klaumann, T., 305
Kleffner, F., xiii
Klein, H., 307
Knepflar, L., 92
Knippen, J., 276, 287
Knowledge trees, 265, 266
Kopelman, R., 74, 76, 84
Kotter, J., 14, 233
Kreb, R., 32
Kreitner, R., 6, 7, 47–48
Krikorian, C., 75, 136
Krueger, K., 35
Kruger, J., 47, 49, 74, 85, 163, 165–166
Kuechler, C., 304
Kwiatkowski, J., 13, 81, 156

Ladany, N., 136, 237
Lafferty, J., 277, 278
Laird, B., 309
Langellier, K., 138
Larson, L., 121
Latham, G., 8, 48, 198, 221, 239
Latting, J., 76
Leadership, 10–17
    continuous process improvement, 16, 22, 175, 234–235
    critical thinking, 16–17, 23, 175–176
    relationship to supervision tasks, 23–24
    styles of, 11–14, 20–21
    value-driven, 14–15
Leadership Grid, 12
Leadership skill, 14
Lecomte, C., 74
Ledford, G., 13
Lee, C., 48, 238
Leebov, W., 16, 175
Legal issues
    for average clinicians, 172, 177
    for marginal clinicians, 166–167

Leiter, M., 234–235
Lesson plan preparation, 257
Levering, R., 15
Levy, P., 229
Lewis, B., 10, 237
Lichtenberg, J., 128
Liddle, B., 166, 171
Lieber, R., 9
Life-cycle model, 12, 13, 152–153
Life-cycle theory of leadership, 7
Lifelong learning, 62, 160, 219, 261, 280
Lincoln, M., 304
Linnan, K., 334
Lipton, M., 4, 14
Listening, active, 138–139
Literature review
    on feedback, 73–77
    on group supervision methods, 303–308
    on performance objectives, 47–48
    on role-playing, 333–336
    on simulation, 343–346
    on supervising clinical training, 152–154
    on supervisor professional growth, 272–278
    on supervisory conferences, 119–120
Locke, E., 8, 48, 221
Lockyer, J., 229
Loganbill, C., 335
Logemann, J., 22, 32, 96, 123, 194, 223, 258
Logue, O., 197, 198
Loiselle, J., 306
Long, L., 136–137
Longhurst, T., 194
Looby, E., 128
Loop induction feedback strategy, 87–88
Lopes, J., 334
Lougeay-Mottinger, J., 80, 81–82
Lowe, T., 227, 228, 230
Low Inference Self-Assessment Measure (LISAM), 32
Lubinski, R., 235
Ludington, J. R., 161, 249, 252, 272
Ludlow, B., 307
Lyter, S., 74, 76, 90

Macias, D., 334
Madan, A., 334
Madill, H., 156
Magee-Bender, L., 87
Maier, H., 334, 335
Makiney, J., 229
Managed care, 278–279

Manatt, R., 74, 228, 229–230, 232, 239–240, 283–284

Manning, D., 305

Manning, R., 74, 76, 84

Marginal clinicians, supervision of, 162–167

Marks, F., 333

Martin, T., 157

Marx, R., 276–277

Maslow, A., 5–6, 7, 18, 236–237

Mawdsley, B., 13, 20–21, 33, 125–126, 153, 164, 313, 316, 318, 321–322

May, A., 92

McAllister, L., 153, 304

McBride, M., 86, 132, 139

McCanse, A., 12, 21, 125–126

McCarthy, M., 334

McClelland, D., 7

McCrea, E., 34, 35, 61, 78, 135, 137, 248, 250, 253, 272, 279–280, 285, 287, 316, 318, 319, 321–322

McCrea Adapted Scales for the Assessment of Interpersonal Function in Speech Pathology Supervision Conferences, 35, 61

McCready, C. V., 189–190

McCready, V., 75, 136, 137, 274

McDonald, J., 153

McElroy, M., 160, 282

McFarlane, L., 78, 159–160, 173, 189, 194, 195, 196, 197, 205, 210, 274

McGarity, D., 306

McGill Guidelines for Tape Analysis, 88

McGregor, D., 6

McLeod, S., 86, 126, 180–181, 250, 262

McNeill, B., 275

McNichol, J., 237

McQuillen, J., 344

Meetings. *See also* Conferences, supervisory
in supervisor professional growth, 284–285

Mehta, S., 345

Mentors, 236

Mercaitis, P., 85, 86, 103, 121, 122, 123, 159, 255, 264

Meyer, S., 92, 257

Michalak, D., 307, 308, 313, 329

Microsupervision, 304

Miller, F., 235

Miner, A., 35

Mirroring, 226, 322. *See* Pacing.

Mitchell, M., 156

Modified teaching clinic (MTC), 317

Modifying behaviors, in supervisor professional growth, 283

Morrison, E., 135–136, 137, 171, 226, 253, 278

Moses, N., 16–17, 136, 139, 156, 175–176, 254, 285

Mosher-Ashley, P., 345

Moskowitz, M., 15

Moss, S., 223, 258

Motivation, 5–10
application of principles to speech-language pathology and audiology, 18–20
how to motivate, 5–7, 18–20
relationship to supervision tasks, 23–24
theories of, 5–7, 20
what motivates, 7–9, 20
workplace philosophy and examples of, 9–10

Motivators, 6–7, 237–239

Mouton, J., 12

Mowry, G., 333

Muma, J., 122

Munson, C., 305, 334–335, 336, 337

Murray, H., 7

Muryn, M., 334

Narrative feedback, 78–79

Natalle, E., 138

National Student Speech, Language, Hearing Association (NSSLHA), 18

Negative perceptions of supervisor behavior, 182–183

Nelson, B., 8, 10, 200, 238, 239

Nelson, C., 175–176

Nelson, G., xiii, 274

Nelson, M., 121, 132–133

Networking, in supervisor professional growth, 284

Nicholas, L., 35

Nicholls, J., 21

Nichols, K., 138

Nichols, P., 344

Nonverbal analyses, 33, 34

Nonverbal communication, in supervisory conferences, 138

Oakley, K., 229

Objective feedback, 84–85

Objectives. *See* Performance objectives

Observation strategies, 77–78, 89–90
structured observation, 77–87, 89–90, 200, 223–224
in teaching clinic method, 309, 312
therapy observation, 265

O'Connor, E., 34
Olsen, H., 308, 313, 329
Oratio, A., 35
Organizational climate/culture
     acculturation to, 195
     leadership and, 10–17
     motivation and, 5–10
     supervision and, 4
     value of strong, 240
Organizational effectiveness, 231–240. *See also*
          Leadership; Motivation
     characteristics of successful workplaces, 231–236
     job satisfaction and, 197–198, 236–240, 280
Orphen, C., 239
Outstanding clinicians, supervision of, 172–178
Overbaugh, R., 343

Pacing, verbal, nonverbal, in supervisory
          conferences, 133–135, 141, 202, 225
Paixao, M., 343
Parsons, M., 32, 76, 90, 91, 275
Passaro, P., 198, 201
Patel, K., 334
Peake, T., 275
Peaper, R., 121, 122, 126, 264
Peer assistance strategy, 307
Peer coaching, 307
Peer learning, 304
Peer supervision, 265–267
Pennington, D., 306
Performance documentation, 201–202
Performance evaluation, 227–231
     bias in, 157–158, 227–228
     format and content of, 230–231
     portfolio assessment, 229
     supervisor-driven, 229–230
     three-sixty evaluation, 228–229, 283–284
Performance objectives, 47–62
     competent performance, 196
     examples of, 49–51, 221–224
     identifying, 48–49
     literature review, 47–48
     relationship to supervision tasks, 62
     selecting, 49
     setting, 199–200, 235–236
     in supervisee preparation, 256–257
     as supervisory tool, 29–31
     tasks relevant to, 29, 62
     undocumented, 60
Perkins, J., 85, 86, 103, 159, 255
Perkins, W., xiii

Perlstein-Kaplan, K., 80, 81–82
Peroff, L., 82, 83, 258
Perry, W. G., 16–17, 23
Peters, T., 15, 19, 175, 231
Pfeiffer, J., 75, 90–91
Phillips, J., 8, 221, 277
Pickering, M., 89, 120, 122, 133, 135, 136, 137,
          147, 159–160, 171, 175, 226, 253, 282
Pickett, A., 198
Pietranton, A., 237
Pistole, M., 305
Pitts, J., 176
Planning
     preconference, 123–132, 225
     in teaching clinic method, 309
Podsakoff, P., 74
Polkinghorne, D., 128
Pollack, M., 334
Popp, G., 9
Portfolio assessment, 229
Positive perceptions of supervisor behavior, 182
Post-test data, 32
Potter, R., 74
Powell, D., 305
Power Cluver, E., 320
Power-deFur, L., 32, 217
Practicum
     for supervisee preparation, 255–261
     for supervisor training, 287
Praise, 10
Preconference planning, 123–132, 225
     by supervisee, 131–132
     by supervisor, 123–131
Prescott, T., 35, 55, 88, 263–264
Price, C., 306
Price, K. R., 161, 249, 252, 272
Problem identification, 281
Problem-solving
     and supervisor professional growth, 286–287
     in teaching clinic method, 310, 312, 313, 316
Productivity. *See* Leadership; Motivation;
          Organizational effectiveness
Professional development
     of supervisees, 261–267
     of supervisors, 271–300
     teaching clinics in, 317–318
Professional growth within organizations, 3–26
     leadership, 10–17
     motivation and, 5–10, 18–20, 23–24
     relationship to leadership tasks, 23–24
     tasks relevant to, 3–4, 23–24

Professionalism, 197, 260
Profile type data collection, 36–40, 41, 51, 53, 55, 57
Proxemics, 138
Prudhomme, M., 87, 107
Psychology, group supervision in, 305–306

Rabinowitz, F., 334
Radaszewski-Byrne, M., 192, 196
Rassi, J., xiii, 92, 119, 159–160, 274, 282, 335
Rating scales, 33, 79–84
Reading, in self-guided growth, 282
Redmond, K., 35
Reflection
    conference, 120
    self-reflection, 264, 283
    in supervisor professional growth, 282
Reid, D., 32, 76, 90, 91, 275
Reiman, A., 33, 306
Relapse prevention strategy, 276–277
Report writing, 259–260
Research-directed development, 288–289
Resick, C., 47–48
Rewards, 237–239
Richardson, J., 306
Rieke, S., 334, 345
Rigrodsky, S., 135–136, 137, 171, 226, 253, 278
Ringwalt, S., 161, 249, 252, 272, 279–280
Robbins, P., 307
Roberson, L., 239
Roberts, H., 237
Roberts, J., 34, 75, 79, 122, 123, 136, 140, 153, 248, 253
Robertson, P., 276
Rockman, B., 49, 129, 130, 132
Rockman, M., 156
Rodgers, T., 95, 217, 221, 228, 230
Rogero, E., 87, 107
Rogers, C., 61
Rogers, T., 14, 21
Role identification, 197
Role-playing, 199, 331–376
    examples of, 339–343
    impact of, 335–336
    implementing, 336–338
    literature review, 333–336
    nature of, 333
    relationship to supervision tasks, 338–343
    tasks relevant to teaching supervisory skills through, 331, 338–343
    thoughts about, 332
    use of, 333–335

Romero, D., 82, 220, 222
Rosenthal, D., 48
Rosenthal, R., 156
Runyan, S., 85–87, 94, 112, 304

Saari, L., 8, 48, 221
St. Louis, M., 306
Salary
    determination of, 94–95
    as motivator, 7, 237–239
Sama, L., 74, 76, 84, 91
Satisfiers, 6–7
Sbaschnig, K., 82, 83, 126, 154, 158, 317, 319
Schalk, M., 82, 83, 258
Schatz, J., 13, 81
Scherer, J., 14, 21
Schermerhorn, J., 157
Schill, M., 89
Schmitt, J., 157–158
Schmitz, H., 92
Schmoker, M., 48
Scholten, I., 318, 320
Schubert, G., 35, 309
Scudder, R., 13, 20–21, 125–126, 153, 157–158
Seal, B., 85–87, 112, 304
Seating arrangements, for supervisory conferences, 129–131
Seigel, J., 333
Selective verbatim recording, 33, 34, 201, 224
Self-actualization, 5, 19–20, 235, 237
Self-directed growth, 262–267, 282–285
Self-esteem, 18–20, 74, 237, 238
Self-evaluation, 160, 264
Self-guided growth of supervisors, 282–285
Self-reflection, 264, 283
Self-supervision, 122, 155, 254, 319–320
Sells, J., 128
Seltzer, H., 35, 122–123, 140, 153, 248, 251, 253
Semrau, L., 344
Sequential type data collection strategy, 31, 39, 40–44
Sexton, T., 32
Shank, K., 34, 122, 320
Shapiro, D., 16–17, 32, 34, 35, 122, 123, 136, 139, 156, 175–176, 254, 259, 261, 263, 283, 285, 313, 316, 319, 321, 322
Shatz, J., 156
Shaw, K., 8, 48, 221
Shellenbarger, S., 216
Shingo, S., 16, 19–20
Showers, B., 48, 218

Showers, G., 334

Shriberg, L., 13, 80–81, 82, 156

Sign systems, 33

Simmons, K., 13, 81, 156

Simulation, 331–376
  literature review, 343–346
  nature of, 333, 343
  relationship to supervision tasks, 346–347
  simulation game, 347–348
  simulation orientation, 348–374
  tasks relevant to teaching supervisory skills
      through, 331, 346–347
  thoughts about, 332

Site selection, for supervisory conferences, 129

Situational leadership, 12–14, 24

Skau, K., 86, 132, 139

Skinner, B., 7–8

Sleight, C., 320

Slocum, J., 238–239

Smallwood, N., 236

Smith, A., 6

Smith, K., 33, 34, 35, 79, 93, 94, 122, 123, 140, 153,
      163, 196, 229, 248, 251, 253, 263, 274, 283

Smith, M., 13, 81, 156

Smith's Adaptation of the Multidimensional
      Observational System for the Analysis of
      Interactions in Clinical Supervision, 35

Snadden, D., 229

Socha, L., 74

Social work, group supervision, 304–305

Socratic approach, 251

Sommer, R., 130

Southwest Airlines, 15

Spangler, L., 138

Spitzer, D., 10

Stevens, D., 276

Stoffman, D., 9

Stoltenberg, C., 275

Stone, D., 74

Stone, E., 74

Stout, S., 238–239

Strang, H., 344

Strasser, S., 239

Strauss, L., 334

Strike-Roussos, C., 128–129, 253, 273, 278

Student-Supervisor Self-Exploratory Training, 88

Successful workplaces, 231–236

Supervisee(s)
  acculturation of, 158–160, 179
  characteristics of, 156–157
  diagnosis, 129–130, 132, 141, 160, 237, 281
  diagnosis form, 130

expectations for conferences, 120–122
  experience with feedback, 76–77
  feedback involvement of, 86–87
  goals in supervision process, 220–221
  impressions of, 157
  interviews of, 217–218
  introduction to data collection, 45–47
  observations of, 89–90
  preconference planning by, 131–132
  professional growth of, 261–267
  supervisor diagnosis of, 129
  in supervisor preconference planning, 128–129
  training of. *See* Supervisee preparation

Supervisee preparation, 219–220, 247–270
  context for, 248
  overview of, 249–250
  practicum components, 255–261
  professional growth in, 261–267
  relationship to supervision tasks, 267–268
  supervision continuum in, 251–254
  supervisory process and, 254–255
  tasks relevant to, 247–248, 267–268

Supervising clinical training, 151–187
  of average clinician, 167–172
  of beginning clinician, 158–161
  continuum of supervision, 154–156, 161, 169,
      171, 173
  of externship experience, 178–181
  feedback about supervision experiences, 180,
      181–183
  literature review, 152–154
  of marginal clinician, 162–167
  of outstanding clinician, 172–178
  relationship to supervision tasks, 183–184
  supervisee characteristics, 156–157
  supervisee impressions, 157
  supervisor beginning thoughts, 152
  supervisor bias, 157–158, 227–228
  tasks relevant to, 151–152, 183–184

Supervising in the workplace, 214–244
  organizational effectiveness, 231–240
  performance evaluation, 227–231
  relationship to supervision tasks, 240–241
  supervision implementation, 219–227
  supervision process, 215–219
  tasks relevant to, 214–215, 240–241

Supervising speech-language pathology assistants,
      188–213
  approved tasks for assistants, 208
  competencies, 206–208
  conferences, 202
  decision matrix for monitoring, 210–213

goals and strategies for attainment, 196–198
guidelines for, 189–195
organizational acculturation, 195
performance documentation and appraisal, 201–202
relationship to supervision tasks, 202–203
sample curriculum, 205
scope of practice, 189–191
supervisory tools, 198–201
tasks relevant to, 188–189, 202–203
Supervision process, 215–227
benefits of, 226–227
implementation of, 219–227
job initiation, 218–219
role definition of supervisor, 215–217
supervisee interview, 217–218
in supervisee preparation, 254–255
Supervisor(s)
beginning thoughts on clinical training, 152
bias of, 157–158, 227–228
later thoughts on clinical training, 178
preconference planning by, 123–131
professional development of. *See* Supervisor professional growth
role definition of, 215–217
Supervisor-driven evaluation, 229–230
Supervisor professional growth, 271–300
conference analysis form, 296–297
continuum of supervision, 273, 281, 282, 284
formal supervisor training, 285–288
literature review, 272–278
promotion criteria, 293–295
relationship to supervision tasks, 289
research-directed development, 288–289
self-guided growth, 282–285
state of the art, 278–281
tasks relevant to, 271–272, 289
Supervisory conferences. *See* Conferences, supervisory
Supervisory models, xiv–xvi
Supervisory style, 155–156, 253
Supervisory tools and techniques, 198–201
accountability and, 223
audiotape, 200
data collection, 29–47, 199, 222–223
demonstration therapy, 164, 199
joint planning and role-playing, 199
objective setting, 199–200
selective verbatim recording, 33, 34, 201, 224
structured observations, 77–87, 89–90, 200, 223–224
videotape, 88, 200, 223

Swanson, D., 89
Sweda, J., 319, 320
Synthetic Economy for Analysis and Simulation (SEAS) project, 345–346
System for Analyzing Supervisor-Teacher Interaction, 35

Tallies in data collection, 33, 34, 36, 54–56, 58–60
Target behavior, 32
Tarnopolsky, O., 345
Task-Maturity Model, 13
Tasks of Supervision (ASHA)
data collection, 29, 62
feedback, 73, 95–96
history of, xiii–xiv
leadership, 23–24
motivation, 23–24
performance objectives, 29, 62
professional growth within organizations, 3–4, 23–24
role-playing, 331, 338–343
simulation, 331, 346–347
supervisee preparation, 247–248, 267–268
supervising clinical training, 151–152, 183–184
supervising in the workplace, 214–215, 240–241
supervising speech-language pathology assistants, 188–189, 202–203
supervisor professional growth, 271–272, 289
supervisory conferences, 118, 142–143
teaching clinic, 303, 322–323
Taylor, C., 86, 87, 159, 160, 255, 264
Taylor, M., 74, 156
Teacher education, simulation in, 343–344
Teach for America program, 229
Teaching clinic method, 88, 303–330
adaptations of, 315–318
advantages and disadvantages of, 319–320
alternate uses of, 318–319
closing thoughts, 321–322
components of, 308–315
literature review on group supervision, 303–308
new directions in, 307–308, 314–315
relationship to supervision tasks, 322–323
research summary, 320–321
tasks relevant to, 303, 322–323
training materials, 326–330
Teamwork, 232–233
Tebb, S., 305
Teitelbaum, S., 181, 183
Terrio, L., 87

Theory X, 6

Theory Y, 6, 19–20, 24

Therapy implementation, 258–259

Therapy observation, 265

Thies-Sprinthall, L., 33, 306

Thomas, M., 229

Thompson, P., 236

Thornton, G., 217, 345

Three-sixty evaluation, 228–229, 283–284

Tihen, L., 121

Till, J., 35

Tillema, H., 229

Time sampling in data collection, 33

Timing of feedback, 91–92

Todor, W., 74

Toews, J., 229

Training. *See also* Professional development; Role-playing; Simulation; Supervisee preparation; Supervising clinical training; Teaching clinic method

    formal supervisor, 285–288

    nature and effects of, 272–274

    for teaching clinics, 311–312

Truelove, B., 223

Tryon, G., 156

Tsolis, A., 306

Turnover, 235

Tziner, A., 239

Ueberle, J., 120

Ulrich, S., xiii, 33, 35, 122, 248, 263, 274, 283

Underwood, J., 35

Underwood Category System for Analyzing Supervisor-Clinician Behavior, 35

University of Alberta, 159–160

UTD Competency Based Evaluation System, 81–82

Vail, C,, 307

Vallon, J., xiii, 274

Value-driven, 14–15, 21–22, 313–314

Values, workplace, 233

VanDemark, A., xiii, 274

Verbal communication, in supervisory conferences, 133–135

Verbal feedback strategies, 90–91

Verbatim recording, 33, 34

Viadya, V., 334

Videotapes. *See also* Teaching clinic method

    in professional development process, 263

in supervisor professional growth, 284

    as supervisory tool, 88, 200, 223

Villareal, J., xiii

Vincelette, J., 276, 287

Violato, C., 229

Wagner, B., 112, 121, 136

Wall, B., 36–37, 40–41, 45, 47

Walz, G., 32

Waterman, R., 15, 19, 175, 231

Watkins, C., 275, 276

Wayne, S., 254–255

Weber, J., 344

Weil, M., 334

Weinrich, B., 264

Weiseth, C., 318

Welch, N., 87

Weller, D., 313

Weller, R., 35

Welling, R., 87

Wells, K., 335

West, J., 335

Whiston, S., 32

White, L., 48

White, P., 221, 230

Wienke, W., 307

Wilber, M., 138

Wilbur, J., 138

Wilkins-Canter, E., 76, 78, 84, 86, 90

Williams, C., 126, 154, 158

Williams, L., 313, 316, 317, 319, 321

Williams, M., 333

Wilson, B., 91

Wilson, J., 87

Wisconsin Procedure for the Analysis of Clinical Competence (W-PACC), 13, 81–83, 156

Wittkopp, J., 75, 91, 121, 164, 199, 220

Wolf, K., 32

Wood, C., 333

Wood, R., 344

Workplace

    philosophy of, 9–10

    supervising in. *See* Supervising in the workplace

W-PACC (Wisconsin Procedure for the Analysis of Clinical Competence), 13, 81–83, 156

Written material, feedback on, 92–94

Zahorik, J., 153

Zins, J., 277–278

Zuber, A., 10